The Joan Palevsky Imprint in Classical Literature

In honor of beloved Virgil—

"O degli altri poeti onore e lume . . ."

—Dante, *Inferno*

The publisher and the University of California Press Foundation gratefully acknowledge the generous support of the Joan Palevsky Endowment Fund in Literature in Translation.

THE CARE OF THE BRAIN IN EARLY CHRISTIANITY

THE CARE OF THE BRAIN IN EARLY CHRISTIANITY

Jessica L. Wright

UNIVERSITY OF CALIFORNIA PRESS

University of California Press
Oakland, California

Cataloging-in-Publication Data is on file at the Library of Congress.

ISBN 978-0-520-38767-6 (cloth : alk. paper)
ISBN 978-0-520-38768-3 (ebook)

Manufactured in the United States of America

28 27 26 25 24 23 22
10 9 8 7 6 5 4 3 2 1

CONTENTS

ACKNOWLEDGMENTS

This book would not have been possible without the care, attention, and nurturing of many people, only a fraction of whom I can name here.

Most immediately, I want to thank Eric Schmidt and LeKeisha Hughes at the University of California Press, as well as the anonymous referees, whose patience, guidance, and feedback has been unparalleled. Also fundamental to the entire project are my doctoral advisors: Brooke Holmes, Brent Shaw, Catherine Conybeare, and Christian Wildberg. Your probing questions and your belief in this project carried me forward through seemingly impossible stretches.

Formative to my thinking on medicine and religion in late antiquity was my early involvement in ReMeDHe, the working group in Religion, Medicine, Disability, and Health in Late Antiquity, and I remain immensely grateful to Kristi Upson-Saia and Heidi Marx for inviting me in so early in my own work. Also critically important were the Program in the History of Science, Medicine, and Technology and the Center for the Study of Religion at Princeton University. Working across disciplines has for me meant feeling always like an outsider: I am grateful for the friends and teachers I found in these spaces. In particular, I want to acknowledge the contributions to my way of thinking made by Emily Kern, Jenny Rampling, Katja Guenther, and Keith Wailoo.

During the writing of this book, I have been housed by a number of different institutions—Princeton University, the University of Southern California, the University of Texas at San Antonio, and Sheffield University. The material, intellectual, and interpersonal support that each institution offered has been vital to the completion of the project. I am especially grateful to Jill Fleuriet and Şerife Tekin for their engagement with and support of my work, Jonathan McLellan and Jessica Nowlin for welcoming me to San Antonio, and Constanze Güthenke, Khristina Gonzalez, and Lisa Bitel for consistent encouragement and advice. Beyond the institutional structures, this work has also been nourished through the mentorship and friendship of Helen Morales, Mike Chin, Nancy S. Rabinowitz, Shelley Haley, and Tina Shepardson.

Audiences at numerous conferences, workshops, and universities have sharpened and enriched my thought through their questions and suggestions—in particular: Princeton University; University of Maryland, College Park; Dartmouth College; Occidental College; Carleton College; Oberlin College; University of Toronto; University of Texas at San Antonio; Trinity College Dublin; University of California, Santa Barbara; University of California, Los Angeles; and Colby College.

My students during this time have also shaped me, and none more so than those I taught through the Prison Teaching Initiative. Their friendship, their acts of solidarity, and their poetry remade my understanding of what it means to teach and what it is to live an intellectual life.

Many friends and loved ones have sustained me, put up with me, fed and housed me, and read or listened to my work over these years. Among those closest to this project are Becky Jinks, John Boopalan, Ester Jamir, Sophie Holmes, Mathura Umachandran, Naomi Williams, Emery Pearson, Anna Diemar, Katie Kleinhopf, and the whole Tin House crew (especially Nadine Monem, who wrote with me during the final stages). Others who have sustained and cared for me over the years of writing include Philippa Gullett, Hartley Miller, Helen Thomas, Helena Duncalf, Patrick Stockwell, Veronica Diaz, Amers and Sam Goff, Jill Stockwell, Tom Sapsford, Eyo Ewara, Jo Reyes-Boitel, and my Metanoia cohort.

Lastly and most of all: my family has offered unconditional support and patience through years of distraction, including long periods of time overseas. My parents, my stepmother, and my sibling have each in their own way contributed to making me—and this book—what we are. Mel Webb was there when this book began. Helen Flint has borne witness to its conclusion.

This book is for my grandmother, Dorothy Wright.

ACKNOWLEDGMENT OF PREVIOUS PUBLICATIONS

Chapter 3 draws upon material from my chapter "Ventricular Localization in Late Antiquity: The Philosophical and Theological Roots of an Enduring Model of Brain Function," in *Imagining the Brain: Episodes in the History of Brain Research*, edited by Chiara Ambrosio and William Maclehose, 3–22, Elsevier, 2018.

Chapter 4 draws upon material from my article "The Brain as Treasury and as Aqueduct: Metaphors of the Brain in Theodoret of Cyrrhus," *Studies in Late Antiquity* 2.4 (2018): 542–66.

Chapter 5 draws upon material from my article "John Chrysostom and the Rhetoric of Cerebral Vulnerability," *Studia Patristica* 81.7 (2017): 109–214. It also draws upon material from my chapter "Brain, Nerves, and Ecclesial Membership in John Chrysostom," in *Revisioning John Chrysostom: New Approaches, New Perspectives*, edited by Chris de Wet and Wendy Mayer, 361–409, Brill, 2019.

Chapter 6 draws upon material from my article "Preaching Phrenitis: Augustine's Medicalization of Religious Difference," *Journal of Early Christian Studies* 28.4 (2020), 525–53.

Chapter 7 draws upon material from my chapter "Are We Our Brains? How Early Christianity Shaped Western Ideas about Power, Morality, and Personhood," in *Embodied Difference: Divergent Bodies in Public Discourse*, edited by Jamie A. Thomas and Christina Jackson, 37–58, Rowman & Littlefield, 2019.

Introduction

In the early fifth century C.E., the bishop Augustine (354–430) responded to a letter that criticized his agnosticism with regard to the origin of the individual soul.[1] The crucial question was this: were all souls generated from Adam, or did God make a new soul for each human? Augustine professed not to know. His correspondent had accused him of being as ignorant as a cow if he could not give an account of his own soul. Augustine responded that the relationship between body and soul was a mystery to all:

> From what part of the body does that which they call the *hēgemonikon* [the governing part of the soul] rule over the rest? Is it from the heart or from the brain? Or is it divided, with movement ruled from the heart and perception from the brain? Or are perception and voluntary movement both from the brain, while the involuntary pulsation of the blood vessels is from the heart? And if these two faculties are governed from the brain, why does it perceive even unwillingly, but does not move the limbs unless it wills?[2]

Given human uncertainty over how the heart and brain operate, Augustine reasoned, it was surely unsurprising that the soul itself was obscure.

As his questions slyly reveal, Augustine was not so ignorant. The organ of the governing part of the soul was a stock question in ancient philosophy and regularly appeared in theological texts.[3] Theodoret of Cyrrhus (c. 393–457) mapped out an overview:

> How far they have differed amongst themselves regarding the location of the *hēgemonikon* is simple to map out: Hippocrates, Democritus, and Plato have stated that it is seated within the brain, Strato in the space between the eyebrows,

> Erasistratus the doctor in the region of the cerebral membrane, which he terms the *epikranis*, Herophilus in the brain's ventricle, Parmenides and Epicurus in the torso as a whole; Empedocles, Aristotle, and the Stoics collectively allocate the heart to it. And among these, again, some place it in the ventricle of the heart, others in the blood, some in the pericardium, and others in the diaphragm.[4]

The Stoic concept of the *hēgemonikon* referred to one of eight parts of the soul, the others being the five senses, reproduction, and speech.[5] The *hēgemonikon* was the center of consciousness, responsible for thought, sensation, and voluntary motion. Consisting of *pneuma* (refined air), it extended outward from the heart like an octopus or a spider, activating and governing the rest of the creature.[6] By the second century, the term had become generalized and could be applied to the ideas of thinkers far beyond the chronological and intellectual reach of the Stoics.[7] The Presocratic philosopher Heraclitus, for example, had certainly never heard of the *hēgemonikon*. Nor, in all likelihood, had Plato or Hippocrates. Nonetheless, "What is the organ of the *hēgemonikon?*" could be answered with reference to anyone with an opinion about the bodily processes responsible for mental activity.[8]

By late antiquity, the central sites of the *hēgemonikon* were all located in either the head or the torso.[9] These two clusters are typically identified as "encephalocentrism" (the brain is the organ of the *hēgemonikon*) and "cardiocentrism" (the heart is the organ of the *hēgemonikon*).[10] Plato and the medical writers (Hippocrates, Herophilus, Erasistratus) were among the foremost authorities cited in favor of encephalocentrism.[11] Aristotle and the Stoics were most prominent in arguments for cardiocentrism.[12] Most late antique theologians, including Theodoret, preferred the brain.[13] In this, they followed Plato (explicitly) and the second-century physician Galen (implicitly).[14] This was in spite of the lack of scriptural corroboration: Jesus was never recorded instructing his disciples to "Love the Lord your God with all your brain, with all your mind, and with all your strength"—nor did God "examine our brains" for signs of evil.[15] Instead, scriptural authorities centered the heart.[16] Augustine addresses this discrepancy in his treatise *On the Trinity:*

> Some, therefore, have reckoned that [the mind] is blood, some the brain, and some the heart—not in the way that Scripture says, *I will confess to you, Lord, with all my heart* (Ps 9:2), and *You shall love the Lord your God with all your heart* (Dt 6:5), where the word is being applied catachrestically or metaphorically, from body to soul. Rather, they are thinking just about that part of the body we observe when viscera are torn apart.[17]

Augustine saw that parts of the body might represent aspects of the soul and psychic experience. He sought to separate this rhetorical technique from arguments about how the soul operated through the substances and organs of the body. To help his reader grasp theories about the soul/body relationship, he called to mind an everyday experience: observing "the viscera . . . torn apart," in a marketplace, for example, or at war. He was pressing back against a rising tide: during late antiquity, medical understandings of the brain as organ of the *hēgemonikon* gained symbolic power in discussions of what it meant to be a human being—rational, but embodied; vulnerable, but capable of ruling over the earth. Among Augustine's contemporaries, the brain was both medical concept and rhetorical tool.

I have begun with the question of the *hēgemonikon* in part because it was the most prominent debate about the brain in late antique society. Also, however, it draws attention to a key theme in this book as a whole: the concept of the brain as a governing organ. *Hēgemonikon* means "that which governs." Within Stoic thought, it was the coordinator of the other parts. By late antiquity, and in part through the work of Galen, the *hēgemonikon* had become conflated with Plato's *logistikon* ("that which reasons"). As organ of the *hēgemonikon-logistikon,* the brain became an increasingly human organ, responsible not only for self-governance but for governance over others also. The fusion of ideas about reason and governance in the brain within early Christian thought forms an unexplored but crucial stage in the history of the brain as the putative key to what it means to be human. How this process unfolded in the images and arguments of early Christian texts is the focus of this book. The goal is to better understand what lies beneath our own fascination with the brain as the center of our power, and how our concepts and imaginings of the brain have in consequence shaped what we imagine power to be, how we understand it to operate through our bodies, who gets to have it, and who does not.

THE ROOTS OF BRAINHOOD

We are living in the aftermath of the era of the brain.[18] Across academic and lay scientific discourse, we learn that gender is constituted in the brain, that gut inflammation produces brain chemistry conducive to depression, and that functional magnetic resonance imaging technology, which records the magnetic properties of blood flow in the brain, can represent our thoughts and actions, as well as where and why they take place.[19] In accounts of trauma, therapeutic focus has come to focus on the brain and nervous system, a shift that Catherine Malabou has described as "cerebrality," in opposition to the Freudian focus on sexuality and the genitals.[20] The boom in psychopharmaceuticals has fostered the development of what Nikolas Rose calls "neurochemical selves."[21] In the words of neurobiologist Dick Swaab, we are our brains.[22]

Philosophers and neuroscientists have argued that our assumption that the brain is identical with the human subject must be understood historically. Some claim that it is a holdover from Cartesian dualism, out of place in materialist neuroscience.[23] Fernando Vidal has provided a more specific and compelling etiology, arguing that the identification of the human self with the brain arose within seventeenth-century Europe out of the convergence of philosophical materialism with psychological theories of personal identity and the reconceptualization of soul not as animating force but as intellect.[24] He names the resultant phenomenon "cerebral subjectivity" (sometimes, more colloquially, "brainhood").[25] Crucially, Vidal understands cerebral subjectivity to be ideological, insofar as it is bound up in the classical liberal prioritization of an autonomous and rational human subject, a position that pretends to the absence of interdependency within human communities and that excludes from full citizenship and sometimes selfhood those who are dependent or whose cognitive capacities are perceived as nonnormative or impaired.[26] Rather than understand cerebral subjectivity as the sticky residue of dualism within the otherwise materialist discipline of neuroscience, Vidal argues that cerebral subjectivity in fact generated the discipline of neuroscience—that is to say, the identification of the self with the brain produced the brain as an object of scientific investigation.

When it comes to the period prior to the seventeenth century, historians of the modern brain are typically rather vague. Skipping from Galen (second century) to Descartes (seventeenth century), Vidal argues that the anatomical brain had little relevance to the concept of the human person in the intervening period. The Galenic brain "functioned as a factory and storehouse of the animal spirits," such that "animal spirits" and humors "determined a person's character."[27] Fluids and gases, not anatomy, were the key. As such, the brain itself bore no relation to the self.

In this argument, Vidal represents a general consensus. We tend to think of the brain as modern. By this I mean secular and scientific: scientific, insofar as neuroscience owes its development to the scientific method and the invention of modern technologies, such as microscopes and electricity; secular, insofar as it promises a materialist account of mental activity and so displaces the theoretical need for a soul. The brain is so modern, in fact, that we imagine it as a high-tech object—a computer with its own hardwire and circuitry; before that, it was envisioned as other kinds of up-to-date technology—a movie theater, a tape recorder, a writing pad, a loom.[28] As such, the brain appears antithetical to the period and the cultural landmarks that fall within the scope of this book: late antiquity, the rise of early Christianity and the so-called collapse of the Roman Empire, and the narrowing of intellectual activity to a theological frame, to the exclusion of disciplines such as philosophy, astronomy, and biology. This is reflected in the fact that late antiquity is often passed over in histories of the brain, despite the fact that this period saw important developments in the concept of the brain, both in expert and in popular discourse.

As we saw above, the brain played a central role in ancient and late antique discussions of what it meant to be a human being. A central goal of my analysis is to begin the work of connecting our (quite detailed) knowledge of ancient Greek medical ideas about the brain with our (extremely detailed) knowledge of early modern European medical ideas about the brain, focusing in particular on the critical moment when early Christian intellectuals established themselves as central social and political authorities within the Roman Empire. I will argue that the concept of the brain was a powerful tool in their explorations of what it meant to be human and to hold power over others. In so doing, I seek to dig down beneath Vidal's seventeenth-century genealogy of the cerebral subject to expose the premodern and Christian root system beneath. Early Christianity, as I argue through the course of this book, shaped modern self-identification with the brain as agent and instrument of governance over self and others.

Early modern knowledge about Galenic theories of the brain was filtered through influential late antique preachers and theologians, each of whom had their own theologically inflected ideas about the role of the brain in human personhood. Like Galen, late antique Christian intellectuals considered the brain to be the organ of the rational soul. Unlike Galen, they willingly departed from the constraints of medical theory to examine the role of the brain in accounts of salvation, church-building, and ascetic practice. It is valuable, therefore, to contextualize modern and early modern notions of brainhood in terms of their early Christian antecedents. The voices of late antique theologians—as loud as Galen's in sixteenth- and seventeenth-century Europe—presented the medical concept of the brain as a tool for thinking about the human being and the soul, so laying the foundations for the identification of brain with human self that came to dominate Western science and philosophy. By examining how preachers and theologians made use of the brain, we can glimpse the early Christian interests and obsessions that haunt our conceptions of the brain as the organ of the self.

LATE ANTIQUITY AND THE HISTORY OF MEDICINE

Late antiquity typically refers to the transitional period between ancient and medieval worlds.[29] Within the history of the Mediterranean and its adjacent regions, it is fundamentally tied to the disintegration of the Roman Empire and the rise of Christianity and Islam as politically powerful, monotheistic religious systems. Often it is understood as a time of crisis and decline, although the work of cultural historians in recent decades has amply demonstrated the vibrancy and adaptability of late antique culture and society.[30] The chronological boundaries of this period are debated, in particular because "late antiquity" elaborates a periodization rooted in Greco-Roman history and encompasses elements beyond the purely chronological: as Hervé Inglebert has argued, it tends to refer to a geographical region (the territory of the Roman Empire), specific themes (for example, religious transformation), and a negative value judgment (the "late" of late antiquity refers to the longstanding perception of the period as one of cultural decadence and political fragmentation).[31]

Some follow Peter Brown's *The World of Late Antiquity* in identifying the period as c. 150–750.[32] Others focus more narrowly on c. 200–600 or some period within that frame, especially if working more closely on an aspect of the Roman empire.[33] Still others recommend that we should instead pursue first millennium studies, which offers a more arbitrary window that is not centered around Greece and Rome.[34] The scope of this book is, roughly speaking, c. 200–600, with the central focus falling on the fourth and fifth centuries, during which period Christianity transformed into the dominant religion of the imperial elite, in part through the investment of elite intellectuals who drew upon medical and scientific knowledge to formulate authoritative statements about what it meant to be a human and a Christian.

Within a traditional, classicizing view of the ancient Mediterranean world, late antique culture has often been understood as inferior and imitative of what had come before, a belief that was expressed already in late antiquity itself.[35] Until quite recently, the period was cast as the gateway to the so-called Dark Ages, and it was assumed that Christian preachers and intellectuals abandoned the coolly rational scientific investigations of classical Greece and Rome, insisting instead upon theological dogma.[36] There was a widespread perception, slow to change, that medicine in particular stagnated after Galen (c. 130–215/16).[37] Historians have pushed back on this view in recent decades, paying close attention to late antique medical culture on the one hand and to Christian intellectuals' engagement with scientific and medical ideas on the other in order to establish richer intellectual and popular histories of medicine during this period of transformation.[38] It has become clear that late antiquity was a period that valued the work of intensively studying, repackaging, and repurposing ancient (indeed, already "classical") works across a wide range of intellectual disciplines. These acts of organization neither excluded existing scientific ideas nor functioned solely as vehicles that incorporated classical material whole and transmitted it in pristine form to the medieval world. Instead, the intensive engagement with the past that we see in late antique intellectual culture indicates ongoing negotiations between varied sources and authorities. These negotiations filtered and reshaped medical and scientific ideas about humans and their environments for late antique audiences and medieval readers.

At the root of the assumption that late antique Christian authors stood in the way of science is the presumed genealogical connection between ancient Greek "science" (that is, the study of the natural world) and modern science (that is, the set of disciplines and methods that emerged in seventeenth-century Europe). This connection, which is embedded in twin narratives of the "Greek miracle" (that is, the exceptionalism of ancient Greece as a site for the invention of, among other things, philosophy, science, and medicine) and European "inheritance" of Greek culture, has meant that ancient Greek (and only ancient Greek) science has traditionally been included in histories of the science, including histories of the brain, as though science were an invention of the Greeks that found its fulfillment in early modern Europe.[39]

As historians have long pointed out, this narrative betrays its intellectual roots in European hegemony, insofar as it frames the activity of medieval Arab-Islamic thinkers as the vehicle in which Greek knowledge was ferried into the European Renaissance.[40] It also raises the question of what we mean when we use the word "science." Does it refer to a culturally specific activity invented in early modern Europe? In this case, the ancients cannot have practiced science since it did not yet exist. Is it, rather, an umbrella term that is useful for describing various cross-cultural practices of seeking and making knowledge about the natural world? If so, then the whole opposition between (Greek) science and (Christian) religion collapses, since this kind of science can (indeed, often does) include theistic understandings of the natural world.[41] The resilience of narratives of connection between ancient Greek and modern Western science is rooted in the projects of European colonialism and white supremacism, insofar as both have called on connections to the classical world for the legitimacy of cultural and political dominance.[42] Closer attention to the wedge of Christianity that is lodged between ideas of ancient Greek and modern science as rational, secular projects reveals the lie in the conventional arc from Greek miracle through Christian decline into early modern European rebirth: by historicizing scientific objects, furthermore, we can begin to denaturalize them and so contribute to the work of building a pluralistic science studies that does not take a single epistemological frame or conceptual system as its center of gravity.[43]

What, then, did "science" look like in late antiquity? The rise of Christianity as an imperial religion certainly shut down forms of religious and intellectual pluralism within its sphere of influence, but it did not bring about the "decline" of science so much as transform and adapt scientific projects and knowledge to new ends. By tapping into the transformations that late antique Christian authors wrought upon existing medical ideas about the brain, it is possible to interrupt the imagined evolutionary progression between ancient Greek and modern, Western science and also to grasp the theological pressures that shaped some key scientific objects as they were taken up by early modern European scientists.

This shift in narrative from decline to transformation is common within late antique studies. It is now generally understood that late antiquity was a moment of social, political, religious, and cultural transformation in the Mediterranean world. During this period, Christianity became first a legal and then a compulsory religion within the Roman Empire. Bishops, priests, and holy men became ambassadors between rulers and cities, rich and poor, human and divine. Theological debates burned like wildfires, resulting in depositions, excommunications, and exile. Fundamental to these controversies was the contested status of the human body, which was rejected as a site of corruption and sin but also celebrated as the medium of both the incarnation and the resurrection, as well as of spiritual practices such as ascetic training.

Within this book, science refers to the cross-cultural and transhistorical project of examining and describing the world, with a focus on the "natural" world, that is, living bodies and their environments.[44] While I do distinguish between medical, philosophical, scientific, and theological approaches in late antique culture, I follow Heidi Marx in the basic premise that late antique intellectuals worked across disciplines to study both natural and supernatural phenomena: in late antiquity, science did not exist as an intellectual discipline defined in opposition to theology; rather, the study of the natural world was integrated with theological investigation.[45]

Like Galen, late antique Christian intellectuals considered the brain to be the organ of the rational and governing soul, the *hēgemonikon*. They followed medical authorities in describing the brain as a soft and vulnerable organ that received sensory impressions, stored memories, and initiated voluntary motion. When a person displayed signs of madness, they held the brain responsible. They explained to their congregants that the brain was connected to all the other parts of the body through the nerves, which carried *pneuma* from the brain into each individual part, establishing a network that relied on the integrity of the brain to function. In the majority of their references to the brain, late antique Christian authors borrow from medical ideas, occasionally expanding or elaborating the figurative language associated with these ideas to support their own rhetorical agendas. This is significant because Christian pastoral texts, especially homilies and sermons, enjoyed a far wider circulation than medical treatises among late antique and medieval audiences. Late antique Christian writings were an important vehicle for transmitting medical ideas about the brain outside of expert medical communities.

Furthermore, unconstrained by the scope or genre expectations of medical authors, late antique Christian preachers and theologians were in a position to appropriate the brain as a flexible tool in their rhetorical arsenal. The brain governed the body just as humans governed the earth and God governed the cosmos. The brain was physically vulnerable compared to other parts of the body, in the same way that the human being was physically and psychically vulnerable in comparison to other animals (that is to say, vulnerable to attack and to temptation). Christian individuals needed to take care of their brains through appropriate behaviors (for example, moderate fasting) in order to ensure that their rational souls could operate freely and effectively, so enabling the kinds of self-control important to spiritual health. At the same time, the brain was not in the same category as the soul: injury to the brain could not actually compromise salvation since the brain was merely bodily matter. These tensions shaped the concept of the brain as it was transmitted to medieval and early modern audiences.

Early Christian reception is a key, albeit understudied, moment in the history of the brain; in similar ways, the brain is a particularly crucial concept to explore when considering early Christian engagement with medical expertise and the body more generally. This is because the brain was typically understood as the node that connected the material and mortal body to the immaterial, immortal soul. It is also because, contrary to common assumptions about stagnation in late antique medicine, a new theory of brain function was developed during this period. The earliest extant witnesses to the model of brain function known as ventricular localization come from the late fourth and early fifth centuries, chiefly from the works of theologians, although they were almost certainly drawing from medical texts or acquaintances. According to ventricular localization, discrete faculties of the soul, such as memory, operate through, or dwell within, ventricles (that is, "little stomachs") within the brain. Ventricular localization was to become one of the longest-enduring models of brain function in human history, and it paved the way for subsequent frameworks that highlighted localization, such as phrenology. Its dominance was assured in part because of its centrality in influential Christian texts.

The brain is also an interesting object of examination within the study of early Christianity because it became a figurative resource to aid in exploring key questions and debates, especially in relation to governance, reason, salvation, and their relation to human vulnerability. As I will explore, early Christian authors developed imaginative strategies for incorporating the brain into accounts of what it meant to be part of political and spiritual communities: the brain as a king, the brain as Christ, the brain as a drunken man—these images developed out of early Christian efforts to tap into and to control the potential of the brain. In the same way that metaphors tend to reflect underlying conceptual structures and assumptions about how the world works, the elaboration and repetition of new metaphors about the brain influenced perceptions of its shape and functions.

Finally, the philosophical questions of early Christian writers set the stage for centuries to come: To what extent is the brain responsible for moral judgement? Is a person who suffers from brain-based mental illness responsible for their actions? Is the soul contained within the brain, or does it rather exist externally, playing the brain like some kind of flute or lyre? These questions were not new to Christian authors, but Christian theological debates made them newly pressing, and it was through sermons and homilies that they were to filter down to later audiences.[46] In late medieval and early modern Europe, when the brain came to the center of attention with the translation into Latin of texts such as Nemesius of Emesa's *On the Nature of the Human Being* and Galen's *On the Usefulness of the Parts*, the context in which it invited investigation and fresh theorization was contoured around philosophical questions that had been motivated by early Christian concerns.

APPROACHES TO THE BRAIN

Previous studies of the brain in ancient Mediterranean thought have focused on medical and philosophical texts, almost exclusively with a view to the psychological functions of the brain.[47] Theories of the brain's role in cooling the body or absorbing excess fluids and descriptions of the brain's texture and internal structures have rarely received attention, and often they have been dismissed as erroneous.[48] The distinctive contribution of this book is to explore the brain as a cultural object that had a wide range of functions and that took shape across several hundred years and in a range of social and intellectual contexts. In this, I follow Roberto Lo Presti, who framed his study of the Hippocratic treatise *On the Sacred Disease* as "a kind of archaeological operation" intended to contribute to the "epistemological history of the brain: the history of its constitution as an object of knowledge," not by seeking out the exact forerunners to modern neuroscience in ancient medicine, but by sketching out "the epistemological presuppositions and discursive rules that rendered such [modern] theories and scientific investigations possible."[49] Whereas Lo Presti takes a single text as his lens, the scope of this book is a cultural moment: the emergence of Christianity as a legitimate and then dominant religion within the late Roman Empire and the upsurge in Christian leadership drawn from the educated elite, who brought with them both extensive knowledge of philosophical and medical theories of the body and an investment in the cultural capital of these theories as a kind of currency that circulated through rhetorical performances.

Early Christian preaching constituted a major passage-point in the transmission of medical ideas, including ideas about the brain, into the early medieval world. Late antique texts that incorporated references to the brain did not function as refrigerators (to borrow from Nutton's historiographical critique) but like microwaves, blenders, and paring knives that recycled, reshuffled, and reshaped existing medical knowledge for new rhetorical and pedagogical programs.[50] Rather than focusing on the authors who knew most about the brain or who represent the closest possible access to cutting-edge medical ideas, this book works more in the mode of reception studies, exploring how ideas were ferried out of ancient medicine into other realms of thought.[51] In this, I seek to open up the ancient concept of the brain for study as a cultural object that straddles expert and nonexpert discourse.

By taking early Christianity as my focus, I have sought to show how the work of hammering out ideas about power, salvation, and embodiment toward the legitimation of a newly powerful religion shaped the brain into the kind of conceptual object that could come to represent selfhood—in particular, the kind of selfhood that depends upon modes of control and reason for its existence and its value. I borrow the term "conceptual object" from Brooke Holmes' study of the emergence of the "physical body" as separable from the human subject, "an object of and an impetus to thought and imagination."[52] Like Holmes, I seek to defamiliarize an object that "has remained largely external to our critical apparatus" to the extent that ancient accounts of the brain are typically assessed on their level of "accuracy" (that is, their degree of proximity to current ideas). In this, I also follow other historians of the body in borrowing tools and strategies from medical anthropology to decenter modern biomedicine as the exclusive or dominant framework of knowledge.[53] This shift in perspective is a matter both of historical method (insofar as it attempts to examine ancient texts and ideas on their own terms) and of politics since it is part of a broader movement to challenge the imposition of imperialist scientific systems of managing and regulating bodies.[54]

My approach to the history of the brain more particularly is grounded in critical neuroscience, a transdisciplinary field of research that analyzes how and why the brain has come to play a central role in scientific explanations of human behaviors.[55] An explicitly political field, critical neuroscience seeks to expose the values, moral frameworks, and ideologies that underpin neuroscientific research and popular engagement with the brain, especially those that equate understanding the brain with understanding what it means to be human.[56]

Core to this work is the argument that the centrality of neuroscience to current explanations of what humans are and how we operate is an artifact of cultural, political, and economic practices rather than a reflection of the centrality of the brain itself to human subjective experience.[57] This is not to deny the efficacy of neuroscience or the accuracy of the "brain facts" that it produces. Rather, it is to analyze "the ways in which, and conditions through which, behaviors and categories of people are naturalized" and, further, to examine "how these 'brain facts' are appropriated in various domains in society."[58] Following this rubric, the present book analyzes how early Christian intellectuals appropriated "brain facts" that circulated within medical and philosophical literature in order to establish the natural status and moral value of specific behaviors (for example: moderate asceticism) and categories of people (for example: the spiritual athlete).

At the heart of critical neuroscience is the work of "reinscrib[ing] the objects and practices of neuroscientific knowledge back *within* the webs of social, cultural and historical context to which they are always inevitably subject."[59] This is explicitly *not* a social constructivist vision, but instead understands the brain and neuroscience itself to be entangled with one another and with other material stuff, discourses, practices, and problems.[60] Similarly, my project in this book is not to assert the falsity of claims that the brain is crucial to cognition, moral judgement, and self-control. Rather, it is an attempt to make legible the historical moment at which the brain became a way of talking about the importance of vulnerability and control to what it meant to be human. This work *is* grounded in the premise that the brain could have been otherwise, that we certainly might have been otherwise, had it not been for the particular norms that Christianity established during the dawn of its imperial ascendancy. The alternative possibilities that I imagine for the brain are both conceptual and material: how we think about the brain changes the brain, as many others have pointed out, both because it affects how we treat the brain (for example, how we nourish it, how we exercise it, how we manipulate its activity) and because thinking itself is a fundamental process through which the brain transforms.

The body is a fundamental theme in the study of late antiquity.[61] With their focus on asceticism, celibacy, demons, martyrdom, resurrection, and the relationship between flesh, spirit, and soul, late antique religious experts set the terms for theories and experiences of embodiment within medieval Europe, leaving a legacy that in many ways still remains. The focus on how these religious experts incorporated and elaborated upon medical knowledge is more recent, reflecting the rise of humanist approaches to the sciences in recent decades. The study of medicine and religion in late antiquity has opened up new avenues of research, highlighting the interdisciplinarity of late antique intellectual activity and the depth of technical knowledge that lies behind apparently casual remarks and tropes that have to do with the body and its well-being.

A key question within this field is how to interpret medical metaphors in religious texts.[62] This question is salient within critical neuroscience also. Metaphors of the brain often encode ideas about the relationship between the brain and the mind or self.[63] When metaphors change or contradict one another, this may reflect the different aspects of the brain/self/mind relationship, theoretical pluralism, or the liminal quality of the brain's role as mediator between different planes of being.[64] As Jan Slaby and Suparna Choudhury write in their programmatic essay, it is necessary to ask how "certain metaphors begin to frame, and even shape, our understanding of the brain," indeed, how they "become tenable in the first place."[65]

Given the figurative tendencies of early Christian texts, these questions might already be considered fundamental to the chapters that follow, regardless of the metaphors in question. Yet, within the study of medicine and religion, the interpretation of metaphors is especially crucial. The central structuring metaphor within early Christianity was that of healing as salvation.[66] This image served as a lynchpin in a conceptual network that supported the elaboration of metaphorical and conceptual associations across various domains, most obviously the theological, but also the moral and the political. Preachers and theologians, borrowing from philosophers, identified themselves (and Christ) as physicians of the soul and their work as healing their audiences of sin.[67] Any reference to medical knowledge, including the concept of the brain, in early Christian texts must be interpreted in light of these fundamental metaphors.

Christian references to medical concepts have often been dismissed as mere ornament or idiom. Yet, they are basic windows into and tools for shaping experiences of embodiment and relationality.[68] Metaphors reveal what speakers expect their audience to already understand and have the capacity to imagine, "the horizon of possibilities for thinking and acting" within a cultural and intellectual context.[69] Within this book, I follow other late antique historians in drawing on conceptual metaphor theory (CMT) as a useful framework for making legible the thought-worlds that metaphors imply.[70] According to CMT, metaphorical expressions (metaphors that are encountered in texts or speech, for example, "follow your path") can be analyzed to reveal conceptual metaphors (underlying conceptual structures, for example, LIFE IS A JOURNEY).[71] While the reductive tendencies of CMT invite debate, its central claim—metaphors reflect habits of thought—is widely accepted, and the theory has opened new avenues for research into late antique history by encouraging the reinterpretation of metaphors not as ornaments but as indicators of "an underlying way of thought" that is largely preconscious.[72] This approach is reflected in a growing body of scholarship that investigates medical metaphors in late antiquity.[73]

CMT has proved attractive to and useful for late antique historians not only because it enables the analysis of metaphors as evidence for the history of thought, but also because of the importance that it gives to the body. According to Lakoff and Johnson, the body is a fundamental source of metaphors: the conceptual metaphor GOOD IS UP, for example, assumes the body as a point of departure.[74] Embodied experience produces metaphors—both metaphorical expressions and their underlying (and typically implicit) metaphorical concepts. This resonates with the body metaphors (especially metaphors that connect body to society) that wend through late ancient discourse. When transferred from a linguistic to a historical approach, CMT, with its focus on embodiment, offers tools for analyzing not only how bodily experience directs metaphorical concepts, but also how metaphors structure and illuminate the experiences of ordinary embodiment. This takes us beyond the fundamental claims of CMT. As Kristi Upson-Saia writes, "Late ancient Christians' medical metaphors [were] more than just a conceptual or linguistic frame to borrow. . . . Religious authors were borrowing medical ideas to think about early Christians' material bodies (both their anatomy and physiology) so that they could describe what ailed their congregants and prescribe material, ritualized interventions that would restore them to full health."[75] Metaphors reveal habits of thought that are often unconscious, but they are also used to navigate and manipulate bodies. Greek philosophers had developed the popular metaphorical expression that *philosophy is medicine for the soul.* Late antique Christian theologians and preachers transformed this metaphor into an argument that Christianity is medicine for the soul and the body also.

When interpreting metaphors of the brain in late antique texts, it is important to consider the understanding of figurative language within ancient rhetorical theory and Christian exegesis also. In the arguments that I construct throughout this book, much turns upon the interpretation of complex metaphor and, crucially, upon the question of whether an account of the brain is to be understood in literal or figurative terms, to the extent that such a binary can be applied. This raises the further question, however, of the extent to which late antique audiences would have thought about this distinction, and indeed of what frameworks they had in place to make sense of the medical metaphors that they encountered within sermons and other texts.

In his *Institutes of Oratory*, Quintilian introduced metaphor as follows: "Let us begin, then, with that which is both the most frequent and the most beautiful by far—that which I call *translatio*, but which is known in Greek as μεταφορά."[76] As Averil Cameron has argued, figurative language was especially important in early Christian rhetoric, not only as a "beautiful" artifact, but also as a tool for illuminating the mysterious and unknowable qualities of the divine, by "presenting the audience with a series of images through which it was thought possible to perceive an objective and higher truth."[77] This use of metaphor to illuminate the unfamiliar through the familiar could be understood not only in terms of transformed perception or revelation, but also as the relocation of the observing subject. In his commentary on *Song of Songs*, Gregory the Great wrote that allegory (which ancient rhetoricians often defined as a kind of metaphor) "makes something like a machine [*machinam*]" by which the soul "might be lifted [*leuetur*] to God."[78] In other words, if metaphor is, etymologically, a "carrying across," then, when integrated into allegorical interpretation, it functioned as a lever that lifted the soul out of the mortal, bodily realm and into the realm of the divine.

The fourth century was a period of contestation regarding the value and veracity of allegorical and literal interpretations of the Judeo-Christian scriptures.[79] In the late twentieth century, scholars in late antique studies and Patristics began to challenge the conventional view that fourth-century exegetes were divided into the "Alexandrians," who dealt in allegory, and the "Antiochenes," who offered only literal interpretations.[80] While there were exegetes who identified with each camp, the terms are perhaps better understood as "fighting words," leveraged in order to "justify one's own reading and denigrate that of the other."[81] The stakes in this exegetical battle were high, but the result was not that one mode of reading prevailed; rather, through polemical sermons and orations, pamphlets and tracts, late antique congregants were trained to distinguish layers of figurative and literal meaning within scriptural imagery.[82] Exposure to a range of competing interpretations—all of which drew upon a range of reading strategies, and many of which deployed both figurative and literal exegesis—schooled late antique audiences in the practice of discerning multiple meanings within a single image, even within a single word.[83] Late antique audiences and readers were expected to apply these interpretative practices not only to images in the Judeo-Christian scriptures, but also to those developed by contemporary Christian authors. Trained in rhetoric and in exegesis, preachers wove literal and figurative threads into a mode of speech that worked upon its audience through its connection between multiple images and planes of meaning. When we encounter metaphors of the brain in Christian texts, we should assume not only that these metaphors can function as tracers for underlying conceptual structures but also that late antique audiences engaged in sophisticated strategies of interpretation in order to construct their own understanding of what it meant to have a brain and what this then meant for the work of being human.

REASON, REGULATION, VULNERABILITY, AND THE BRAIN

"From what part of the body does that which they call the *hēgemonikon* rule over the rest? Is it from the heart or from the brain?"[84] When Augustine raised these questions in his letter to the layperson who had challenged him regarding his ignorance about the origins of individual souls, he was drawing on commonplace knowledge to dismiss his opponent. The brain entered late antique consciousness as a probable, if problematic, answer to the question, *What is the organ of the governing part of the soul?* A core argument of this book is that early Christian authors built on the foundation of this question to present the brain as crucial for governing both the self and others, a capacity that was tied to reason (as we might expect) and vulnerability (which we might not). This triangle of governance, reason, and vulnerability shaped the brain into the kind of object that could become a "cipher for the self" in early modern European science, and it also naturalized certain norms and expectations related to human and especially Christian identity. This is in part because, as I will argue, the brain became identified with the human being, both in the metonymic sense (the individual brain could stand in for the individual human) and in the sense that brains themselves became humanized, representing the distinctive characteristics that guaranteed the claim to a unique human capacity for rulership and salvation.

In a letter to his brother Peter, Gregory of Nyssa writes of humankind as follows: "How, you might ask, has such a creature been allotted governance over everything? . . . The apparent neediness of our nature is the occasion for domination over all things that are under our control."[85] The brain echoed this paradox: it was soft, delicate, and in need of physical protection; yet it was also the governing organ within the microcosm of the animal body—and not merely in spite of, but also because of, its weakness. Softness was the foundation for sensitivity. Intelligence required vulnerability. This oxymoron—strength in weakness—served to explain the apparent disconnect between the Christian theory that God had designed human beings perfectly for their role as governors and stewards of the created world and the obvious weakness of human bodies in comparison to other animals. It also warned listeners of their limitations as mortal, embodied beings. The brain, as the instrument of the distinctively human capacity for reason, became a kind of model and metonym for the way in which physical vulnerability could simultaneously produce and constrain the intellectual qualities that enabled hierarchical power and control.

Early Christian authors used medical ideas about the brain not only as conceptual and figurative tools to explore what it means to be human, but also to instruct their congregants and readers in proper Christian behavior. Preachers bolstered their condemnation of drunkenness, for example, by hinting at the effects of alcohol on the brain. At the same time, excessive ascetic practices (for example, avoidance of sleep) were criticized on the grounds that they could damage the brain and so undermine the purpose of ascetic practice in the first place.

This emphasis on cerebral vulnerability motivated conformity to behavioral standards by representing the limits and the techniques of self-governance. The brain became a material signifier of human vulnerability and therefore of human dependence on God. It is no coincidence, then, that it is in the early Christian period that we see a sudden multiplication of anthropomorphizing metaphors of the brain: the brain as king, the brain as priest, the brain as a drowning man. These metaphors reflect the proximity between the brain and the human being in early Christianity—a proximity that was, I argue in this book, a precursor and foundation for subsequent identifications of the individual human self with their brain. The aspects of human identity associated with brainhood in early Christian thought were rationality, regulation (over self and others), vulnerability, and the capacity for spiritual sickness and healing.

CHAPTER SUMMARIES

Chapter 1 begins by examining the circulation of medical knowledge outside of expert contexts in late antiquity. This work is a necessary foundation to grasp the significance and the limits of references to the brain in Christian literature. Through parallel analyses of Christian and non-Christian sources, I argue that medical knowledge about the human body carried cultural capital in late antiquity and was in the process of being transformed into more accessible and portable forms. References to the brain in early Christian texts reflect broader cultural frameworks and values.

Whereas the first chapter offers social and cultural context for the analyses that follow, chapter 2 provides historical context, surveying ideas about the brain that circulated prior to late antiquity. The purpose of this is threefold: first, to sketch out the range of intellectual resources that Christian authors may have accessed in their representations of the brain; second, to explore how psychological and nonpsychological models of the brain coexisted, sometimes even within the same account, in ancient medicine and philosophy; and third, to show, nevertheless, how the psychological model of brain function (the brain as the organ of the governing part of the soul) became dominant in the centuries leading up to late antiquity. This last point is important because it suggests why the brain was such a potent symbol for late antique Christian authors.

Chapter 3 continues the work of the second chapter in examining theorizations of brain structure and function, but it pays particular attention to late antiquity. My argument in this chapter shows how a close reexamination of the sources within their Christian context might transform our understanding of the history of medical concepts of the brain. As this chapter explores, the longest-enduring model of brain function emerged in the fourth century C.E. and was transmitted almost entirely through the writings of two late antique bishops. This model, which is called ventricular localization in the study of ancient medicine and cell theory in medieval or early modern studies, ascribed a discrete faculty of the soul to each "ventricle" or "cell" that earlier anatomists had identified within the brain. These faculties depended on the movement of *pneuma* through the ventricles of the brain and the associated nerves. Historians of the brain have long asserted that ventricular localization is not a true model of brain function, since the brain seems to operate merely as a container for the *pneuma*. I argue in this chapter that if we interpret ventricular localization in light of the late antique metaphor of the body and brain as instruments of the soul, then we can set aside the modern binary between brain substance and hollow ventricles and understand the ventricles, *pneuma*, and cerebral structure to be working in collaboration with one another in the manner of a flute or a lyre. That is to say, by examining the early Christian sources for ventricular localization in closer detail, it becomes possible to see the limitations in the modern concept of the "brain" (qua solid body) as a tool for assessing late antique theories and to lay the foundations for more nuanced analysis.

Chapter 4 marks a turn from explicit theorization of how the brain works to interpretations of its figurative appearances in early Christian rhetoric. The focus of the chapter is the central metaphor of the brain as a governing agent within the human body. In late antique Christian writings, I argue, we see the emergence of varied and elaborate anthropomorphizing of the brain in different governing roles. These metaphors suggest a tightening association between the brain and the human being as bodies that govern self and (through self-governance) others. As I turn to in the following chapters, this capacity for governance was both enabled and constrained by vulnerability.

Chapters 5 and 6 examine the rhetoric of cerebral vulnerability in early Christian texts. By this, I mean the ways that Christian authors used medical and philosophical discussion of the brain's physical delicacy as a tool for talking about the psychological vulnerabilities and mortality of human beings. Chapter 5 demonstrates that Christian preachers used the physical vulnerability of the brain to construct persuasive arguments for ascetic practices, especially fasting, avoidance of alcohol, and minimal use of perfumes. Chapter 6 argues, in turn, that preachers and theologians used the brain-based mental illness phrenitis to build arguments against reliance upon asceticism, especially excessive asceticism, as a tool for salvation. Through this two-pronged argument, I show how the vulnerability of the brain could stand in for the limits of human self-determination as embodied, rational beings.

What was the theological advantage to early Christian authors of emphasizing cerebral vulnerability? Chapter 7 turns from the pastoral mileage available in this rhetoric to its implications for Christian anthropology. Through an examination of the use of comparative anatomy in Christian discussions of the human being, I argue that the emphasis on cerebral vulnerability as a sign of human dependence on God was part of a broader appropriation of the brain as symbol of the human being in late antique Christian thought. This "humanization" of the brain served a theological and pastoral agenda and laid the foundations for the identification of the brain with the individual human subject in subsequent medical and philosophical thought.

Specifically, this conception of the human being was of a creature that governs and can be saved. The early Christian brain required a particular kind of care (moderate ascetic practices) in order to tend to its vulnerability in a way that would continue to allow for reason, salvation, and control over the self and the rest of the created world.

CHAPTER I

The Circulation and Performance of Medical Knowledge in Late Antiquity

In his treatise *On Prayer,* the learned monk Evagrius of Pontus (c. 349–399) describes the demonic causes of the eight *logismoi* (thoughts) that distract the monk from prayer. Among the most dangerous of these is vainglory, which affects only the perfected monk, whose "mind prays purely, unerringly, and truly." This happens, Evagrius writes, when "the demons creep in no longer from the left but from the right." The effect of vainglory in this instance is specific: the monk sees "an appearance of God in a form customary to the senses," and therefore supposes that "he has finally achieved the purpose of prayer." The vision arises first because of the passion of vainglory, and second "because of the place in the brain that is touched and palpated in its blood vessel by the demon." Evagrius goes on to connect these two causes: the passion of vainglory is provoked by the demon, which "kindles" the place in the brain that it touches, and "bends the light around the mind at will."[1]

Evagrius integrates demonic and naturalistic components into his explanation of the passions.[2] Composed of *pneuma* (air), which was also the instrument or substance of the soul, demons could enter through the nose as terrible odors, and not uncommonly caused illnesses through their interference in human bodies.[3] What is striking in this example is Evagrius' description of how demons manipulate the brain. By "touching" and "kindling" the region of the brain and its associated blood vessel, the demon distorts the monk's sensory faculties, summoning a false vision of God. This explanation is grounded in the popular medical concept of the brain as the organ responsible for enabling and synthesizing bodily sensations. It also reflects a development in fourth-century medical theory, that is, the localization of specific cognitive functions such as sensation in discrete regions of the brain. Indeed, Evagrius invokes the very logic used by medical writers to establish the spatial localization of cerebral functions: any given cognitive dysfunction is caused by damage to a distinct part of the brain, and therefore the functions of different parts can be elucidated through controlled damage to them. Symptoms such as hallucination or vainglory reveal interior corporeal disruption.

Late antique Christian authors such as Evagrius used medical knowledge about the brain in order to establish their therapeutic expertise with regard to the soul. In order to persuade their congregants and readers to trust them as "physicians of the soul," preachers and theologians incorporated the brain not only as an "instrument of the soul" (as it had long been understood in medical and philosophical discourse), but also as a mechanism for the influence that the body could have upon the soul.[4] The passion of vainglory, according to Evagrius, was caused by demonic pressure upon the brain. Asterius of Amasea (c. 350–410), a close contemporary and neighbor of Evagrius, describes a similar bodily process in his *Homily on the Holy Fast:* abstaining from food reduces "the palpation of arteries" and "the darkening of the brain through the influx of vapors" that is caused by regular digestion.[5] Other factors thought to compromise the brain and its cognitive functions included physical trauma, strong odors, drunkenness, indigestion, lack of sleep, and environmental conditions (too hot, too cold, too wet, too dry). These concerns derived from the tradition of learned, naturalistic medicine that originated with the Hippocratic authors in the fifth century B.C.E. and that remained a dominant paradigm for explaining bodily processes and dysfunction in late antiquity. While Christian preachers and theologians borrowed the title "physician of the soul" from Greco-Roman philosophers, they paid closer attention than philosophers to medical theories about the brain. Where ancient physicians focused on nonhuman agents of disease causation and therapy (for example, yellow bile), and ancient philosophers on human agency (for example, greed), ancient preachers and theologians sought a synthesis that might allow them to account for and control the physical conditions of the human will.[6]

Late antique knowledge and expertise were constructed and confirmed through speech acts and practical demonstrations by individuals within a broader social context, that is, self-authorizing behaviors that were validated by the community.[7] Since there were no degree-granting institutions, experts were necessarily self-made, often through the support of networks that comprised patrons, teachers, fellow students, and friends. Knowledge was interdisciplinary, focusing on objects of study (the human body), rather than on disciplines (medicine, philosophy, theology), although disciplinary difference did matter when it came to distinguishing courses of study or claiming exclusive expertise.[8] Anatomical literacy, I will argue, enabled preachers to assert their authority as experts on the care of human souls. As the organ of the soul, the brain was central to this project.

The emergence of imperial Christianity in the fourth century created a class of ambitious intellectuals tasked with teaching the wider population and catering to the elite in order to establish anthropological and therapeutic authority. This chapter explores the social and intellectual conditions in which these intellectuals developed and projected expertise with regard to the medical concept of the brain. First, I explore the usefulness of medical knowledge at elite dinner parties in late antiquity. I argue that medical expertise was a valued commodity, but of a different kind than canonical *paideia*. This difference, I suggest, made it attractive material for late antique Christian intellectuals seeking to establish their authority without seeming indebted to the so-called "pagan," or "Hellenic," tradition. Second, I consider the role of "iatrosophists" in popularizing medical knowledge, following an argument made by Chris de Wet that late antique preachers should be understood as iatrosophists of the soul.[9] Finally, I introduce late antique medical texts as a context for understanding not only where Christian authors acquired their knowledge about the brain, but also how their own writings might have been interpreted through the lens of contemporary medical publications. In sum, I argue that the prominence of technical information about the brain in late antique Christian texts reflects a broader cultural context in which expert medical knowledge carried intellectual capital and substantiated intellectual authority, even as the tradition of medical experimentation and novel theorization began to erode. The heightened focus on the brain in late antique Christian rhetoric responded directly to the potency of medical expertise, particularly with regard to the brain, in late antique society.[10]

MACROBIUS AND AUGUSTINE: MEDICAL KNOWLEDGE AT ELITE DINNER PARTIES

In the mid-fifth century, Macrobius Ambrosius Theodosius wrote a dinner-party dialogue that purported to record conversation among historical senatorial figures at a celebration of the Roman festival of the Saturnalia. The host of the dinner party, Vettius Agorius Praetextatus, had died in 384, and the dialogue is apparently set shortly prior to his death, perhaps in 382, the last Saturnalia before the emperor Gratian ended state subsidies for civic cults.[11] Likely writing after 430, when a Theodosius who might be identified with our author served as praetorian prefect of Italy, Macrobius perhaps drew upon the surviving corpus of letters between Praetextatus and his acquaintances to animate the traditional form of the sympotic dialogue.[12] While portions of the dialogue are adapted from earlier texts, such as Aulus Gellius' *Attic Nights*, the particular guests and their convergence at the Saturnalia are Macrobius' own creation.[13] As in many examples of the genre, the senators are joined by a physician, the historical Dysarius, who answers questions about the digestive system, drunkenness, and the brain.[14] Through Dysarius, Macrobius' *Saturnalia* offers an ideal portrait of the medical expert at work in his late antique social context. Considered "a key text for any evaluation of the intellectual interests of the elite of late fourth- and early fifth-century Rome," this work offers an apt entry-point into the valuation and circulation of medical knowledge in late antique society.[15]

Macrobius describes an ideal dinner party of historical figures, "a highly idealized and highly stylized republic of learning."[16] During the first six books, the conversation circles around questions of traditional *paideia* (elite education): Virgil, etiquette, Roman law, the heavenly spheres. As Macrobius illustrates, *paideia* was not merely a matter of accumulating knowledge; as the glue that held the aristocracy together, it was also a process of subject formation that entrenched cultural ideals and social hierarchies.[17] Following a rebuke by Praetextatus, the young man Avienus learns to avoid the appearance of arrogance in the company of his elders, while the disruptive guest Evangelus prompts "reinforcement of the consensual styles of analysis" shared among the other discussants.[18] Status was established and confirmed through proper use of *paideia* in social situations. As an outsider to the Roman elite—an uninvited guest, a Greek, a medical professional—Dysarius contributes little to this initial discussion.

Only in the last extant book of the dialogue does the host, Praetextatus, turn the conversation away from a heated discussion of insults to "subject matter suitable for a dinner party—and not only about food, but also whatever has to do with the nature of the body and other such things," suggesting as he does so that Dysarius might be called upon as the authority among them.[19]

The remainder of the book is devoted to medical topics, with Dysarius fielding one question from each guest in turn. Dysarius is pressed to address a range of traditional topics, including diet, digestion, the composition of foods, wine, and blushing. His most detailed anatomical discussion, however, is reserved for the nervous system and the brain, in response to questions by the boorish Evangelus, who asks first how dizziness occurs, and then, when Dysarius explains dizziness in relation to the brain, how the brain can be thought to function as the organ of sensation, given that the cerebral substance itself is insensitive to touch.

The division of material in the *Saturnalia*, between traditional *paideia* in books 1–6, where Dysarius barely speaks, and medical knowledge in book 7, where Dysarius is the central authority, reflects the cultural division between these two modes of learning. Medical expertise circulated as intellectual capital in late antique society. As Heidi Marx and Kristi Upson-Saia have argued, "basic medical logic was a requisite of Greek *paideia* and a subject which the Roman aristocracy, including Jewish and Christian elites, integrated and absorbed."[20] Nevertheless, as the figure of Dysarius illustrates, medical knowledge was not traditional *paideia*—it is not the senatorial elites who establish their authority and connections by discoursing on the brain, but the outsider, the Greek physician. This perhaps explains why early Christian authors felt so free to include medical learning in their pastoral and theological texts: it exhibited their learning and cultural competence, but avoided the more contentious literary content on display earlier in the *Saturnalia*.[21] Preachers, many of whom had benefited from extensive rhetorical education, might choose not to quote Demosthenes or Cicero, but they could—with or without citation—offer a detailed description of, for example, the double membranes that shelter the brain from the friction of the skull.[22]

Macrobius' *Saturnalia* illustrates how expert medical knowledge about the brain could circulate outside of professional medical contexts. It reflects an idealized literary and intellectual culture in which the human body was a topic of learned conversation and in which physicians such as Dysarius wielded the authority of expertise. While it is unlikely that the dialogue directly reflects actual conversations among the intellectual elite of late antiquity, it does indicate their interest in human anatomy and physiology, especially as it related to elite activities, such as feasting, drinking, and philosophizing. This is further corroborated by the fact that the text itself is a vector for medical knowledge. While Macrobius represents the dissemination of medical knowledge among nonexperts as taking place in the intimate and immediate context of an elite dinner party, the very medium of his account reveals the textual basis for the circulation of medical knowledge in late antiquity. Dysarius is a trope, based ultimately on the figure of Erysimachus in Plato's *Symposium*, and the questions put to him—as well as the answers that he provides—are drawn largely from anthologies of sympotic conversation, such as Plutarch's *Table Talk*, as well as from philosophical and medical handbooks, such as the *Physical Problems* and *Medical Problems* that are spuriously attributed to Alexander of Aphrodisias.[23] Such handbooks proliferated in late antiquity, providing a quick reference guide for nonexperts, such as Macrobius, to present expert knowledge from a range of technical fields.[24] Macrobius offers not (or not only) a window into late antique small talk, but an indication of the cultural capital attached to medical knowledge about the human body, and a glimpse of the learned physicians who moved in upper-class circles.

Dysarius was also a historical figure, an acquaintance of the senator Symmachus, who wrote letters of recommendation on his behalf.[25] In these letters, Symmachus refers to Dysarius as "professor of medicine," and as holding the highest place among "professors of healing," phrases that Macrobius echoes in the first book of the *Saturnalia*, when Dysarius is introduced as one "who at that time seemed to stand out at Rome among the others who professed the art of medicine."[26] The letters of Symmachus indicate that Dysarius both practiced medicine under elite patronage and served as a teacher of medicine, albeit perhaps to his patrons rather than to aspiring professionals. While Macrobius fictionalizes the relationship and the *Saturnalia*, further, is structured by the conventions of the genre rather than by observation, the figure of Dysarius nonetheless offers insights into the role of fourth-century learned physicians—such as Vindicianus (c. 340–400) and Oribasius (c. 320–400)—in the late antique imagination.

Dysarius' description of brain anatomy and function may have served a pedagogical function, summarizing medical knowledge for a nonexpert audience; however, it is unlikely that it was intended as a surprising or controversial account. Macrobius presents his reader with a familiar image of the brain as the organ of sensory function (*cerebro quasi omnes corporis sensus gubernanti*), the habitation of the soul (*habitatio eius in cerebro est*), and the root of the nerves, which Dysarius describes as operating in yoked pairs (*syzygia*), a Greek medical term.[27] He uses common metaphors: the brain "governs" (*gubernet*), as if over a city (a twist on the Platonist metaphor of the rational soul governing from the head), or steers (*gubernet*), as if over a ship (thus the spinal marrow, which extends from the marrow of the brain, is described as the "ship's keel," *navi carina*).[28] The mechanism by which the brain performs its sensory and governing functions is Galenic: *spiramentum* (breath, translating the Greek word πνεῦμα, commonly translated into Latin as *spiritus*) gathers in the cavities or ventricles of the brain (*in cavernis cerebri*) and flows from these cavities into the nerves, endowing all the parts of the body with sensory power.[29] Dysarius' account of the anatomy and function of the brain reflects a medical consensus that had been in development since the nervous system was charted during the Hellenistic period, and it is likely that he expected his audience to be familiar with his account, at least in its broad strokes. Even the question that Evangelus puts to Dysarius—how can the brain be the organ of sensation, if cerebral matter itself is insensitive?—was already familiar. This was Aristotle's objection to the encephalocentric model, and Dysarius' answer presupposes a Platonist framework: the brain has no need of sensation in itself, because it is the dwelling-place of the soul, while sensation belongs to bodily parts.[30]

The account of the brain that Dysarius gives to his senatorial audience in Macrobius' *Saturnalia* is similar in detail and focus to the briefer allusions to the brain in fifth-century Christian pastoral and theological texts. Evangelus' question regarding how the insensitive brain might be responsible for sensation moreover establishes the basic problem with which late antique Christian intellectuals grappled: how can the material brain be the organ of the immaterial soul? That question, which came in many different guises, lay at the root of much ambivalence regarding the brain in late antique Christian discourse. Whereas Evangelus was chiefly concerned with weaseling out a possible contradiction in Dysarius' theory, Christian authors worried that the brain might contain—and so constrain—the soul, that damage to the brain might compromise the integrity of the soul, and that the functions of the brain might render the soul theoretically unnecessary. In some cases, as we will see in subsequent chapters, they worked hard to weaken these risks by denying or minimizing the role of the brain; in other cases, they highlighted these very risks in order to reinforce their own lessons about the care of the body and the implications of bodily self-discipline for the health of the soul. As Macrobius reveals, these late antique preachers and theologians were speaking to audiences already familiar with the framework of the brain, and with the problems and potential that it held.

Early in the fifth century, perhaps fifteen or twenty years before Macrobius wrote the *Saturnalia*, the pagan aristocrat Rufius Antonius Agrypnius Volusianus attended a party at which the conversation turned controversial.[31] After discoursing on the well-trodden paths of rhetoric and philosophy, one guest challenged the others to branch out into an explanation of Christian theology. In particular, he questioned the doctrine of the incarnation: Could "the lord and ruler of the world" really have been held within a woman's body? Why would an almighty god have subjected himself to an insignificant body and all of its inconvenient necessities, such as sleep, appetite, and sensation? Volusianus, who was not yet a Christian (although he had several prominent Christian relatives), wrote to the bishop Augustine for intellectual guidance.[32] Augustine responded with a series of analogies intended to demonstrate how the greatness of God could be "not by mass, but by power"; among the analogies he uses to illustrate this argument is the brain: "From a single point, and as if from the center of the brain, [he] divides all the senses into a fivefold distribution."[33]

Volusianus was son of Ceionius Rufius Albinus, one of the senatorial guests in Macrobius' *Saturnalia*.[34] The conversation that he reports to Augustine is situated within a very similar cultural and intellectual environment to that recreated by Macrobius some two decades later. When Augustine uses the brain to explain the contradictions of incarnational theology, he is speaking within a social context that included the participation of medically informed intellectuals who considered the brain to be a central and relevant problem in understanding human nature.

Macrobius' *Saturnalia* illustrates how expert medical knowledge about the brain could circulate outside of professional medical contexts. While the dialogue is conventional and idealized, it nonetheless reflects a social milieu in which the intellectual elite might gather at a dinner party and discuss, in heated and perhaps not entirely sober fashion, the workings and capacities of the human being. In some instances, they perhaps wrote to learned physicians to clarify points of disagreement; with regard to theological questions, however, bishops such as Augustine served as sources of authority. Augustine's choice to answer a theological question with reference to the functions of the brain suggests the cogency of medical knowledge as a resource for persuasion and the establishment of authority in late antique intellectual culture. It also offers a glimpse of how innovative Christian rhetoricians such as Augustine incorporated the brain into their theological toolkit.

In the *Saturnalia*, Dysarius holds total authority when it comes to the human body: there is no Augustine present to offer his own, layperson's account. Only in one instance does the Greek philosopher Eustathius offer a counterargument: when Dysarius states that a plain diet is easiest to digest, Eustathius argues that a varied and moderate diet is the key. Dysarius responds to Eustathius' arguments by drawing a firm line between their areas of expertise: his reasoning is based on medical training, while that of Eustathius is based on rhetorical skill. This distinction was a common method of gatekeeping in ancient medical and philosophical discourse, and we will encounter it again in the following section, where we will examine the professionals who seem to mediate between the position of Dysarius (physician) and Augustine (rhetorician), the iatrosophists described by Eunapius of Sardis as the most prominent teachers of medicine in the late antique Mediterranean world.

PREACHERS AS IATROSOPHISTS

Iatrosophist was the term for rhetoricians who disseminated medical ideas to the public, and who may or may not have practiced medicine themselves. I argue in this section that we might understand Christian preachers who engaged with medical themes as learning from and operating in the mode of the iatrosophists.[35] This raises the question of how audiences might have heard Christian preachers when they launched into discussions of human anatomy or framed their sermons as therapeutic, guiding their congregants in healthy practices of the soul. What kind of authority did preachers carry with their audiences when they introduced medical themes? Were they believable as experts on the body, or were their references to the brain understood in purely rhetorical or figurative terms? In order to address these questions, we need to turn to the cultural phenomenon of iatrosophists at large.

The Second Sophistic rhetorician Dio Chrysostom (c. 40–115) offers a caustic account of medical orators: "The kind of lecture I mean is like a spectacle or parade, similar to the exhibitions of so-called physicians, who, sitting on high in the center, explain the connections of joints, the combination and juxtaposition of bones, and other such things: ducts, breaths, and excretions."[36] Such figures, Dio reports, draw admiring crowds, but they are inferior to the "genuine physician," who leaves the pleasures of rhetoric aside, and instead performs the difficult work of displeasing the patient for the sake of health: "He provides instructions in what patients must do, and he prevents patients from eating or drinking what they want, and he takes hold of abscesses and cuts them out of the body."[37]

Rhetoric had always been a core part of the learned medical tradition.[38] Hippocratic physicians gained clients and patronage through public speech, and the influential physician Galen of Pergamon reported competitive exegetical and anatomical demonstrations, in which a physician could be tested by his rivals before a large crowd.[39] Alongside this there developed a tradition of disparaging medical authors or orators for excelling in rhetoric instead of medical practice. This tradition manifested in late antiquity as a perceived split between the elite iatrosophists, who lectured in the intellectual centers of the late Roman Empire, and practicing physicians, who devoted themselves to healing the sick, and who studied and taught through apprenticeships.[40] Whatever the historical truth of this division at the level of professional competence, it clearly reflects the high cultural value of medical discourse in late antique intellectual culture.[41] It was imaginable that a man could build a highly successful public career based on talking about medicine alone.

Eunapius of Sardis (born c. 345/6) records in his *Lives of the Philosophers and Sophists* the careers of famed medical sophists of late antiquity: Zeno of Cyprus, Magnus of Nisibis, Oribasius of Pergamum, and Ionicus.[42] "Doctors," Eunapius writes, by way of introduction, "also flourished during this period," referring with the title *doctors* both to physicians trained in rhetoric and to rhetoricians trained in medicine.[43] The most important in his account are Zeno of Cyprus, Magnus of Nisibis, and Oribasius of Pergamon.

Zeno of Cyprus established a school, perhaps in Athens, which is the chief location of Eunapius' earlier biographical subjects, or Alexandria, which was famous as a center of medical education.[44] According to Eunapius, Zeno lectured on and practiced medicine, and his illustrious pupils pursued different paths: some became rhetoricians, some physicians, and others both.[45] Among these was Magnus of Nisibis, judged to be better at rhetoric than healing, as both Eunapius and the Byzantine physician Theophilus Protospatharius report—indeed, Eunapius goes so far as to say that Magnus persuaded patients who had been cured by other physicians that they were still unwell.[46] Perhaps because of his rhetorical excellence, he was given a public school in Alexandria, and Eunapius reports that people traveled from far away, either to admire him (θαυμάσαντές, lit. "to treat him as a wonder") or to study.[47]

Oribasius of Pergamon (c. 320–403) had the most enduring influence among Eunapius' iatrosophists.[48] As personal physician to Julian, he played a part in making Julian emperor and went into exile after Julian's death. He also wrote several works that excerpted, anthologized, and summarized earlier medical authorities, above all, Galen. In some places, he cites different authorities by name and by text; elsewhere, he centonizes Galen's work, stitching together sentence fragments from different texts to present a smooth and condensed account of the human body, its functions, and its diseases.[49] While the medical professors at Alexandria shaped the medical curriculum for centuries to come, focusing it entirely around Hippocrates and Galen, Oribasius fixed the content and the limits of medical literacy across a broader population—those who might not have the resources to study original medical treatises, but who sought an accessible and encyclopedic overview.[50] Oribasius provided a map for lay readers of medical texts in late antiquity and after.

Iatrosophists provide a cultural reference point for the incorporation of medical knowledge about the brain into sermons by fourth- and fifth-century preachers: it was not unexpected for audiences (especially but not only among the educated elite) to learn about the anatomy, physiology, and illnesses of the body through public speeches—just as it was fairly common for these same audiences to learn about the care of the soul from philosophers.[51] The incorporation of anatomical and physiological information into sermons made sense within the landscape of late antique rhetoric. It also made sense in light of the new political power that learned physicians wielded in late antiquity, serving as ambassadors and advisors to rulers within and beyond the Roman Empire.[52] Oribasius' emperor-making career may have been unusual, but it fit into a social pattern that made medical education attractive even to students who did not intend to enter the medical profession: medical students might enter the imperial administration, become professors themselves, or, in some cases, take up leadership roles within the church.[53]

Iatrosophists also offer a glimpse of how the intellectual elite of late antiquity may have developed lay medical expertise.[54] An idealized example of this is provided by Gregory of Nazianzus in his eulogy to Basil of Caesarea, which he delivered in the early 380s.[55] Gregory and Basil had studied philosophy and rhetoric at Athens together, while Gregory's brother Caesarius was studying medicine at Alexandria.[56] According to Gregory, Basil obtained universal knowledge, transcending the narrow fields of study by which more mundane experts were defined.[57] Gregory lists areas of study in which Basil excelled (astronomy, geometry, mathematics), culminating with his mastery of medicine.[58] Motivated by his own sickness and his desire to tend to the health of others, Basil studied not only the rules of therapeutic practice, but also the principles behind medicine, and its theories.[59] Basil's motivations for studying medicine reflect the ideal concerns of the late antique Christian nobleman: he learns how to take care of his own body, and the bodies of the afflicted in his care.

Lay medical expertise demonstrated self-sufficiency and self-discipline complementary to the philosophical therapeutics of the soul. Intellectuals who extended their range to encompass medicine were assumed to focus first on therapeutic practice, rather than on the principles behind it. In his appetite for knowledge, according to Gregory, Basil has exceeded the fundamentals. We might take as illustrative the Latin work *On Medicines* by the Gallic aristocrat Marcellus of Bourdeaux.[60] This compilation of medical letters (for example, from Hippocrates to the Hellenistic king Antiochus) and recipes (for example, how to create a eunuch without using a knife) was perhaps written after a career as *magister officiorum* in the court of Theodosius I. The work, which is dedicated to Marcellus' sons, does not offer an explanation of how or why medicines work, but instead advertises itself as a handbook of recipes gathered from far and wide for the sake of healing.[61] This is the ordinary level of medical knowledge that, according to Gregory of Nazianzus, at least, Basil has surpassed. Gregory's rhetoric of excess reveals the high social value attached to theoretical medical knowledge as a marker of the advanced intellectual.

Eunapius, like Basil, strove for lay medical literacy beyond the basics of practical knowledge. In a four-volume work addressed to him, Oribasius locates Eunapius among the *philiatroi* who seek instruction on readily accessible remedies for use "on the road, in the fields, or when no doctor is present."[62] As in Gregory's account of Basil, Oribasius flatters Eunapius through reference to his extensive understanding of medical theory: "but you have progressed in the theory of the art further than is normal for *philiatroi*."[63] In keeping with Marcellus, however, Oribasius sticks to practical remedies, avoiding explanation of anatomical or physiological theories, and only occasionally touching upon the principles behind the humoral theory of disease. Like Gregory, Oribasius emphasizes the practical focus of ordinary *philiatroi* in order to exaggerate the intellectual prowess of his addressee.

The early Christian figures who are central to this monograph—those who talked in detail about the brain—did not undergo medical training, at least so far as we know.[64] Gregory of Nyssa never studied abroad, and the formal education of Ambrose, Augustine, and John Chrysostom was limited largely to rhetoric, literature, and, eventually, theology.[65] Yet, these preachers and bishops had colleagues, family members, acquaintances, and congregants who had pursued formal medical training, who were familiar with expert medical texts, and who practiced medicine professionally. At least when addressing the more well-off members of their communities, late antique Christian authors could well expect a level of medical literacy. This is the background that we must imagine when they introduce the anatomy of the brain, diagnoses of brain fever, or analogies between sensory function and ecclesial duty into their works. While many among their audience members might have had only a superficial knowledge of what they were talking about, their elaborate metaphors were intended to have pedagogical force and would have been legible to educated listeners, as well as those who had not enjoyed the luxury of an education, but who had heard medical rhetoricians speak in public spaces.

Like many forms of knowledge in late antiquity, medical education was developing into a text-based mode of study.[66] More accessible texts, such as the summaries of Oribasius, the pharmacological compilation of Marcellus, and the translations of Caelius Aurelianus, were in demand, perhaps for physicians without the resources to study the longer and more theoretical works of Hippocrates and Galen.[67] At the schools of medicine in Alexandria and other major intellectual centers, lectures provided students with line-by-line commentary of canonical medical works.[68] Texts had always been important within the learned medical tradition, but in late antiquity, the evidence points toward wider interest in accessible medical texts, as well as a new focus on medical rhetoric. In his *Medical Collections*, Oribasius centonized Galen and anthologized a range of earlier texts. Few other medical authors survived, except in encyclopedias and handbooks. Late antique iatrosophists and the authors of the "derivative" texts that flourished in late antiquity set the limits of medical literacy for the postclassical world.[69] In the following section, I turn to this third and final mode of the transmission of medical knowledge in late antiquity in order to sketch out both the kinds of written sources that early Christian authors might have consulted and also the textual culture within which their own accounts of the brain circulated.

MEDICAL TEXTS IN LATE ANTIQUITY

During the fourth century, the market for medical handbooks and commentaries rapidly grew. The eleventh-century physician Ibn Riḍwān wrote:

> In the time of Oribasius, when kingdoms became dominated by Christianity, Oribasius thought of reviving the art [of physic] and compiled his popular *Compendium* for the laity, thus familiarizing the Christian kings with [the contents of] medicine. Paul [of Aegina] followed his path, and when their successors saw these two compendia, they have continued until the present time to compile their own.[70]

Besides Oribasius' *Medical Collections* (written in Greek), the fourth century also saw the publication of the Latin text *On Medicines* by the lay author Marcellus of Bordeaux, several Latin works by the North African physician Vindicianus (made famous by his brief appearance in Augustine's *Confessions*) and his student Theodorus Priscianus, who was an imperial physician in Constantinople, Latin adaptations of Greek medical texts by Vindicianus' compatriot and contemporary, Caelius Aurelianus, and a Latin gynecological text by another North African medical author known as Mustio.[71] Subsequent centuries would see the publication of commentaries on the works of Hippocrates and Galen out of lectures at medical schools in Alexandria, Athens, and Ravenna, as well as the influential but neglected *On the Construction of the Human Body* by the leading Byzantine physician Theophilus Protospatharius (Greek), the *Twelve Books on Medicine* by Alexander of Tralles (Latin), and the encyclopedic work titled *Sixteen Books on Medicine* by Aëtius of Amida (Greek).[72]

These texts received little scholarly attention until recent decades, since they were considered nonliterary and largely derivative.[73] Their sole historical value was thought to lie in their preservation of earlier formulations and ideas.[74] There was (it was thought) little to be gained in the way of medical developments or the history of ideas from the content of late antique medical texts. Beginning in the 1980s, this approach began to be reversed. Across the study of ancient medicine and philosophy, scholars have increasingly recognized the need to contextualize fragments within their extant text, creatively arranged, adapted, and deployed in service of the "secondary" author's agenda—that is, the quotations from Galen and Lycus that Oribasius incorporates into his encyclopedia must be read as part of Oribasius' project, and not simply as fragments, purified through excision from their late antique context.[75] As Catherine Osborne wrote with regard to Presocratic fragments in the works of Hippolytus of Rome: "Reading an embedded instead of a fragmented text we read it as a functioning and meaningful system, governed by the preoccupation of an interpreter whose interests we can assess, rather than a set of disjointed parts, detached from the context in which they might mean something."[76]

Editorial work is a selective enterprise that can illuminate the intellectual (and, here, the medical) cultures of its time. Late antique medical writers curated existing material in service of their own ends. The turn to handbooks, textbooks, and translations in late antique medicine reveals for us what authors and audiences of this period valued in the writings of their predecessors and how they used components from medical and philosophical traditions to enact new projects.

The derivative form of late antique medical texts also indicates a new social and intellectual function. The movement to translate, condense, organize, and compile reflects a new interest in popularizing and disseminating technical knowledge. What had been available only in Greek began to be written or rewritten in Latin. Encyclopedias systematized centuries of work into handily organized summaries that referred readers back to original sources. Handbooks condensed and arranged arguments, and letters sought to survey the most important things the intellectual (expert or nonexpert) ought to know. Physicians had long written treatises and letters addressed to a single layperson, but medical authors in late antiquity worked to make medical knowledge accessible to new audiences.[77] The development of medical metaphors in late antique Christianity was fed by a wealth of accessible medical material. Preachers and theologians who incorporated medical terminology and concepts into their work did not need a formal education in medicine to engage with medical ideas beyond a superficial level.

Despite the fact that it summarizes extensive medical knowledge about the human body, the extensive letter *On the Constitution of the Human Being* (traditionally rendered as *On the Making of Man*) by the Cappadocian bishop Gregory of Nyssa is not counted among late antique medical texts, being marked as Christian theology rather than ancient medicine.[78] Indeed, for the first twenty-nine chapters of the letter, Gregory deals with philosophical and theological questions about the rational soul (can it be contained within any physical body?), the phenomenon of death (what kind of bodily damage causes the soul to depart?), and the resurrected body (will resurrected bodies have sexual organs?).[79] Yet, in the final—and longest—chapter, Gregory turns to a topic more fitting to medical discourse: the precise construction of the human body.[80] Interpreting this text in light of the late antique trend toward synthesis of medical knowledge both sheds light on Gregory's motivations in composing this final chapter in the first place and also suggests how his text might have been received. In particular, it reveals the role of accessible textual accounts in the circulation of knowledge about the human brain (and the body as a whole) and the advantages for early Christian authors of participating in the production of such texts. My discussion of this work will also serve as an introduction to key themes and elements in late antique accounts of the brain.

One might learn about the precise construction of the human body, Gregory writes, through self-examination, or by reading the books of those who have devoted themselves to such studies, whether through dissection, conducted in order to reveal the arrangement of the internal organs (we might think, for example, of Galen's influential work *On Anatomical Demonstrations*), or through theoretical explanation of the purpose for the existence of each part (as illustrated in Galen's *On the Usefulness of the Parts*).[81] For those, however, who wish the church to become teacher of such things—"so that they might depend on no external voice"—Gregory has prepared a short (διὰ βραχέων) account of such things, which occupies the sixteen pages that follow.[82] Gregory does not situate himself among the experts who understand human anatomy and physiology through autopsy. Instead, his authority is staked in his ecclesial credentials and, albeit implicitly, in his textual research.

Gregory articulates a central strategy in late antique Christian discourse about the human being, that is, the incorporation of expert medical knowledge into theological texts for the purpose of establishing the authority of the church regarding the nature, fate, and purpose of human beings. He also suggests a central source of information: medical texts. While books were fundamental to late antique higher education, we have little information about what medical texts late antique Christian authors were reading. For the most part, they provide technical medical information without citation, or at best with a mention of "medical experts" as their source.[83] Gregory's acknowledgement that medical knowledge might be gained through books is unusual. It echoes his earlier discussion of whether the mind should be located within the heart or the brain, where he explains that "those investigating the natural causes of such things" and "those who have devoted their time to anatomical observations" have developed a theory of brain-based sensory function.[84] While Gregory might claim the authority to speak about the human body for the church and for himself, he nonetheless acknowledges his reliance upon medical and scientific professionals, whose expertise circulates in textual form.

Gregory provides a typical late antique summary of ancient medical theory that draws on Aristotelian, Platonist, Stoic, and Galenic sources and focuses especially on the contributions of the internal organs, specifically the brain, the heart, and the liver.[85] Fundamental to the operation of all organs is balance and harmony between the four qualities (hot and cold, dry and wet), as well as between softness and hardness.[86] The brain, Gregory notes, contributes to life in a special degree, like the foundation of a building; this is clear from the fact that damage to the cerebral membrane is followed by death.[87] Yet, the heart and the liver furnish the brain with the power through which it animates the body.[88] Blood (from the liver) and *pneuma* (from the lungs and heart), rarefied to pure vapors, nourish the brain, such that it might anoint the cerebral membrane and so enable the faculty of voluntary motion. In a striking passage, he compares the brain to a "charioteer," guiding voluntary motion via the muscles and bones.[89] The brain and cerebral membrane were also responsible for sensory function, as we learn earlier in the letter, when Gregory writes that "the cerebral membrane is the foundation of the sensory organs ... having folded the brain within itself and being anointed by the vapors rising from it."[90]

In one key detail, Gregory's description of the brain does diverge from the standard Galenic account: that is, his identification of the cerebral membrane as the root of the sensory nerves, rather than the brain itself. This reflects the variety of medical perspectives available in late antiquity, and it seems to owe something to Galen's predecessor, Erasistratus of Ceos, who had indeed argued that the sensory nerves were rooted not in the brain itself, but in the membrane that surrounds it.[91] While late antique medicine is often usefully described in broad-brush terms as "Galenism," it is more probable that late antique theologians, preachers, and physicians drew upon a range of different authors and (often contradictory) theories.

Overall, however, Gregory demonstrates a familiarity with a concept of the brain that resonates across late antique medical and theological texts. When early Christian preachers and theologians talk about the brain, they tend to emphasize its importance in sensory function and voluntary motion; they often mention the cerebral membrane; they assume that the brain is nourished by some combination of blood and *pneuma;* and they frequently refer to the vapors that rise from the depths of the body into the cavities of the brain. Just as Gregory refers to the brain as a charioteer, guiding the movements of the other bodily parts, various of his contemporaries identified the brain with the ruler of a city or the governing part of the soul. Gregory's account of the brain reflects a shared body of knowledge.

While Gregory's account of the brain is representative of a common trend, his comparison of the brain to a charioteer is unique. The metaphor alludes to Plato's *Phaedrus*, where the rational part of the soul serves as charioteer over the irrational appetitive and sensitive parts.[92] It seems, therefore, to attribute to the brain a function that Plato associated with the rational soul, directly contradicting Gregory's insistence earlier in the treatise that the rational and governing soul must be immaterial, permeating the whole body and using no single organ (heart or brain) as its instrument.[93] We might interpret this contradiction as inconsistency on Gregory's part. Alternatively, it is possible that the metaphor of the brain as charioteer simply belonged to a separate realm of discourse. Debates about the soul were philosophical (chapter 12 of Gregory's treatise), while theories of brain function were medical (chapter 30).[94] Their convergence in the popular question of where in the body the *hēgemonikon* might be found was a consequence both of philosophical summaries that incorporated medical positions and of the extensive argumentation published by the medical author Galen, who used anatomical and logical demonstrations to "prove" that the brain must be the instrument of the governing soul. Gregory's apparent contradiction might be better interpreted as a reflection of how the brain gained traction as a conceptual object across different intellectual communities and traditions, and, most importantly for us here, how Christian rhetoricians such as Gregory could draw on material from these various traditions to serve a range of purposes, accepting different versions of the brain according to whichever tradition or field was most salient in any given instance.

Gregory's summary of the "precise construction" of the human body contributes to a broader movement to make anatomical and physiological narratives about the human being available to a nonexpert audience. Its categorization as theological is determined by the professional status of its author (bishop), the earlier chapters of the letter, and the theological agenda of the whole. If it circulated apart from the main body of the work, this chapter might be considered a typical late antique medical text: compressed, heterogenous in its influence, clearly inspired by Galen, and focusing above all on the question of animation and the body/soul relationship. In fact, it is likely that it did hold influence as a source of medical knowledge—enough, at least, that the lengthy treatise *On the Nature of the Human Being*, which was written by the bishop Nemesius of Emesa around the end of the fourth century and which contained more detailed discussion of the human body, including in particular the anatomy and function of the brain, was transmitted under Gregory's name during the medieval period.[95] This was not simply because Gregory was a more famous author; rather, it reflects the ways that Gregory had situated himself as the mouthpiece of ecclesial summaries of medical expertise.

CONCLUSION

In the wake of the legitimation and then enforcement of Christianity, fourth- and fifth-century Christian authors scrambled to establish themselves as authoritative teachers, political advisors, civic patrons, and, indeed, physicians. The incorporation of expert medical knowledge into Christian texts was a strategy to reinforce anthropological authority (that is, expertise regarding what it means to be human) and therapeutic legitimacy (the power to instruct audiences in practices conducive to health, that is, salvation). Yet, while the medical emphasis in their writings is distinctive, the medical knowledge that they wove into theological and pastoral arguments would not have seemed out of place: to the contrary, it fit into a wider recognition of the cultural capital that traveled in medical accounts of the human body. Important to such accounts was the brain, which embodied key tensions in late antique Christian anthropology.

Across late antique Christian literature, the brain appears as the organ of rational thought and self-governance. This is in spite of the fact that the Jewish and Christian scriptures gave this role to the heart and in fact did not once so much as mention the brain. What preachers said about the brain, and how they said it, was shaped by their social and intellectual context, as well as by their pedagogical responsibilities. In a world where dinner party guests might ask visiting physicians to explain the puzzle of the insensitive brain's sensory function, where iatrosophists taught future rhetoricians and politicians as well as future physicians, and where medical handbooks were a growing industry, the references to the brain in late antique sermons, letters, tractates, and poems were intended to speak to a knowing audience. When preachers and theologians talked about the anatomy of the brain, they were participating in an intellectual economy that privileged expert knowledge about the human body and that considered anatomical knowledge to hold answers about the soul.

This chapter has sketched out a general topography of lay engagement with the brain in late antiquity, in order to provide a context and foundation for the analysis of rhetorical manipulation of the brain in sermons and theological texts of the fourth and fifth centuries. As I have argued, medical knowledge about the brain was already in circulation as a vehicle for cultural capital, such that Christian authors were not so much introducing new expertise or a new trope as speaking to an existing interest, drawing on common cultural resources, and redeploying a popular concept to serve their rhetorical and pedagogical programs. For the most part, they did not undertake formal training in medical theory, although those who pursued higher educational opportunities may have listened to medical lectures. Their knowledge about the brain, while sometimes quite technical, was drawn from resources accessible beyond the medical profession—learned conversation, public lectures, and accessible texts. As such, their own discussions about the brain were continuous with and expanded upon the existing thought-world of their audiences, at least those who had access to other texts or other forms of public speech.

CHAPTER 2

The History of the Brain in Ancient Greek Medicine and Philosophy

The previous chapter explored how the medical concept of the brain circulated in late antiquity. It detailed different channels through which Christian authors and their audiences might have gained knowledge about the brain, and it demonstrated the significance of the brain in late antique and Christian understandings of the human being. But when late antique Christian intellectuals studied medical and philosophical theories of the brain, what precisely did they learn? The present chapter traces ideas about the brain in ancient Greek medicine and philosophy from Presocratic references (c. 600 B.C.E.) through to the extensive writings of the medical author Galen of Pergamum, who flourished during the second century C.E.[1] Across this span of almost one millennium, understandings of the brain underwent significant transformation. Unlike in contemporary medicine, however, where research tends to lose validity with age, ancient medical research gained authority through the passage of time. The chronological organization of this chapter does not, therefore, reflect a progressive increase in credibility, although it does chart the increasing role of the *hēgemonikon* (the governing part of the soul) in shaping ideas about the function and anatomy of the brain. Rather, I have organized the material chronologically in order to indicate the accretion of new material over time.

The narrative that I offer here also reflects ancient understandings of the history of ideas about the brain. For example, as discussed in the introduction, the concept of the *hēgemonikon* emerged in Stoic thought, but was rapidly generalized and could be mapped onto the opinions of prior authors without explanation. Given the paucity of early material and our reliance upon ancient secondary sources (for example, polemical quotations), my narrative here can only suggest a limited account of how ideas about the brain transformed across time. What it can offer with more certainty is a series of snapshots reflecting how ancient and late antique authors and audiences constructed the history of the brain as a conceptual object.

Most modern scholarly accounts of the history of the brain in ancient Greek medicine and philosophy operate through a psychological lens.[2] That is to say, they are primarily interested in the question of how body and soul are thought to interact (what is the organ of the *hēgemonikon?*), and the brain enters the picture merely as one possible theoretical tool. There are few studies that focus on the brain for its own sake, and there is not yet any study that surveys ideas about the brain in close detail and for its own sake from the Presocratic philosophers through to Galen. This focus on the psychological debate has led to a narrower picture of the brain than was available to late antique audiences. Missing in particular are the aspects of the brain that had nothing to do with its governing powers. For example, modern discussions of the brain in Hippocratic medicine typically focus on texts that affirm its role in cognition but ignore the significance of phlegm and flux. While this chapter does trace the emergence of the brain as the organ of the *hēgemonikon*, it also attends closely to the brain as the material stuff within the head. As we will see, these two versions of the brain developed alongside one another in ancient thought, sometimes merging and at other times parting ways.

PRESOCRATIC PHILOSOPHY

Many late antique theologians and their readers, as well as the more highly educated preachers and congregants, would have been familiar with what is perhaps the most widely cited testimony to Presocratic interest in the brain. This comes from the end of Plato's *Phaedo*, in which Socrates is preparing for his own death. Asked to support his claim for the immortality of the soul, Socrates compares his own idealist approach to the materialist explanations offered by earlier philosophers. "When I was a young man," Socrates says, "I was wonderfully keen on that wisdom which they call 'investigation into nature.' For I thought it splendid to know the causes of everything, why it comes to be, why it perishes, and why it exists."[3] Among which, he includes the following: "Is it blood, or air, or fire through which we think, or none of these, but rather the brain that provides us with the senses of hearing and sight and smell—from which arise memory and opinion, which, when they become stable, give rise to knowledge?"[4]

The Presocratic philosophers—the *phusiologoi,* "investigators of nature," as they were sometimes known—were committed to physical explanations for the natural world, including cosmological, biological, and psychological phenomena.[5] Of particular interest are the accounts of thought and sensation that they offered.[6] As Socrates suggests, the brain was prominent in Presocratic theories of sensation—at least insofar as we can trust the philosopher Theophrastus of Eresos (371–287 B.C.E.), who is responsible for most of what we know of such theories.[7] Thought, meanwhile, tended to be explained in terms not of organs but of substances, in particular, blood (Empedocles of Acragas) and air (Diogenes of Apollonia).[8]

The most celebrated Presocratic theorist of the brain is Alcmaeon of Croton (c. 500–420 B.C.E.).[9] A Greek-speaking city in southern Italy, Croton was home to a Pythagorean school of philosophy and was also a thriving medical center.[10] Alcmaeon himself may have been a Pythagorean, although most judge this unlikely; more plausible is the suggestion that he was a medical practitioner, but this is also a matter for speculation.[11] What we do know is that he was later recalled as the earliest proponent of what was to become the "encephalocentrist" account of the body/soul relationship, that is, the view that the soul operates through the brain.[12] According to the fifth-century compiler Stobaeus, the philosopher Aëtius (first to second century C.E.) recorded that "Alcmaeon [said that] the *hēgemonikon* is in the brain, and therefore one smells by means of this [organ] dragging odors through the airways."[13]

The attribution of this view to Alcmaeon is certainly anachronistic: the Presocratic "soul" (ψυχή, *psuchē*) was not the governing agent that it would become in later philosophy.[14] The claim perhaps reflects the extent to which subsequent thinkers used arguments about sensation to identify the primary organ of the soul. What the claim does seem to indicate accurately is Alcmaeon's attention to the brain as the central organ of sensory function, which we find reported in Theophrastus also: "All the senses are joined somehow to the brain, so are incapacitated if it is moved or changes position. For it obstructs the passages through which the senses [operate]."[15] The clearest example Theophrastus provides is smell, which arises when odors are drawn in through the nose along with air (πνεῦμα, *pneuma*), and so travel up to the brain.[16]

In his discussion of Alcmaeon's theory of smell, Lloyd writes, "Here as elsewhere, Alcmaeon evidently imagined the process of sensation as involving the transport of πνεῦμα to the brain."[17] As we will see later in this chapter, the medical concept of the nervous system developed out of the basic model that Lloyd extrapolates here: sensations are carried to the brain via passages or channels, through the medium of *pneuma*. In addition, as we shall see in later chapters, this *pneuma*, which covered a range of technical meanings in Hellenistic medicine and philosophy, was further adapted by early Christian authors to describe the third member of the Trinity, the *hagion pneuma* ("holy spirit").[18] At stake in Lloyd's claim, then, is the question of whether Alcmaeon anticipated two of the most influential theories of Mediterranean antiquity: the central nervous system and the Christian concept of the Holy Spirit.

The model that Lloyd delineates emerges with greater clarity in later Presocratic philosophy. Diogenes of Apollonia (fl. c. 440–430 B.C.E.), the last of the Presocratics, attached both sensation *and* thought to the air (ἀήρ) that circulated through channels within the body.[19] Theophrastus writes: "Diogenes attaches sensation, just like life and thought, to the air (τῷ ἀέρι)."[20] For example, smells are absorbed by the brain through the air that surrounds it, so long as the air is "in proportion" to the odors and the brain in its proper state of spongelike porosity—in Diogenes' words, "loose and open because of the ducts."[21] The ducts (φλέβια) were fundamental to Diogenes' vision of the human body as being crisscrossed by passages that enabled the circulation of air, thereby supporting life itself.[22] These ducts ran not only between the brain and the sensory organs, as suggested by Alcmaeon (and by Lloyd), but also within the brain itself. They remained a central structure within explanations of sense perception in Greek medicine and philosophy throughout antiquity, as we will see.[23]

Too little remains from Presocratic writings to fully determine a general "Presocratic" understanding of the brain.[24] It is clear, however, that later philosophical and medical authors located the roots of encephalocentrism in Alcmaeon's physiological theories about sensation, and that they considered the concepts of *pneuma* and of sensory channels—so vital across a range of later medical, philosophical, and theological contexts—to have significant Presocratic antecedents, especially in the work of Diogenes of Apollonia. Presocratic philosophers would never have framed their investigations in terms of the question "What is the organ of the *hēgemonikon?*" Nevertheless, they could be retrospectively inserted into popular genealogies of encephalocentrism. This reconstruction, available to late antique Christian intellectuals and their audiences, is just as important for our purposes as what Presocratic philosophers actually thought about the brain. By late antiquity, this was how they were remembered.

THE HIPPOCRATIC CORPUS

The legendary physician Hippocrates of Cos (c. 460–370 B.C.E.) is said to have been contemporary with the later Presocratics, although several texts included in the Hippocratic corpus date to the fourth and even third centuries B.C.E.[25] While these texts did not come to be classed as "Hippocratic" until long after they were written, their transmission as a unified body of medical material warrants treating them as such, especially as a representation of late antique knowledge about what Hippocrates, the most influential medical authority in antiquity, had to say about the brain.[26] Among their shared features, the most prominent is an emphasis upon naturalistic explanations of disease as the consequence of interactions between different stuffs within the body and between the body and the environment.

According to Hippocratic writers, the brain was filled with phlegm.[27] This was one of the main bodily humors theorized by Hippocratic authors, sometimes set in opposition to bile, and eventually canonized in the quartet of phlegm, blood, yellow bile, and black bile.[28] Each of the humors was associated with a season (phlegm was predominant in winter) and with bodily qualities (phlegm was cold and wet).[29] The brain too was imagined as a cold and wet organ: as the author of *On Fleshes* (c. 450–400 B.C.E.) describes it, "the brain is the mother-city of that which is cold and viscous, while the mother-city of oiliness is heat; for when heat is applied, the very first thing to liquify becomes oil."[30] The brain leaked phlegm into the vessels that ran throughout the body, so causing chest infections, seizures, ulcers, and other painful conditions.[31] The author of *On Diseases* 2 narrates the process by which the brain first absorbed and then released its phlegm: "The tonsils, the undersurface of the tongue, the gums, the tongue, and all other such things that are naturally here suffer disease on account of phlegm. For phlegm descends from the head, and the head attracts phlegm from the [lower] body; [the head] attracts [phlegm] whenever it is heated, and it is heated by food, the sun, drinking, and fire."[32] This pathological flow of phlegm and its responsibility for various diseases is commonly known as "flux theory" or "catarrh."[33] It was caused by the accumulation of moisture from all over the body within the head, which was imagined as functioning like a kind of "cupping instrument," a medical instrument that was used to manipulate fluids within the body.[34] The brain, being soft and "wool-like," absorbed this moisture and then redistributed it through safe channels, such as the eyes, nose, and mouth, thereby preventing the body from becoming excessively wet.[35]

In addition, some Hippocratic texts understand the brain to be responsible for reason, behavior, and emotional experience, as well as perception.[36] The most famous account of this view is the treatise *On the Sacred Disease*, which argues against supernatural explanations of the "sacred disease" (often identified in modern literature as epilepsy), in favor of a naturalistic etiology that depended on the concept of flux.[37] According to this text, intelligence is carried into the body by air breathed in from outside.[38] This air travels first to the brain and then to other parts of the body, enabling perception, thought, and voluntary motion.[39] Sometimes, however, the passages of the air are blocked by the influx of phlegm.[40] When this happens, the patient "becomes voiceless and chokes, and foam runs out of the mouth, and the teeth clench together and the hands contract, and the eyes roll around, and the patient is no longer conscious, and for some also a stool passes below."[41] The reason for these symptoms is twofold: if phlegm floods the vessels, then it blocks the passage of air, thereby preventing thought, perception, and motor control; if phlegm remains trapped within the brain, however, it "agitates" and "melts" the brain matter, preventing *both* the brain *and* the senses from being "steady," and thereby impairing the brain's interpretive function: "We become mad because of moisture; for whenever [the brain] is moister than natural, it is necessarily moved [κινέεσθαι], and, being moved [κινευμένου], neither sight nor hearing remain still [ἀτρεμίζειν] . . . but while the brain remains still [ἀτρεμήσῃ], the human being is intelligent [φρονέει]."[42] The verb "to be still" does double-duty here, describing the condition of both the brain ("while the brain remains still") and the powers of sensation ("neither sight nor hearing remains still"), reflecting the materialist understanding of cognitive function and mental illness in the Hippocratic corpus. While *On the Sacred Disease* is the earliest explicit account of the encephalocentrist position, insofar as it represents the brain as the site of consciousness and the organ responsible for motor command, it does not in any way suggest that the brain was the instrument or domicile of the soul; instead, the brain serves as interpreter of the passing air.

The description of the brain as "agitated" (κινέεσθαι, κινευμένου) recalls Alcmaeon's warning that "if [the brain] is moved [κινουμένου] or changes position," it blocks the sensory passages (by obstructing, according to Lloyd, the flow of *pneuma*). The focus upon cerebral distress in relation to the blockage of vessels echoes a less prominent Hippocratic text, *On Glands*.[43] According to this work, disease occurs when the brain does not release its "natural fluxes" to, for example, the orifices in the face, the throat, the spine, and the hips.[44] If flux gathers, then the brain itself might be "stung" and "prone to much disturbance [τάραχον πολὺν ἴσχει]," such that "the mind loses reason and the brain suffers spasm and ulcerates the person as a whole. . . . the intellect is disturbed [ἡ γνώμη ταράσσεται] and [the patient] survives disordered in thinking and disordered in seeing, tolerating the nature of the malady with gaping grins and strange visions."[45] Once again, the repetition (τάραχον, ταράσσεται) emphasizes the bond between brain and intellect (the brain is "prone to much disturbance . . . the intellect is disturbed"), highlighting the physicality of thought as a function of the brain.

Presocratic philosophers and Hippocratic medical authors shared a common approach: psychological phenomena, like everything else in the natural world, were explained in physical (i.e., "natural") terms, where *phusis* (φύσις, "nature") was understood as the ordered material world, for which rules of stability, growth, and transformation could be articulated. In fact, the distinction between "physical" and "psychological" is a modern one, unrecognizable to the Hippocratic authors themselves, for whom the *psuchē* was a material object, subject to natural/physical laws.[46] Within this picture, the brain—for some early medical authors, at least—was responsible for cognitive and sensorimotor functions. If it was troubled or damaged in any way, then these functions were also disturbed.

And troubled the brain was, above all by the accumulation of phlegm. Based upon observation of goats, the author of *On the Sacred Disease* writes that "the brain is eaten away by the phlegm and dissolves, and the dissolved part becomes water, which surrounds the outside of the brain and washes around it."[47] The natural association of the brain with phlegm—the wettest and coldest of the humors—was also the source of its troubles. The very function of the brain in relation to the balance of bodily substances was to accumulate moisture for safe redistribution (the "natural fluxes")—in this respect, the brain was like a gland, being "white and loose textured, just like glands," and providing "the same benefits to the head" as glands elsewhere, that is, "giving relief from moisture and sending the excess from the fluxes away out to distant parts."[48] Yet, this proper function could lead to the destruction of the brain itself, and was the cause of many other diseases being attributed to the brain.

The brain performed two functions within the Hippocratic body: it moderated the distribution of phlegm and other moisture, and it enabled perception, thought, and motor control. We think of these functions as of different orders, the somatic and the psychic, and indeed authors of later antiquity often focused on one kind of function to the exclusion of the other. In fifth-century medicine and philosophy, however, the distinction was not salient. Both the regulation of phlegm and cognitive activities operated on the bodily plane. When the phlegm got out of control, the cognitive faculties were affected.

CLASSICAL PHILOSOPHY

Philosophers of the fourth century radically redrew this landscape. In the passage from Plato's *Phaedo* examined above, Socrates recalls the different kinds of explanation that earlier philosophers provided for thought (fire, blood, and air) and perception (the brain). These physical explanations stood in contrast to Socrates' account of the soul as an immaterial and immortal entity, the locus of the true self, which separates from the body upon death.[49] The dialogue, which is set in 399 B.C.E. on the day of Socrates' execution, marks a new era of investigation into the nature of the human being. The dominant questions shifted from how human bodies think and perceive to how the soul (which thinks and perceives) operates through the body, and in which bodily part it resides. This question was to remain fundamental in later thought, regardless of whether the soul was conceived of in material or immaterial terms.

The two most influential philosophical writers of the classical period were Plato (428/427–348/347 B.C.E.) and Aristotle (384–322 B.C.E.). While Aristotle studied under Plato, the two had quite different philosophical approaches and ideas, and their followers developed into different schools: the Academicians, Middle Platonists, and Neoplatonists, following Plato, and the Peripatetics, following Aristotle. Yet, the standard curriculum in philosophy required students to read works by both Plato and Aristotle, and by late antiquity an "eclectic" approach had developed, generating accounts of the brain and soul that combined approaches and concepts distinctive to each philosopher and philosophical school.[50]

Plato

Plato considered the human soul to be an immortal, immaterial entity, separable from the body, and divisible—at least theoretically—into three parts:

the rational part (λογιστικόν, *logistikon*, responsible for thought and judgment), the spirited part (θυμοειδές, *thumoeides*, responsible for emotions and feelings), and the desiderative part (ἐπιθυμητικόν, *epithumētikon*, responsible for desire).[51] In his cosmological dialogue, the *Timaeus*, Plato maps this tripartite soul onto the body: the divine and rational part of the soul is contained within the head, the spirited part in the heart, and the desiderative part in the liver. This division is cast in explicitly political terms: the spirited part, Plato writes, is "settled nearer the head [sc. than the desiderative part], between the midriff and the neck, so that it might listen to reason and together with it restrain by force the desiderative part of the soul, should the latter at any time refuse outright to obey the dictates of reason [λόγος] coming down from the citadel."[52] Situated between the rational and the desiderative parts, the spirited part of the soul mediates between ruler and unruly populace. This psychological function is mapped onto human anatomy and cast in architectural terms. At a report from reason (λόγου) of threat to or wrongdoing by any bodily member, spirit (θυμοῦ) sensitizes the body through the blood vessels connected to the heart, where the spirited part resides. For this reason, "they established the heart . . . as the guardhouse" within the body.[53] The governing role that Plato assigned to the *logistikon* allowed later authors to identify Plato's *logistikon* (located in the head) with the Stoic *hēgemonikon* (located in the heart) in order to frame Plato's *Timaeus* as an intervention in the debate regarding the question, "What is the organ of the governing part of the soul?"

Notably, however, Plato does not identify the brain itself (like the heart or liver) as the domicile of the *logistikon* but assigns this part of the soul to the "head." This is perhaps because he subsequently assigns a separate role to the brain, as the portion of marrow—the primary substance out of which the human body is formed—destined to receive the "divine seed": "And, having molded into a sphere that portion of the marrow that was, just like a field, to contain the divine seed within itself, he called it 'brain' [ἐγκέφαλον]."[54] Whereas the "head" suits the political metaphor of the rational soul that governs affect and desire, the "brain" serves as an organic metaphor of the soul that takes root. While Plato does not explain the relationship between this "divine seed" and the *logistikon*, they are likely the same thing: earlier in the text, Plato described the *logistikon* as "the immortal principle of the soul."[55] In addition, both the "divine seed" and the *logistikon* are intentionally separated from the mortal parts of the soul: the lower gods construct the neck as "an isthmus and boundary between the head [that is, the location of the *logistikon*] and the chest [that is, the location of the *thumoeides* and the *epithumētikon*]."[56] Meanwhile, the demiurge separates the portion of marrow intended for the "divine seed" from the remaining marrow, which is destined to contain the "mortal part of the soul," and which forms the cores of the bones.[57]

According to *Timaeus*, the brain is chiefly associated with the divine and immortal qualities of the soul, rather than with its governing role.[58] Yet, Plato's image of the head as citadel was to become a key feature in later discussions of the brain as the organ of the *hēgemonikon*. Plato repeats this image toward the end of *Laws*, where the "Athenian stranger" compares the political state to a human being. Every living thing, he argues, contains some preservative force: above all, the soul contains the mind, and the head contains the senses, and therefore "the excellence of these two [the soul and head] clearly provides salvation for all animals."[59] Within the city, the preservative force is the council of elders, which the speaker compares to the mind, and the young scouts and guards, which the speaker compares to the senses. "Is there a way," the Athenian stranger asks, "for our city to become like the head and the senses of rational beings?"[60] For the guards, positioned at the crown, keep watch and "transmit perceptions to memory, informing the elders—those likened to mind—of everything that happens in the city."[61] In this way, the guards and the elders together preserve the state. Once again, there is no mention of the brain. Memory and sense perception are distributed among individual agents commissioned by the state to perform fixed tasks. The physiology behind these faculties goes unexplained.

Subsequent authors synthesized the metaphors from *Timaeus* and *Laws* to describe the senses that surround the acropolis of the skull as "spear-carrying" guards, borrowing language from Plato's description of the heart. By the second century C.E., the metaphor became a proof for the encephalocentrist position that the brain is the organ of the soul, since the *hēgemonikon* (or, in some cases, the brain itself) rules from within the acropolis of the skull, guarded on all sides by the senses. Chapter 4 examines this tradition and its importance for the emergent conception of the brain in late antiquity. For now, what I want to emphasize is the absence of the brain from Plato's account of the body-as-city, despite the importance of this Platonist metaphor in subsequent arguments for encephalocentrism. Even though Plato himself did not argue that the brain was the domicile or instrument of the *logistikon* (and certainly not of the *hēgemonikon*, which was not yet a common concept), he became associated with this perspective through the appropriation of his body-as-city metaphor in subsequent debates. By late antiquity, Plato was all but synonymous with the argument that the brain is the organ of the soul. So Jerome, discussing Plato's tripartition of the soul in his Commentary on Ezekiel, remarks that "many, following Plato, locate wisdom in the citadel of the brain."[62] The syncretic image became a shorthand for Platonist encephalocentrism, grounded in basic anatomical observation (the sensory organs are, after all, mostly in the head) and justified through political analogy.

Aristotle

Although a pupil of Plato, Aristotle disagreed with his teacher in many regards, not least of which was the function of the brain. Far from being the site of the rational soul or mind, the brain was, for Aristotle, responsible primarily for cooling the heat of the heart, while the heart itself both mediated sensations and controlled movement.[63] Aristotle's explanation for how the brain carried out its cooling function was based upon the principle that the brain itself was the coldest part of the body, and drew further on a combination of the medical understanding of the brain as a source of phlegmatic flux (Aristotle was, after all, the son of a physician), on meteorological knowledge, and on the common analogy between the human body and the earth.[64]

> Therefore, just as moisture that is evaporated by the sun's heat, when it arrives in the region above, is cooled down by the chill of that place and, being condensed, is carried back down, becoming water again, the superfluous vapors [in the body] are condensed into phlegm through the rising of heat to the brain. This is why fluxes appear to originate from the head. Those vapors that are nutritive and not diseased, being condensed and carried back down again, cool the heat.[65]

The brain cooled the lower parts of the body by condensing hot vapors into rain. As in Hippocratic thought, Aristotle's brain was a cold organ and the central site for the accumulation and redistribution of moisture.[66] As such, it was responsible for the growth of hair (because hair, like grass, is nourished by moisture) and also the source of human seed.[67] Unlike the authors of *On the Sacred Disease* and *On Glands*, however, Aristotle rejected any suggestion that mental function might be enabled or compromised by the condition of the brain.[68]

Although Aristotle's understanding of brain function was dismissed in later medical and philosophical thought, the subsequent generation of medical scientists made substantive use of his explanation of how the heart governs motor activity in their theorization of the central nervous system.[69] According to Aristotle, the movement of animals is governed by their "unmoved mover," that is, the soul, whose source or principle (ἀρχὴ, *archē*) is situated "in the heart."[70] The intermediary between the soul's command and the body's movement is desire.[71] According to Aristotle, this intermediary must be embodied, and the bodily medium is connate *pneuma*, the same gaseous substance that we found in Presocratic and Hippocratic writers.[72] Being elastic in quality, Aristotelian *pneuma* changed with the expansion and contraction of the heart, particularly in response to images, sensations, and ideas.[73] By affecting the sinews (νεῦρα, *neura*), *pneuma* controlled the movement of the limbs—just as puppets, Aristotle explained, are moved by altering the tension of their strings.[74]

Two concepts central to Aristotle's explanation were to remain fundamental in later accounts of motor and sensory activities as functions of the brain. These concepts were *pneuma* and *neura*. Connate *pneuma* (*pneuma sumphuton*, sometimes translated as "innate *pneuma*") was an air-like substance produced by the heart. This *pneuma* performed similar functions to the gaseous substance known under various names in earlier medical and philosophical writings, enabling animal life, thought, perception, and voluntary motion.[75] As theories of brain function developed, *pneuma* was to retain a central function.

By *neura*, Aristotle means the connections between the motivating heart and its associated limbs, including sinews, tendons, and muscles. The *neura* conduct movement by stretching and tensing, a mechanism enabled by the *pneuma*. Yet, Aristotle did not explain how the *neura* themselves were connected to the heart, which was generally known as the point of convergence for arteries and veins, rather than for *neura*.[76] In later medical accounts, as we will see, the *neura* became increasingly sophisticated theoretical entities that did not simply and mechanically transmit the force of *pneuma* but were somehow activated by *pneuma* in order to conduct sensory and motor functions as material extensions of the brain.

Aristotle's theory of brain function is often set in opposition to the "encephalocentric" model of Plato and, subsequently, of Galen. Yet, Aristotle developed key concepts that were to become important in later models of the brain as responsible for sensation, voluntary motion, and reason. The theorization of the brain as organ of the *hēgemonikon* was not a smooth progression or discovery, but rather was constructed out of parts recycled and repurposed from preexisting and oftentimes conflicting accounts.

LATE CLASSICAL AND HELLENISTIC MEDICINE AND PHILOSOPHY

In his account of the Greek "discovery" of the nervous system, Friedrich Solmsen writes that "it did not occur to Aristotle to specify channels in which the πνεῦμα might flow to the limbs (or to the sense organs); yet this question was soon to present itself again, was to dominate the discussion of the medical researchers, and was to find its way also into the philosophical speculations."[77] This question of how *pneuma* mediated between the embodied principle or source (*archē*) of psychological activity (the heart or the brain) and other parts of the body was taken up with enthusiasm by late classical and Hellenistic medical and philosophical experts. The development of a durable account can be described in four main components: (1) The medical practitioner Praxagoras of Cos (c. 340–280 B.C.E.) envisions the arteries rooted in the heart as narrowing into *neura*.[78] (2) Hellenistic medical scientists Herophilus of Chalcedon (c. 335–280 B.C.E.) and Erasistratus of Ceos (c. 304–250 B.C.E.) dissect the human brain and demonstrate its connection to the *neura*, which they use to account for all sensory and motor function.[79] (3) The Stoic philosopher Chrysippus (c. 279–206 B.C.E.) theorizes *pneuma* as the substance of soul, and so provides a physical account of the *hēgemonikon* (the governing part of the soul) as operating out of the heart.[80] (4) Medical authors, most prominently Galen of Pergamon (c. 130–215/6 C.E.), transfer *pneuma* as the instrument or substance of soul to the brain, where they envision it operating through the sensory and motor *neura* (nerves).

Praxagoras of Cos

Praxagoras of Cos was born in the late fourth or early third century B.C.E.[81] He had diverse medical interests, writing on subjects including nosology, anatomy, and therapeutics.[82] Nothing remains of his work but testimonies and fragments; from these, however, it appears that Praxagoras was familiar with the writings of Aristotle. Ancient authorities identify him as the teacher of Herophilus. Despite the loss of his works, it is clear that he served as a central connection between the Hippocratic writers and Aristotle, on the one hand, and Hellenistic medical scientists, on the other.[83] In his theories about *pneuma* and its operation through the *neura*, Praxagoras was a formative influence.

Based on what evidence survives, Praxagoras appears to have claimed that inhaled *pneuma* nourishes the soul.[84] Warmed and refined within the heart, the *pneuma* then travels outward through the arteries, which gradually dwindle into structures that look like *neura*, that is, Aristotle's cord-like structures that control bodily movement.[85] This theory was an attempt to bridge the gap within Aristotle's model of voluntary motion between the heart, with its innate *pneuma*, and the sinews, which were understood as binding the limbs together but in no way connected directly to the heart.[86] Subsequent medical authors mocked Praxagoras' theory as unrealistic, but it was nonetheless influential, laying the groundwork for an account of sensorimotor function via the *neura* that were traced through dissection back to the brain.[87]

Hellenistic Medical Scientists

The "discoverers" of the nervous system were Herophilus of Chalcedon and his younger contemporary, Erasistratus of Ceos.[88] As is the case for most Hellenistic scientific writing, only fragments and testimonies remain. Herophilus and Erasistratus became the most famous of the medical scientists working in Ptolemaic Alexandria, where—for a short period, and to the distress of later ancient commentators—human bodies were available for vivisection.[89] Herophilus famously mapped out the inner structure of the brain and the pathways of the *neura*, which he explained as enabling not only motor (as in Aristotle) but also sensory activities, through the operation of the *pneuma*.[90] According to Herophilus, *pneuma* comes into contact with the *neura* through the "ventricles," a series of hollow spaces within the brain that were often understood in architectural terms as containers or vats. Herophilus identified three or four ventricles within the brain: two at the front, one in the rear, feeding down into the spinal marrow, and perhaps a third between them—although some claimed that this was no more than a passageway.[91] According to Herophilus, the rear ventricle (third or fourth, depending on whether the middle ventricle is counted) was the locus of the soul.[92]

Building on the work of Herophilus, Erasistratus distinguished more clearly between sensory nerves, which he considered to be hollow and rooted in the cerebral membrane, and motor nerves, which he identified as solid and rooted within the brain itself.[93] This differentiation did not become widespread, although it does crop up occasionally in nonmedical sources from late antiquity, indicating that it was still in circulation.[94] It represents an early attempt to explain in material terms how *neura*—previously a term that meant something like "sinews"—could be responsible for sensory function as well as motor control. The need for a plausible explanation of this functional plurality motivated further research into the *neura* and their connection to the brain.

By rerouting the *neura* through the brain and making them directly susceptible to *pneuma*, Herophilus and Erasistratus developed the conception of the nervous system that was to structure medical understandings of the relationship between brain, body, and soul in late antiquity. While we lack any complete or even sizable original documentation of their accounts of brain anatomy, physiology, and function, it is clear from what remains that their work formed the foundation for all that was to come after in ancient medical conceptions of the brain.

Stoic Psychology and Physics

The Stoic philosopher Chrysippus, influenced perhaps by Praxagoras, took the theory of a soul being nourished by *pneuma* one step further.[95] According to Chrysippus, all things in the cosmos are permeated by *pneuma* that moves inward and outward at different levels of tension (*tonos*).[96] Inanimate objects are permeated by *pneuma* of the least tension (*hexis*, "holding," i.e., that which makes things cohere and gives them their qualities).[97] Plants are sustained by *pneuma* at a slightly higher level of tension (*phusiskon*, "natural"). Nonrational animals require an even higher level of tension (*psuchikon*, "psychic, animate"). For the rational human being, the tension of the *pneuma* was described as *nous* ("mind"), and this *pneuma* was considered to be the substance of the soul.[98] Each level of *pneuma* presupposes the lower kinds: *pneuma* permeates the entire human body, but when it passes through the heart, it becomes *nous*; when it passes through the marrow and bones, it becomes *hexis*.[99]

The key testimony to the localization of the *hēgemonikon* in Stoic thought appears in Galen's polemical *On the Opinions of Hippocrates and Plato*:

> The soul is pneuma connate with us, extending as a continuum through the whole body as long as the free-flowing breath of life is present in the body. Now, of the parts of the soul that have been assigned to the several parts, that of them which extends to the trachea is the voice; that to the eyes, sight; that to the ears, hearing; that to the nostrils, smell; that to the tongue, taste; that to the entire flesh, touch;

and that which extends to the testicles, possessing another such logos, is seminal. The part where all these meet is in the heart, being the governing part of the soul (ἡγεμονικόν).[100]

Whereas Plato had divided the soul into three parts (rational, spirited, and desiderative), the Stoics distinguished eight faculties: the *hēgemonikon*, the five senses, speech, and reproduction. *Pneuma* gathered in the heart and spread out through the vessels of the body to operate each of the remaining seven faculties of the soul: speech through the mouth, the senses through their respective organs, and reproduction through the genitals. This cardiocentric model resonates with the Hellenistic medical theory of the nervous system, perhaps because of the influence of medical authors such as Herophilus and Erasistratus on Chrysippus and other Stoics. What the Stoics added—and what in turn informed future developments in medical theory—was the concept of the *hēgemonikon*, a governing center coextensive with the *pneuma*, known as "mind" (*nous*) and responsible for coordinating all the other faculties of the soul.

If the Stoics had a theory of brain function, it has not survived: as in the case of Hellenistic medical scientists, early Stoic writings survived only as fragments and testimonies preserved by other authors, who were often polemical in their presentation of Stoic ideas. Nonetheless, it is clear that the Stoics wielded significant influence in subsequent theorization of the brain. Their concept of the *hēgemonikon* was to become common currency, and in later medical thought it became interchangeable with the Platonic *logistikon*. Also critical was the idea that *pneuma* could be differentiated according to the kinds of functions it performed. Alongside and after the Stoics, there developed within medical accounts several kinds of *pneuma* held to be individually responsible for specific functions of the soul within the human body, in particular, psychic *pneuma* (responsible for cognitive and sensorimotor functions, thought by physicians to flow through the brain, and by Chrysippus through the heart), vital *pneuma* (responsible for life-giving functions, such as the pulse, thought to flow through the heart), and natural *pneuma* (responsible for nutritive functions, such as digestion, thought to flow through the liver).[101]

GALEN OF PERGAMON

In contrast to all earlier medical authors, Galen of Pergamon (c. 130–215/6 C.E.) left a substantial corpus of written material, much of which is plausibly attributed to his name.[102] An imperial physician at Rome, Galen became famous for his anatomical experiments and his therapeutic expertise. His writings, which often synthesized the work and ideas of earlier authorities, became the foundation for "Galenism," the form of learned medicine that spread—with varying degrees of complexity—through late antique and medieval Europe, Byzantium, and the Arab-Islamic world.[103]

Galen addressed various prominent problems in medical theory, but one of his prized arguments offered anatomical proof for the localization of the *hēgemonikon* in the brain, an explicit refutation of the Stoic theory that located the *hēgemonikon* in the heart.[104] Among the earliest texts in which Galen laid out his arguments against Stoic philosophers was *On the Opinions of Hippocrates and Plato,* in which he sought to demonstrate that the greatest of philosophers, Plato, and the greatest of doctors, Hippocrates, agreed upon fundamental principles with respect to the human body and soul.[105] Among these principles was the central role of the brain in human reason and self-governance.

Galen's central argument in favor of locating the *hēgemonikon* in the brain was based on the key premise that "where the source [*archē*] of the nerves is, there the *hēgemonikon* is also."[106] Once this premise had been established, he set about proving through anatomical experimentation that the brain is the source of the nerves. For example, Stoic philosophers had claimed that one indubitable sign of the *hēgemonikon* was rational speech, which was one of the eight faculties of the soul. Zeno of Citium (c. 336–265 B.C.E.) had argued that since the lungs were the physical source of speech, and since the heart was closer to the lungs than was the brain, therefore the heart must be the *archē* from which rational speech, given force by the lungs, was produced.[107] Galen dismissed this "argument by location," and insisted instead that anatomical connection was essential for demonstrating functional connection, with proximity being a peripheral concern.[108] Identifying the nerve that runs between the larynx and the brain as the anatomical connection in question, he designed an experiment to prove his case. Taking a live (and squealing) pig, he opened the animal's throat and ligated the laryngeal nerve.[109] Immediately the animal stopped squealing. Once Galen released the ligation, the animal resumed its cries. Clearly, Galen argued, the laryngeal nerve that descends from the brain carries the impulse for speech to the vocal cords.[110]

Galen conducted other experiments also, which he documented in his handbook *On Anatomical Demonstrations.* While this work chiefly provides instructions for the postmortem dissection of animal bodies, the ninth book, which is dedicated to the brain, includes first the dissection of a brain detached from the body (that of an ox), then instructions for dissection of the brain within a deceased body (an ape), and finally a short description of experiments that one might perform on the brain of a living animal (preferably a pig or a goat) in order to discern its functions.[111] Galen explained the rationale behind this order in the opening chapter: "Knowledge gained from the dissection of dead animals teaches the position of each of the parts, as well as their number, proper substance, size, shape, and construction. Dissection of living animals teaches the functions sometimes at a glance, and sometimes provides premises for working them out. It is clear, then, that it is necessary for dissection of dead animals to come before dissection of living animals."[112] The purpose of book 9, then, is to demonstrate not only the parts of the brain, but their functions also—in particular, sensorimotor functions, and consciousness.

When it comes to the brain of a live animal, Galen first sliced through the skin and the pericranium, then cut away the bone and peeled back the dura mater (that is, the outer cerebral membrane).[113] As Galen argued elsewhere, damage to the dura mater did not impede sensorimotor activities, a refutation of the Erasistratean theory that the sensory nerves were rooted in the cerebral membranes; according to Galen, the only parts of the brain that needed to be intact to ensure sensorimotor function were the cerebral ventricles.[114] In order to demonstrate this, Galen probed or cut each ventricle of the brain in turn:

> Should the brain be compressed on both the two anterior ventricles, then the degree of stupor which overcomes the animal is slight. Should it be compressed on the middle ventricle, then the stupor of the animal is heavier. And when one presses down upon that ventricle which is found in the part of the brain lying at the nape of the neck, then the animal falls into a very heavy and pronounced stupor. This is what happens also when you cut into the cerebral ventricles, except that if you cut into these ventricles, the animal does not revert to its natural conditions, as it does when you press upon them.[115]

Galen does not explain here why damage to the ventricles sends the animal into a stupor. In his more philosophical work *On the Opinions of Hippocrates and Plato*, however, he suggests that it is the escape of *pneuma* that halts psychic processes.[116]

This experiment became the basis for Galen's claim that *pneuma* is the first instrument of the soul.[117] Following medical tradition, Galen identified at least two kinds of *pneuma*. First, the air that was inhaled was refined into "vital *pneuma*" within the heart; second, vital *pneuma* traveled with the blood through the arteries into the brain, where it was pressed out into the cerebral ventricles as "psychic *pneuma*."[118] Gathering in these ventricles, the psychic *pneuma* acted upon (or perhaps entered) the sensory nerves (rooted in the front of the brain, closest to the sensory organs) and the motor nerves (rooted in the back of the brain, closest to the spine). As Rocca has demonstrated, this distribution did not entail the association of specific functions with each ventricle—this development was to come later.[119]

Beyond this, Galen's theory of *pneuma* was nonspecific and sometimes contradictory. Hankinson has suggested that *pneuma* in Galen "functions only as a sort of place-holder."[120] Debru remarks that Galen "considers it [*pneuma*] to be an 'instrument' [*organon*], although he remains non-committal as to the number of types of *pneuma* there are and as to its nature, both subjects of some dispute in his time."[121] This is no casual imprecision. It was precisely the fuzzy definition of *pneuma* that enabled it to play a flexible role in theories of the body/soul relationship in varied medical, philosophical, and theological contexts across more than a millennium.[122] Galen's noncommittal approach to *pneuma* reflected its range of meanings in both technical and popular discourse.

Where Galen did speak with certainty was regarding whether *pneuma* was identical with, or only the instrument of, the soul. This question was of some interest to Galen, as it was to later philosophers and theologians also. At stake in question was whether the Galenic account of the brain was an adaptation of Stoic materialism, merely relocating the *hēgemonikon* from the heart to the brain, or a revision of Platonist idealism, adding medical explanation to Plato's tripartition of the soul and updating Plato's terminology to synthesize the immaterial *logistikon* with the *hēgemonikon*. Plato won out: rather than simply transfer the Stoic concept of the hegemonic portion of the pneumatic soul from the heart to the brain, Galen argued that the *hēgemonikon* governed the body, using the psychic *pneuma* and the brain is its primary instruments. Based on his anatomical experimentation upon the ventricles, Galen suggested the following conclusions:

> It is better, then, to assume that the soul dwells in the actual body of the brain, whatever its substance may be . . . and that the *pneuma* is the soul's first instrument for all the sensations of the animal and for its voluntary motions as well; and therefore, when the *pneuma* has escaped . . . it does not deprive the animal of its life, but rather renders it incapable of sensation or motion. For if the *pneuma* were itself the substance of the soul, the animal would die immediately upon the escape of the *pneuma*.[123]

The loss of *pneuma* inhibits psychic function, but this does not entail the loss of soul itself. The continuous presence of *pneuma* within the cerebral ventricles was not necessary for animal life, although it was required for the activities proper to that life. It was perhaps this loyalty to Platonism in his rejection of the material soul that made Galen's account of the brain and its functions so widely acceptable among Christian authors.

CONCLUSION

This chapter has traced ideas about the brain in Greek medical and philosophical thought from the Presocratics through to Galen, with particular attention to the development of four key theoretical components: phlegm, *pneuma*, ventricles, and nerves. Two central narratives about the brain have emerged: (1) the brain is a soft and moist organ, responsible for the accumulation and redistribution of fluids and vapors, with the goal of achieving a balance of hot and cold, or wet and dry, across the body as a whole; (2) the brain is the organ responsible for cognitive and sensorimotor functions, making it a key player in discussions of human reason and self-governance. Both accounts of the brain remained influential in late antiquity.

The brain was associated with sensory and motor function and even rational thought from very early in the tradition. It was not until the Hellenistic period, however, that it became a consistent and central feature in explanations of human reason and self-governance. This shift was related to new theorizations of the soul in Hellenistic philosophy, in particular the emergence of the *hēgemonikon* in Stoic thought. The Hellenistic period saw multiple attempts to pin down a specific bodily site for the activities of the soul. Across philosophical and medical sources, what emerges is the concept of a network centered around a single organ, through which flows an unending supply of air and, in some cases, blood also. This concept can be traced back to the Presocratic author Alcmaeon, but it was only in the Hellenistic period that it became the subject of systematic exploration and definition.

Whereas Plato's *logistikon* was abstracted from the body, being immaterial and engaged more in reason than governance, the Stoic *hēgemonikon* existed in material connection with the other parts of the soul, extending through the body as a central source of governance and control. As a consequence, the Stoic *hēgemonikon* could be found in animals, while the *logistikon* most certainly could not. By conflating the *logistikon* with the *hēgemonikon*, Galen legitimated his use of animal models for understanding the anatomical underpinnings and correlates of human psychological activity. The manifestations of the *hēgemonikon* in animal subjects became evidence for the *hēgemonikon*—and, by extension, the *logistikon*—in human beings.

The development of ancient brain science did not end with Galen, although the period after his death has been called the "black hole" of ancient medicine.[124] Few subsequent medical works survive the third century, and between the fourth and sixth centuries, as we saw in chapter 1, medical writing in both Greek and Latin was often "derivative" in form—translations, encyclopedias, summaries, and commentaries dominated the scene. It is a striking testimony to the loss of "original" medical research during this period that one of the most important transformations of Galenic brain science is preserved secondhand, in two Christian texts: *On the Nature of the Human Being*, by the Greco-Syrian bishop Nemesius of Emesa, and *Literal Commentary on Genesis*, by the North African bishop Augustine of Hippo. These two works—the first by an author otherwise unknown, and the second by the most famous author in Latin Christianity—shaped conceptions of the brain over subsequent generations. It is the theory of brain function that these authors report that we turn to in the following chapter.

CHAPTER 3

The Invention of Ventricular Localization

The previous chapter surveyed ideas about the brain across eight centuries of intellectual history from the sixth century B.C.E. through to the second century C.E.[1] The present chapter focuses on a particular moment in the history of ideas about the brain, that is, the development of the concept of ventricular localization, also known as "cell doctrine," in the fourth and fifth centuries.[2] Here, we turn more directly to late antique theological engagement with medical theories of the anatomy of the brain, specifically the localization of discrete psychic faculties in the cerebral ventricles. This theory enabled more precise theorization of how the brain served as the material basis of cognitive functions and therefore also of mental illnesses, such as phrenitis. It also enabled theologians and philosophers working in late antique, Byzantine, Arab-Islamic, and Latin medieval contexts to reconcile the anatomical and physiological teachings of ancient medical science with the concept of the immortal and ultimately separable soul.[3]

There is a conventional narrative that late antique Christian authors initiated a retrogressive movement in concepts of the brain, transferring the cognitive and sensorimotor functions from the brain substance itself to the empty spaces within, and, more precisely, to the *pneuma* that filled those ventricles. To take one example: "Western scholars had no doubts in considering the brain the seat of the human mind's functions although, without exceptions, they persevered in localizing them in the cerebral ventricles and in regarding the animal spirit and not the brain substance as their agent."[4] According to this account, "Western scholars" (that is, late antique theologians and their medieval European readers) compromised the findings of medical science by introducing theological concerns. In order to maintain the immaterial status and integrity of the human soul, they denied the agency of the brain, with "dire and pervasive consequences on the progress of the medical sciences."[5]

In this chapter, I put forward an account contrary to this widely accepted history of late antique Christian marginalization of the brain. I argue that medical accounts of the brain were central to Christian representations of the body and its relationship to the soul. The late antique Christian accounts of cell doctrine that were to become most widely influential in Byzantine, Arab-Islamic, and medieval Latin traditions were themselves drawn from fourth-century medical texts. The tensions between the agency of the brain, the agency of *pneuma*, and the agency of soul that we find in Christian texts in fact derived from tensions within late ancient medicine itself: in particular, the question of how a bodily organ could mediate between the immaterial soul and the material body. This was the question that ventricular localization—a medical theory that proved appealing to theologians—sought to address.

The assumption that theological and anatomical discourses ought to have been separated in antiquity is based on the recognition that their modern relatives, religion and science, occupy distinct and even opposing spheres. In order to understand how brain function came to be imagined in terms of ventricular localization, I argue, it is necessary to examine late antique writings about the brain without applying the modern opposition between science and religion as a lens. While theological, medical, and philosophical writers did each recognize the limits of their expertise (albeit usually only when it suited the limits of their argument), late antique "medical knowing" expanded beyond the boundaries of the genre of medical texts and was transdisciplinary in its scope.[6]

Even if we understand the theory of ventricular localization to be medical rather than theological in origin, however, we must still consider the argument that the importance of the ventricles and the *pneuma* within ventricular localization displaced the brain substance itself, and therefore deemphasized the brain's role in cognitive and sensorimotor activities, that is, the work of the soul. In his important study of "cerebral subjectivity" (that is, the identification of the human subject with their brain), Fernando Vidal distinguishes modern conceptions of the brain as the material of the mind from ancient conceptions of the brain "as a factory and storehouse of the animal spirits," arguing that "it was the qualities of the animal spirits themselves, together with the rest of the humors, that determined a person's character; personality and psychological differences depended on them, not on the mass of tissue that makes up the brain as an anatomical structure."[7] In his summary of ancient views on the brain, he follows the work of Julius Rocca, who concludes his own account of Galen's study of the brain with the following assessment: "Galen's exposition of the ventricular system set in train the concept of 'ventricular dominance' which was not fully reversed until the substance of the brain was explored in the seventeenth century by Thomas Willis, who transferred the functions of the ventricles into the brain substance."[8] This historiographical emphasis upon the brain as a kind of container or a site of production that operates at one step removed from the soul overlooks the triangulation of brain, *pneuma*, and soul in the late antique accounts. The late ancient brain was more closely implicated in human agency—and was a correspondingly more complex and difficult object of thought—than is acknowledged in conventional historical accounts. By reassessing early theories of ventricular localization in late antiquity, we can gain a better grasp of how late antique Christian intellectuals sought to shape understandings of the brain in relation to their theological principles.

The argument of this chapter is that, far from displacing the brain substance from theories of body/soul interaction, ventricular localization represents a complex set of relationships between brain substance, ventricles, *pneuma*, soul, and the activities of the soul (thought, sensation, memory, and movement). The importance of the ventricles does not diminish the contribution of the brain substance: whereas modern scholars tend to interpret the ventricles as *not*-brain, late antique representations of ventricular localization suggest that the ventricles and the brain substance were functionally and structurally interdependent. The dichotomy between brain cavity and brain substance does not apply to late antique accounts of ventricular localization. Their interdependence, I suggest, was conceptualized through the metaphor of the brain as a musical instrument, in particular a flute or a lyre. The ventricles of the brain were not the "abode" of the rational soul, but its instruments (its "organs"). We can more precisely understand how the earliest proponents of cell theory were inviting their audiences to imagine the brain by thinking in terms of a lyre and its collaboration between hollow structure, airflow, and strings in the generation of music.

ANATOMY AND THEOLOGY IN EARLY CHRISTIAN DISCOURSE

Late antique Christian interest in the localization of psychic faculties in the ventricles of the brain was part of a broader picture of theological appropriation and contestation of medical knowledge about cerebral anatomy. One example worth exploring in detail is found in an influential work by a Christian contemporary of Galen, Hippolytus of Rome (c. 170–235).[9] In a brief passage intended to refute the use of brain anatomy as a cosmological model, Hippolytus' *Refutation of All Heresies* reveals a tradition of seeking theological and cosmological significance in medical theories about the brain. It shows that, long before ventricular localization was theorized, the brain could be understood as a bricolage of agential and instrumental parts that served as a site of mediation between material and immaterial planes.

Hippolytus of Rome reveals some of the ways in which cerebral anatomy could inform theological constructions in second- and third-century Christianity.[10] In the extant portions of his *Refutation of All Heresies*, the brain appears six times, as (among other things) an analogy for Eden and a model of the cosmos.[11] In this latter usage, the anatomy of the brain—especially the relationship between ventricles, *pneuma*, and the activities of the soul—served as a privileged site for contesting different theological arguments.

On his first introduction of the brain as a cosmological model (*Ref.* 4.51.10–14), Hippolytus ascribes it to a subsect of those ("heretics") who hold hebdomadal theories of the universe. According to ancient mathematical theory, the hebdomad is the collection of seven mathematical entities out of which all numbers are produced: number, a single number, the squared number, the cubed number, the square squared, the cube squared, and the cube cubed.[12] Early theologians—Hippolytus identifies the famous "heresiarchs" Simon and Valentinus—adopted this system, arguing that all things in the cosmos were produced out of seven things: mind; thought; name; voice; reasoning; conception; and the one who stood, stands, and will stand (Simon); or mind, truth, word, life, human, church, and the Father (Valentinus).[13] While Simon and Valentine are named as chief among those who appropriate mathematical models for hebdomadal cosmology, the authors of the anatomical model go unnamed: "But some," Hippolytus writes, "further try to establish their hebdomads from the medical art: struck by the anatomy [or: dissection] of the brain, they claim that the substance and the power and the paternal godhead of the universe is indicated by the brain's constitution."[14] Just as mathematics provided a mathematical model for the unfolding of all things out of seven, so medicine offered an anatomical model for their arrangement: "For the brain, as the dominant part of the whole body, resides untrembling and without movement [ἀτρεμὴς καὶ ἀκίνητος], holding the *pneuma* within."[15]

Hippolytus' account of hebdomadal descriptions of the brain draws three components from medical tradition. First, the brain dominates the body both in position (it is above the body) and with respect to function (it controls voluntary motion). Second, *pneuma* gathers within the brain, whence it mediates between the brain and the rest of the body. Third, the functioning brain is unmoved. The unmoved quality of the brain ensures the presence of mind (in medical texts, mental health), and also links it symbolically to the unmoved nature of the creator.

Although Hippolytus' summary reflects contemporaneous medical knowledge about the brain, it is unclear how it might illustrate hebdomadal theories of the cosmos. Hippolytus is aware of this gap—indeed, it is an artifact of his selective presentation of material: while the description is persuasive as an anatomical account, it is "a long way from [proving] their proposal."[16] He then goes on to provide an explanation of how far brain anatomy is from any hebdomadal theory of the cosmos:

> For the brain, upon being dissected, has within itself the so-called "little vault," on each side of which are thick membranes, which they call "wings." Moved gently by the *pneuma*, they in turn drive the *pneuma* away toward the cerebellum. The *pneuma*, flowing quickly through a vessel similar to a reed, goes toward the pineal gland, to which is attached the mouth of the cerebellum. The pineal gland, receiving the flowing *pneuma*, transmits it to what is called the "spinal" marrow, whence the entire body has a share in the pneumatic substance, since every artery is hung like a branch from this vessel.[17]

This representation of the brain on the dissection table offers a rare outside view on public vivisections of the kind that Galen made famous. The general structure of the brain and the terminology used reflect medical conceptions about the brain in the second century, including three features of non-Galenic medical theory: the importance of the pineal gland, the notion that the *pneuma* is transmitted from the brain via arteries (rather than nerves), and the claim that the arteries are rooted in the spine. There is nothing in this account that clarifies how or why cerebral anatomy is a false model for hebdomadal theories of the universe. Instead, Hippolytus takes a deep anatomical dive in order to reveal his own superior medical knowledge. There is status to be won in asserting familiarity with medical ideas about the construction of the brain.

We should read this passage, accordingly, as a strategy of exhibition and display. Just as Galen won acclaim through the performance of attention-grabbing vivisections, Hippolytus inserts cerebral anatomy into his text as a kind of ekphrasis of a dissection—that is to say, the detailed description of a dissection as a visual artwork, crafted with care to bring the scene alive for his readers.[18] By using present participles to describe the actions of the "wings" as they move the *pneuma* along (κινούμενα . . . ἀπελαύνοντα), the movement of the *pneuma* itself (διατρέχον . . . διατρέχον), and the work of the pineal gland in transferring the *pneuma* from the brain to the spine (ἐκδεχόμενον . . . ἀναδιδὸν), Hippolytus "zooms in" on the movement of the *pneuma*, "bringing [it] before [the audience's] eyes."[19] The movement of the *pneuma* through the vessels and vaults within the brain is seen in real time, with actions piling on top of one another (ἐκδεχόμενον τὸ διατρέχον πνεῦμα, "[the pineal gland] receiving the flowing *pneuma*"). Hippolytus describes the flow of *pneuma* in process: not one action after the other (first the *pneuma* flows into the reed-like vessel, then the *pneuma* is received by the pineal gland . . .), but all together, each part of the brain in simultaneous and constant operation.

Looking more closely, however, it becomes clear that Hippolytus uses ekphrastic strategies not only in order to inspire awe in his readers, but also in order to critique the persuasive power of display that his opponents rely upon. When Hippolytus introduces the cosmological model of the brain, he explains that its authors looked to medicine for corroboration of their hebdomadal theories because they were "struck [ἐκπλαγέντες] by the anatomy [or: dissection] of the brain." His use of ἐκπλαγέντες situates his own description of cerebral anatomy snugly within the discourse of imperial ekphrasis. According to Longinus (first century C.E.), "the goal [of ekphrasis] in poetry is astonishment [ἔκπληξις]," while in rhetoric the purpose is "vividness" (ἐνάργεια).[20] It is perhaps this distinction—and the traditional suspicion of poetry as persuading its audience of falsehoods—that leads Longinus to observe that, if the ekphrasis is too powerful, then "we are diverted from the demonstration [ἀπὸ τοῦ ἀποδεικτικοῦ] to the astonishment caused by the visualization [εἰς τὸ κατὰ φαντασίαν ἐκπληκτικόν]."[21] When Hippolytus uses the term ἐκπλαγέντες to describe his opponents' motivations, he implies that they have mismanaged anatomical exempla to persuade through astonishment, rather than to establish through proof. As he expands his critique of the cerebral model ("it is persuasive in itself, but is far from their argument") by launching into a detailed description of cerebral anatomy, his point is not to show that cerebral anatomy does not support their model—he gives us no arguments and no detail in this regard—but rather to show that what supports their argument is ekphrasis, a form of persuasive speech that slides all too easily from demonstration to "*emplektika kai taraktika pathe*, 'emotions of amazement and confusion,' which Longinus sees as a way of getting past the censor of the intellect, a way of dazzling us away from factual representation."[22] Hippolytus offers us a glimpse of a shared strategy of incorporating dazzling and even competing anatomical description of the brain into theological arguments. His critique of this strategy as an ekphrastic display, persuading through image rather than evidence, is perhaps even illustrated by his own anatomical account, which does not serve the argument, but stands apart as a marker of medical authority, bearing no clear relation to hebdomadal theory itself.

Close similarities between Hippolytus' description in 4.51 and the account attributed to the Peratae in the following book (*Ref.* 5.17) have led to the general assumption that Peratic writings are likely the source for both passages.[23] The Peratae were an early Christian group identified by Hippolytus as being among the "Gnostics," and known to us chiefly through his polemic. According to Hippolytus, the beliefs of the Peratae centered around the notion of a single cosmos divided into three parts: Father, Son, and Matter. The Son is mediator between Father and Matter, transferring the outflow of *logos* that emanates from the Father to formless Matter, which is thereby transformed into a sensible cosmos that mirrors the divine realm. The brain is offered as a model for this cosmology:

> They offer the anatomy of the brain as a demonstration of these things, likening the brain itself to the Father, on account of its motionlessness, and the cerebellum to the Son, because it is moved and is serpentine in form. They say that this [cerebellum] ineffably and invisibly draws through [or: by] the pineal gland the pneumatic and life-generating substance that emanates from the "little vault." The cerebellum, having collected this [substance], just like the Son, ineffably gives form to matter—that is, the seeds and kinds of things born in the flesh flow into the spinal marrow.[24]

There are four key similarities between the two accounts: First, "motionlessness" (τὸ ἀκίνητον <εἶναι>) is cited as the first characteristic of the brain that makes it an appropriate analogue for the structure of the cosmos. Second, the

Peratic account similarly emphasizes the "little vault" (the ventricular space in the front part of the brain) as the source of *pneuma*, as well as the passage of the *pneuma* into the cerebellum, by means of the pineal gland. Third, the cerebellum is described as "serpentine," evoking a comparison that Hippolytus notes in his earlier account between the "shape of the cerebellum" and "the head of a snake.[25] Fourth, as Hippolytus notes also in book 4, the brain is a source of human seed.[26]

The medical terminology that these passages share indicates a specific analogical connection between the cerebral ventricles and the cosmos. The "little vault" (καμάριον) is the medical term for the front ventricle of the brain, but it is also the diminutive of καμάρα, which, among other things, can mean "vault of heaven."[27] The *pneuma* that flows from this front ventricle/vault of heaven enters the cerebellum (here the Son) by way of the pineal gland. In the more extensive anatomical description given at 4.51, we learn that the pineal gland is not simply a passage through which the *pneuma* passes (διὰ τοῦ κωναρίου), but that the pineal gland actively "receives" the *pneuma* from the reed-like vessel that passes out of the "little vault" and "transmits" it to the cerebellum. The *pneuma* is drawn not so much *through* as *by means of* the pineal gland.

The significance of this detail becomes clearer if we turn to Galen's treatment of the pineal gland in his treatise *On the Usefulness of the Parts*. The pineal gland, Galen explains, stood between the reed-like vessel (in Galen's account, the third cerebral ventricle) and the cerebellum, where some believed that it functioned as "a kind of guardian and steward" (φύλακά τινα καὶ οἷον ταμίαν) regulating the quantity of *pneuma* transmitted.[28] Galen rejects this view, insisting that the pineal gland played no more than a supporting role, holding up certain blood vessels as they bifurcated within the brain.[29] He justifies his rejection of this view as follows: "Since this gland is in no way a part of the brain and is attached not to the inside but to the outside of the ventricle, how could it affect the channel [bearing the *pneuma*], since it is not self-moving [αὐτοκίνητός]? But perhaps they ask what prevents [the pineal gland] from being self-moving?"[30] If it were so, Galen explains, then the pineal gland would be the true brain, and the *enkephalos* itself would be only "a body divided by many channels."[31]

Clearly, Galen's rebuke had not reached the Peratae or the other early Christian theologians who incorporate the pineal gland into their accounts of the brain as a model for cosmic structure. Or, perhaps, they simply do not care. The pineal gland as "guardian and steward," potentially "self-moving," exhibits the intelligent animacy of the components of the universe, a kind of "vibrant matter" both on its own account and, following the arguments of Patricia Cox Miller with regard to "tiny creatures," insofar as it reveals in its own being the presence of the divine.[32] Galen's dismissal of the pineal gland as a major player on the grounds that, if it were a major player, then it would be a self-moving entity and so would replace the brain as first instrument of the soul reflects the slippery conception of the brain (and/or pineal gland) as operating on both bodily and psychic planes. As Hippolytus shows, the brain could be conceived of as an assemblage of quasi-divine, quasi-animate agents (wings, pineal gland, cerebellum) that were also containers and vehicular parts (vaults, reeds, vessels, branches). The power of cerebral anatomy in late antique theological debates lay in part in the ambiguity of the brain as a meeting-point between body and soul.

Hippolytus does not agree with the anatomical evidence that he examines. He scoffs at the idea that one might be so "struck" by the dissection of the human brain that one might use it as a model for illustrating the organization of the cosmos. Yet, he reveals the potency of the dissection and anatomy of the brain in early Christian theological discourse, both as a symbolic representation of immaterial entities (soul, god) and as evidence for how immaterial entities might operate in relation to one another. He also shows how this appropriation of the brain was contested, as its mediatory role threatened to transgress the separation between planes of being (animate/inanimate, body/soul, matter/god).

Brain anatomy was a tool for debating theological issues across different religious groups. It is important to bear this in mind as we consider the surviving theorizations of ventricular localization in late antique medical and theological texts in the following section. When Nemesius and Augustine talk about the anatomy of the brain, as we will explore further in the next section, they are taking part in a diverse conversation about what the anatomy of the brain can reveal about the workings of the cosmos, god, and the soul.

THEORIES OF VENTRICULAR LOCALIZATION

Ventricular localization was one of the most influential developments in the history of the brain. It remained a dominant model for the distribution of cognitive faculties within the brain until the seventeenth century.[33] Yet, little is known about its impact and reception during the fourth century, when it was first described.[34] There are three sources: a sixth-century excerpt from the lost work of the late antique physician Posidonius of Byzantium, who lived during the fourth century; several chapters from a treatise *On the Nature of the Human Being* by the otherwise unknown philosopher-bishop Nemesius of Emesa (perhaps written c. 390, although this date is speculative); and a passage from the *Literal Commentary on Genesis* by another, far more famous, philosopher-bishop, Augustine of Hippo (c. 354–430). A fourth source, the final chapter of a work titled *On the Construction of the Human Being* by the later Byzantine physician Theophilus Protospatharius, has not previously been examined in conjunction with ventricular localization, but reveals an important step in its development. Here, I examine each of these sources in turn.

Medical Theories of Ventricular Localization: Posidonius of Byzantium and Dionysius of Aegae

According to its earliest sources, ventricular localization involved the identification of key faculties of the soul with ventricles inside the brain. For Galen and his contemporaries, these ventricles had been holding places or channels for the *pneuma;* in ventricular localization, a discrete cognitive function became attached to each.[35] There were three or four ventricles altogether (one or two ventricles in the front part of the brain, one ventricle in the middle of the brain, and one ventricle in the rear), but only three faculties. The faculty of imagination or perception was said to operate through the front two ventricles, the doubling of which was thought to match the rule that sensory organs exist in pairs: humans have two eyes, two ears, two nostrils, and two frontal cerebral ventricles. The purpose of this, as Nemesius argued, was to maximize protection—if one organ was damaged, the other might remain.[36]

Posidonius, being the only medical author among the early sources, is assumed to have invented the theory. His account is preserved in the sixth-century medical encyclopedia compiled by Aëtius of Amida. It appears at the beginning of the sixth book of the encyclopedia, the second chapter in a series that discusses diseases of the brain:

> About phrenitis, from the writings of Posidonius. Phrenitis is the inflammation of the meninges around the brain, together with acute fever, and bringing frenzy and derangement of thought. . . . There are many species of *phrenitis,* but these three are the most important: . . . if the front portion of the brain is injured, imagination alone is damaged; if the middle cavity of the brain is injured,

> aberration of thought occurs; but if the rear of the brain is injured at the occiput, memory is destroyed, and the other two faculties also.[37]

Neither Posidonius nor Aëtius set out to explain ventricular localization. Aëtius was writing an encyclopedia of diseases and their treatments, and the excerpt that he culls from the work of Posidonius seems similarly to be nosological in focus. The differentiation of the three most important kinds of phrenitis is explained by the localization of three psychic faculties in discrete portions of the brain. The only explicit indication that Posidonius is describing ventricular localization at all is his reference to the "middle cavity [κοιλίας]" of the brain in relation to the "aberration of thought."

It is possible that, with regard to the "front portion" and the "rear" of the brain, Posidonius was referring to brain substance, rather than to the cavities within. If we consider Galen's famous experiment on the brain of an ox, however, it seems likely that Posidonius did have the ventricles in mind. Galen describes opening up the brain of a living ox and applying pressure to the ventricles one at a time, from front to rear. As discussed in the previous chapter, Galen observed that pressure to or incision of the ventricles from front to rear caused the animal to fall into an increasingly heavy stupor. Posidonius seems to follow this logic, claiming that disturbance to perception (the "front portion of the brain") caused the lightest impairment; disturbance of thought (the "middle cavity") posed a more significant problem; disturbance of memory (the "rear of the brain"), meanwhile, was apparently not serious enough on its own, and Posidonius added that all the faculties were destroyed with injury to the occiput.

The notion that the rear of the brain was most important—that damage to it could entirely ruin the mind—recalls the theory of the Hellenistic medical scientist Herophilus, discussed in chapter 2, that the rear ventricle was dominant. According to Galen,

> those who consider this [sc. the "little vault" that forms a passageway between the front two ventricles and the rear ventricle] to be a fourth ventricle say that it is the most dominant [ventricle] in the whole brain. Herophilus, however, seems to regard, not this [sc. the middle] ventricle, but the one in the cerebellum [sc. the rear ventricle] as dominant.[38]

While the assignment of faculties was a later development, the assignment of dominance to a single ventricle (and debate about which was the most viable candidate) goes back to early dissection of the brain and theorization of its ventricular structure.

The claim that the middle ventricle (Galen's "little vault") governed the others is echoed in Posidonius' association between the middle ventricle and the *logistikon*, that is, in Galen's terms, the *hēgemonikon*. One possible source for this claim that the middle ventricle is most important appears in a text that is difficult to pin down, the *Diktyaka* ("Net-Like [Propositions?]") by Dionysius of Aegae, which is preserved only in synoptic form in the ninth-century *Bibliotheca* of Photius.[39] Dionysius of Aegae has been considered a Hellenistic medical author, working perhaps within the Empiricist tradition, although, as we will see here, what he has to say about the brain calls this dating into question.[40]

According to Photius, Dionysius organized his work in a series of fifty chapters, each of which contained arguments for and against a single proposition about the constitution of the human body. The purpose of these chapters was to train students in dialectic. Chapters 49 and 50 focus on the faculty of thought (διανοητικόν, *dianoētikon*): "49. That the *dianoētikon* is not in the region of the heart but in the region of the head, and vice versa. 50. That the *dianoētikon* is in the region of the middle cavity of the brain, and that it is not."[41] If Dionysius is indeed a Hellenistic author, then this synopsis reveals that the debate regarding whether the middle or rear ventricle dominates long preceded Galen. As Heinrich von Staden and others have argued, however, Dionysius' localization of the *dianoētikon* in any ventricle of the brain at all suggests that the *Diktyaka* might be a much later work, probably post-Galenic, and perhaps even late antique.[42]

Alternatively, it is possible that Photius has reinterpreted Dionysius' Hellenistic thesis through the lens of late antique theories of ventricular localization.[43] This is suggested by a synopsis of the *Diktyaka* that appears earlier in Photius' work: "98. That the *dianoētikon* is not in the region of the heart but in the region of the head, and 99. that the *dianoētikon* is not in the region of the head, but in the region of the heart. 100. That the *dianoētikon* is in the region of the ventricle of the brain."[44] Did Dionysius highlight the importance of the cerebral ventricles in general for cognition (Cod. 185), or did he specify the middle ventricle of the brain (Cod. 211)? The inconsistency of Photius leaves this unclear.

Nor is it the specificity ("middle cavity") alone that links Dionysius to post-Galenic theories of the brain. His thesis about the localization of the *dianoētikon* rather than the *hēgemonikon* or the *logistikon* suggests a connection between the *Diktyaka* and our second major witness to ventricular localization, Nemesius of Emesa. Nemesius, like Posidonius, links the middle ventricle to rational thought. Whereas Posidonius calls this the *logistikon,* Nemesius uses the same word as Dionysius, the *dianoētikon.* As von Staden argues, it seems likely that Dionysius was familiar with the work of Nemesius, or that Photius reinterpreted Dionysius' work through the lens of Nemesius' account of cell theory.

Dionysius of Aegae does not appear in histories of the brain in antiquity: his work is difficult to date, and the theories that he reflects are uncertain. Yet, the culminating chapters of his *Diktyaka* offer a striking indication of the wider cultural significance of the theory of ventricular localization. Photius judges the work to be "a useful book for those training in dialectic practice."[45] (Or, again: "It is not useless for dialectic exercise and knowledge of some received opinions proper to medical theory.")[46] The debate about whether thought operated "in the region of" one particular ventricle within the brain was considered useful dialectic practice (and useful knowledge of medical opinions) outside the scope of medical training. Arguing for and against a proposition was a standard component of ancient rhetorical education. The *Diktyaka* indicate that the possible localization of thought within a cerebral ventricle was a proposition that students might learn to debate.

If Dionysius of Aegae does not make the cut in histories of the brain, Posidonius barely fares better. His account of phrenitis survives in an obscure medical encyclopedia. Like Dionysius, Posidonius is only tenuously dated to the fourth century. His extant account of ventricular localization is in fact a discussion of the varieties of phrenitis that associates regions of the brain with faculties of the soul only in passing. The "middle cavity" is the only ventricle mentioned, and that but once. The reason that Posidonius appears in histories of the brain at all is the similarity of his account to the explicit theorization of ventricular localization in the work of Nemesius of Emesa, who, it is generally assumed, must have taken the theory from Posidonius.

Theological Theories of Ventricular Localization 1: Nemesius of Emesa

Nemesius was a Greek-speaking bishop of Emesa (modern-day Homs) in the Roman province of Syria. It is probable, although uncertain, that he lived and wrote around the end of the fourth century. He is remembered solely for his philosophical text *On the Nature of the Human Being,* which was, for many centuries, attributed to his more famous contemporary, the Cappadocian bishop Gregory of Nyssa.[47] This work is so erudite that commentators have speculated that Nemesius may have trained as a philosopher before being made bishop—indeed, that he wrote *On the Nature of the Human Being* before he converted to Christianity, and only adapted it slightly to conform to the doctrinal expectations of his new role.[48] It is possible, although disputed, that he is identical with—or perhaps a relative of—the Nemesius who served as governor of Cappadocia Secunda during the mid- to late 380s, and who is known through four letters and an epic poem sent to him by Gregory of Nazianzus.[49] In either case, the Nemesius who wrote *On the Nature of the Human Being* was as well-read as Nemesius of Cappadocia Secunda and other elite bishops and administrators of his day. His text, which surveys such topics as the human soul, the elements, the natural faculties, intentionality, fate, and reason, draws upon scriptural authority, Greek philosophical authors such as Plato, Aristotle, and Plotinus, and also medical authorities, whom he subsumes under the name of Galen.[50]

The work opens with a discussion of the soul and the nature of its union with the body. Following a brief account of the elements from which the body is composed, Nemesius turns to the particular manner by which an individual soul operates within its body. He begins by dividing the soul into three faculties: *phantastikon* (imagination, which includes perception), *dianoētikon* (rational thought), and *mnēmoneutikon* (memory). Then he assigns each of these faculties to a ventricle within the brain. Imagination takes as its instruments "the foremost cerebral ventricles, together with the psychic *pneuma* inside them, the nerves rooted in them and steeped in the psychic *pneuma*, and the sensory organs."[51] Thought uses as its instruments "the middle ventricle of the brain and the psychic *pneuma* within."[52] The instrument of memory, meanwhile, is "the rear ventricle of the brain, which they call the *parenkephalis* or the *enkranis*, and the psychic *pneuma* within."[53] This sequence is to be imagined as operating precisely *as* a sequence: "Imagination, therefore, passes on perceptions to thought, while thought or reasoning sends them on, after receiving and judging them, to memory."[54] The ventricles of the brain, the *pneuma* within the ventricles, and the nerves rooted in the ventricles and steeped in the *pneuma* function together as the instruments of the activities of the rational soul.

Like Hippolytus, Nemesius is concerned with the role of demonstrative proof in accounts of the brain and its potential for illuminating the soul. He writes:

> Since we have said that the source and roots of the senses are the frontal cavities of the brain, and the middle [cavity] of thought, and the rear [cavity] of memory, it is necessary to provide a demonstration [ἐπιδεῖξαι], if these things are in such

> a way, so that we might not seem irrationally to believe the things that are said. A sufficient proof [ἀπόδειξις] is taken from the very function of the parts.[55]

This proof, it turns out, relies upon evidence based not upon animal dissection, but rather upon the differentiation of symptoms in mental illness: "When the foremost ventricles are injured in any way, the senses are impeded, while thought remains yet safe. If the middle ventricle alone suffers, then thought is overthrown but the sensory organs remain, preserving sensation according to nature. . . . When it is the *parenkephalis* [sc. the rear ventricle] that suffers, memory alone is lost, without either sensation or thought receiving any harm."[56]

Like (and perhaps following) Posidonius, Nemesius associates impairment of imagination, thought, and memory with damage to specific portions of the brain, and he also takes the mental illness phrenitis as illustration of this relationship, adapting an anecdote from Galen's *On Affected Parts* 4.1–2. A patient suffering from *phrenitis*, having been left without supervision in a room on the second floor of a building outside of Rome, suddenly began to name various glass implements and throw them out of the window. He then picked up a young slave who happened to be in the room with him, asked the passers-by below if they wanted him thrown down also, and, when they jokingly assented, did so. Nemesius uses this story to illustrate the notion that phrenitis might affect thought (the patient acted irrationally) but leave the faculty of perception intact ("for he was aware that the objects were tools and that the slave was a wool-worker").[57] "Through the affections that result in each part," Nemesius concludes, "their activities are impeded: for the creature is damaged with respect to that activity which the part that suffers naturally carries out, just as when the foot suffers we are hindered from walking: for that is the activity of the foot."[58] The comparison of ventricle to foot (ποδὸς) in particular is motivated by the pun inherent in the word "impeded" (ἐμποδίζεται). The pun reinforces the analogy: injury to the ventricle impedes thinking in the same way that injury to the foot impedes walking. In neither case is the soul itself subject to harm. This was crucial to the association between psychic faculties and cerebral ventricles in late antique Christian writings, and we will return to it.

The comparison also recalls a question that Nemesius raises a few chapters earlier, in his discussion of perception: "How, then, does touch belong to the whole body, if we say that the senses are from the frontal cavities of the brain?"[59] The example he gives involves an impediment to walking: "Since it is often the case that, when a thorn strikes our foot, the hairs on our head immediately stand on end, some think that the affection—or the perception of the affection—is sent to the head and in this way perceived."[60] If this were the case, then it would not be "the injured part that hurts, but the brain."[61] Nemesius does not allow that this could be the case. Following Galenic principles, he argues that "it is better to say that the nerve *is* brain."[62] That is to say, the nerve "is a portion of the brain, containing psychic *pneuma* throughout itself, just as iron that has been heated in the fire contains fire."[63]

There are two points to be made here. First, Nemesius seems to hold the view that the sensory nerves are solid, rather than hollow. The relationship between the *pneuma* and the nerves, which represent "portion[s] of the brain," is not that of hollow vessel for psychic fluid, but malleable substance changed by contact with the *pneuma;* the mode in which the nerve contains *pneuma* is that of the infusion or transformation of a solid object.[64] Further to this, what the nerves circulate is not *pneuma,* in Nemesius' presentation of the theory here, but sensory power.[65] While the ventricles of the brain might be hollow containers for the *pneuma,* the nerves of the brain are not. Recall also that when Nemesius names the instruments of each of the three faculties of the soul, he includes the ventricle, the psychic *pneuma,* and the nerves. The labor of perception in particular is distributed across three different components of the brain: the solid nerves, the hollow ventricles, and the *pneuma* that moves between them.

The second point to be made is that Nemesius repeatedly sets the foot and brain in opposition to one another. At stake here is the symbolic opposition between head and foot (most honorable and dishonorable parts of the body, master and slave), which Nemesius attempts to collapse. It is possible that he is directly referencing the corporeal metaphor of social unity familiar from the Pauline epistles: "The eye cannot say to the hand, 'I don't need you!' And the head cannot say to the feet, 'I don't need you!'"[66] Nemesius' contemporary, John Chrysostom (c. 349–407), offers a suggestive analysis of this passage:

> And often, when a thorn is driven into the heel, the whole body feels it and is anxious about it: the back bends over, the stomach and thighs help out, and the hands—rushing forward just like bodyguards [lit. spear-carriers] and attendants—draw out that which has been driven in, and the head stoops down, and the eyes look on with much concern. And so even if the foot has lesser [status] because it is unable to go upward, nonetheless, it has equal [status] because the head leads the way down.[67]

Chrysostom's language, like that of Nemesius, indicates a correspondence between the foot and the head. His description of the hands as "bodyguards and attendants" (δορυφόροι καὶ ὑπηρέται) echoes the common Platonist metaphor of the *hēgemonikon* as king and the sensory organs as its "attendants and bodyguards" (ὑπηρέτας τε καὶ δορυφόρους). Furthermore, John Chrysostom and his student Theodoret of Cyrrhus, who were contemporaries and compatriots of Nemesius, explicitly interpreted the Pauline "head" (as in, "Christ is the head of the church") as a metonym for the brain, focusing in particular on the function of the brain as distributor of psychic *pneuma* through the sensitive nerves rooted in it.[68] According to Chrysostom, if a hand is cut off from the body (that is, if a member of the church is excommunicated), then it can no longer receive *pneuma* from the brain (that is, grace from Christ). If the foot is pierced by a thorn, meanwhile, the whole body attends to it as if it were the head, and indeed the head (that is, Christ) elevates the foot by lowering itself to the earth. Nemesius' hypothetical scenario about a thorn piercing the foot, even as it works out an argument about the function of the cerebral ventricles and the extension of the brain, is also plugged into theological and social debates about the hierarchies and interdependencies between members of the body, including the dependence of human members of the body of the church upon Christ as the brain.

Theological Theories of Ventricular Localization 2: Augustine of Hippo

During the late medieval period, Nemesius' account of ventricular localization transformed medical, theological, and philosophical understandings of the anatomy and function of the brain in northern Europe. Yet, the groundwork had already been laid by Augustine in his *Literal Commentary on Genesis*, an important theological text that is typically dismissed in large-scale histories of the brain as an insignificant or whimsical deviation from the standard account of cell theory. As I will argue here, Augustine's account offers evidence, first, that the theory of ventricular localization circulated in Latin many centuries before the translation of Nemesius' work and, second, that variations of the theory coexisted in late antiquity, offering different degrees of proximity to Galen's own account of the brain.

Augustine, bishop in the city of Hippo Regius in the Roman province of Numidia (modern-day Annaba, in Algeria), was a contemporary of Nemesius. Unlike Nemesius, much of Augustine's work survives—more, in fact, than that of any other ancient Latin author. Prior to his conversion to Christianity,

Augustine had worked as a teacher of rhetoric, and he was familiar with the traditions of Greco-Roman philosophy.[69] It is unclear whether he had read any medical texts, but he nonetheless demonstrated acquaintance with medical concepts.[70] Augustine's *Literal Commentary on Genesis* presents the third major testimony to ventricular localization from the late antique period.[71]

Interpretations of Genesis provided important material for doctrinal disputes, especially regarding cosmology, Christology, and the relation between human beings and the Christian God. Often these interpretations were allegorical, reading scriptural narratives of creation as symbolic theological and cosmological representations.[72] Written toward the end of Augustine's career, the *Literal Commentary on Genesis* was intended to provide a comprehensive account of Genesis in nonallegorical terms. This meant demonstrating its compatibility with ancient medical and scientific authorities.

Book 7 of Augustine's *Commentary* explicates a single verse, Genesis 2:7: "And God fashioned the man with dust from the earth, and puffed into his face the puff of life, and the man was made into a living soul."[73] Augustine interprets the "puff of life" as the entry of *spiritus* (that is, Greek *pneuma*) into the body.[74] In order to explain why this "puff of life" enters "into [Adam's] face," Augustine describes the localization of the psychic faculties within the brain: "The front part of the brain, from which all the senses are distributed, is situated in the forehead; the so-called instruments [*organa*] of sensation are also in the face."[75] The life-bringing *spiritus* proceeds from the face backward into the rear of the skull, which is the source of movement, "in the same way that counsel comes before action."[76] After clarifying precisely how "action" follows "counsel"—not instantaneously, but via the storage and retrieval of information—Augustine outlines a ventricular model: "Therefore, three cerebral ventricles [*uentriculi cerebri*] are described: one at the front, close to the face, which is the source of all sensory power; the second at the back, close to the neck, which is the source of all movement; and the third between them, in which they show that memory thrives [*uigere*]."[77] The "puff of life" that God breathes into Adam's mouth and nose thereby provides a scriptural illustration of the medical theory that psychic *pneuma* travels through the ventricles, from front to back, enabling specific activities of the soul as it goes. The order of the ventricles embodies the order of psychological processes, moving from perception, to recollection, to action. This echoes Nemesius' account, with the exception that Augustine leaves out rational thought and includes voluntary motion.

Like Nemesius and Posidonius, Augustine uses organic mental illness as evidence for his model. According to medical experts, he explains, the "duties" (*officia*) of individual parts fail when the parts themselves are "struck by some illness or injury," while a cure might be effected through repair of the damaged limb.[78] If this language of "duties" sounds suspiciously anthropomorphic—*officia* is the term used by Cicero and later by Augustine's mentor Ambrose to describe the responsibilities of human individuals—then Augustine is quick to stress that the parts are not to be equated with their animate powers: "But the soul acts upon these [parts] as if upon instruments [*organa*] and is not [one] of them; rather, it animates and rules all."[79] Augustine's word for "instruments" (*organa*) is a direct transliteration from the Greek ὀργανα and is therefore probably borrowed from his source, which may have been a medical text or a translation of Plato's *Timaeus*, where the gods bind *organa* within the human head.[80] The "instruments" that Augustine describes are the *spiritus* and the ventricles, which are not, Augustine insists, identical with the soul and its faculties: "The air [*aer*] that infuses the nerves moves the limbs by obeying the will, but itself is not the will; and the middle part of the brain announces the motion of the limbs, to be retained by memory, but itself is not memory."[81] The proof that Augustine provides is the phenomenon of distraction: when the soul's concentration on an idea is "such that it is not free to attend to the middle part of the brain that announces the movement of the body," the person forgets where they are going and passes by their destination.[82] That is to say, failure of memory is not necessarily the fault of the middle ventricle, but can be caused by the distraction of the soul. Here, the middle ventricle appears as an instrument of communication between the body and the soul, which exercises rational thought. It is striking that, once again, the connection examined to clarify the ventricular model is that between the ventricle and the feet, although Augustine is interested not—like Nemesius—in sensory connection between parts of the body (is pain felt in the ventricles or in the foot?), but in motor control between body and soul (is it the ventricle or the soul that remembers the movement of the feet?).

Augustine is marginal to the historiography on ventricular localization, and his description is usually described as an aberration: Frampton calls his account an "interesting variant," and Smith describes it as "a different and perhaps yet more fanciful schematic than the usual tripartite system" than that sketched out by Nemesius.[83] This is for several reasons. First is the rhetorical program of the text: Augustine's account is clearly organized toward a theological goal, that is, scriptural exegesis, whereas Nemesius frames his account as an investigation of the human body. Second is the content of Augustine's account: he does not include rational thought within his version, but replaces it with voluntary motion, shifting memory from the rear to the middle of the brain. This can be interpreted as an adjustment of ventricular localization to further separate the immaterial soul from the embodied faculties of sensation and movement: by narrowing down the functions of the ventricles to those activities which more obviously require corporeal instruments—either the nerves (for sensorimotor function) or the storage of sensory information (as memory)—Augustine designates rational thought as an aspect of soul not reliant upon the instruments of the body.[84] The third reason for the marginalization of Augustine in modern histories of ventricular localization is the fate of the two versions: after Nemesius' text was translated from Greek into Latin in the latter half of the eleventh century, it became the dominant model of cell theory in late medieval and early modern philosophical and scientific texts, despite the long history of Augustine's influence in medieval Europe; as such, it is now taken more seriously by historians.[85]

Augustine is often incorporated as an addendum to Nemesius. Yet, his distribution of the faculties of the soul cleaves closer than that of Nemesius or Posidonius to Galenic medical theory. While Galen did not associate the faculties of the soul with specific ventricles, he did believe that the sensory nerves were rooted in the front part of the brain, and the motor nerves in the rear.[86] Galen's experiments did not seek to prove the localization of thought within the brain (for good reason—all of his experiments were performed on animals, which were assumed to be without the faculty of thought); instead, like Augustine, Galen focused on establishing the sites of sensory and motor functions, and assumed the localization of rational thought by association. Augustine's account is more Galenic than that of Nemesius, but it is usually interpreted as more "fanciful." This is a consequence of reading Nemesius' text as "scientific" and Augustine's as "theological," despite the lack of purchase this opposition had in late antiquity.

From Instruments to Dwelling-Places: Theophilus Protospatharius

The work of the Byzantine medical author Theophilus Protospatharius seems to date to the seventh century, but we have no certain information about his life, his education, or his profession.[87] His anatomical work, titled *On the Constitution of the Human Being*, largely follows Galen, but concludes with an account of ventricular localization. This fourth major source is left out of almost all other histories of the brain; perhaps the brain is difficult to date and so to situate either in any historical context or in the intellectual tradition. Yet, it seems to be the earliest extant theory of ventricular localization that appears in a medical text for its own sake, rather than as an explanation for phrenitis or other kinds of mental illness. Despite the difficulty of dating the text, it rewards examination as an illustration of how medical authors operating within a Christian framework integrated the model of ventricular localization into their accounts of the human being.

The fourth and final book of Theophilus' work focuses on the anatomy of the head. Theophilus opens by presenting a strictly Galenic account of the distribution of the nerves (sensory nerves at the front, motor nerves at the back).[88] The closing chapter, however, repeats the ventricular model of Posidonius and Nemesius, from which voluntary motion is absent:

> The frontal cavities of the brain that are contained by the forehead, then, contain the imaginative part. For, since the three activities—imagination, memory, and thought—are carried out by the psychic *pneuma*, three regions of the brain have been set apart for their abode: the front, the rear, and the middle. Imagination dwells in the front region, therefore, thought in the middle, and memory in the rear.[89]

Theophilus justifies his organization of the ventricles by reference to the same kind of psychological ordering that Nemesius and Augustine describe: imagination (or perception) precedes judgment, which is followed by memory.[90] Despite his inclusion of this model, Theophilus spends more energy defending the localization of the *hēgemonikon* within the head than the assignment of individual faculties to the ventricles. He is concerned above all to prove that "the *hēgemonikon* of the soul" is in the brain rather than in the heart, attributing the latter view, with some puzzlement, to "Homer . . . most other Hellenes . . . and the divine gospel itself."[91] Notably, the major opponents of encephalocentrism no longer explicitly include Aristotle or the Stoics; at the forefront, rather, are the texts fundamental to general education. It seems that Theophilus perhaps expected an audience of intellectuals beyond the medical sphere.

Like Nemesius and Augustine, Theophilus supports the theory of ventricular localization through a discussion of the etiologies of mental illnesses and the parts of the body to which treatments for mental illness are applied. Physicians, he explains, apply "therapeutic ointments, vapor baths, and other remedies to the head, rather than to the heart."[92] A range of illnesses affecting mental function ("dementia, melancholia, mania, epilepsy, coma, phrenitis, catalepsy, lethargy, delirium, amnesia, apoplexy, and paralysis"), Theophilus claims, "arise from the suffering of the brain, when the body [sc. of the brain] itself or the membranes surrounding it become hot or cold or dry or wet, or when the nerves that sprout from it are blocked up for some reason."[93] In this list, it is striking that Theophilus does not invoke phrenitis alone and indeed offers no etiology of mental illness that involves the ventricles in particular. It is the body of the brain, the membranes, and the nerves that are sites of mental illness and that therefore prove the localization of the *hēgemonikon* in the brain.

In tension with this emphasis upon the material components of the brain is the language of habitation that Theophilus introduces into his account of cell theory. The frontal cavities of the brain "contain" (περιέχουσι) imagination, just as the cavities themselves are "contained" (περιεχόμεναι) by the forehead. Three regions of the brain have been set apart for the "abode" (κατοικίαν) of the three psychic faculties, each of which "dwells" (κατοικεῖ) in its own ventricle(s). Whereas Nemesius and Augustine use the image of the instrument, Theophilus prefers metaphors of containment and dwelling. This shift marks a turn from thinking about the ventricles as tools for action to their conception as spaces within which the parts of the soul reside. When modern scholars write that Nemesius "places the *sensus communis* and imagination in the two anterior (lateral) ventricles" or that "Posidonius thus localizes the psychical operations to specific sub-locations within the brain [and] even places one of them, the faculty of reasoning, in the middle ventricle," they are attributing metaphors of containment to the earliest witnesses of cell theory, none of whom actually claim that the faculties of the soul were *located* anywhere in the body.[94]

Theophilus Protospatharius reveals an important conceptual shift toward the metaphor of localization. This shift is generally missing from narratives that see in the work of Augustine and Nemesius an attempt to avoid attributing psychic agency to the material body by locating the faculties of soul within empty cerebral ventricles. Contrary to this account, the early theologians who talked about cell theory considered the ventricles to be instruments rather than containers. Theophilus Protospatharius represents a turning-point toward the metaphor of habitation or containment that was to become pervasive in medieval cell theory.

INSTRUMENTS OF THE SOUL

By treating the ventricles as instruments, Augustine and Nemesius sought to avoid suggesting that the brain might take the place of the soul. Their older contemporary Gregory of Nyssa used the metaphor of the instrument more broadly to signal that no part of the body at all could contain the soul. In *On the Constitution of the Human Being*, which we began to explore in chapter 1, Gregory argued that even though the brain was responsible for sensory and motor functions, it could not contain the mind (*nous*, a term that Gregory used interchangeably with *hēgemonikon*). If it could, then mind might be "squeezed out" by inflammation: "But the intellectual nature does not tend to dwell in the empty spaces within bodies, nor is it squeezed out by the increase of flesh."[95] Instead, Gregory argued that if the brain were injured, then the mind would depart, just as a musician might set aside a broken instrument:

> Since the entire body has been crafted like some musical instrument, it is just like when expert musicians are unable to display their expertise because their instruments, being nonfunctional, do not admit their skill (for an instrument, having deteriorated over time, been broken in an accident, or made useless by rust and decay, remains voiceless and inactive, even when blown into by an expert flautist): so, too, the mind, ranging throughout the whole instrument and touching upon each of the parts in accordance with its intellective functions, works according to its proper nature upon the parts which are disposed according to nature, but with regard to the parts unable to receive its skillful movement, it remains ineffective and unavailing.[96]

The flute transforms the flautist's breath into music, just as the vocal organs turn a person's breath (or *pneuma*) into rational speech. It is possible that Gregory depends here on an explicit comparison between the vocal organs and the flute in Galen's popular anatomical treatise *On the Usefulness of the Parts*.[97] Speech was considered the primary manifestation of reason.[98] When the flute (or body, or brain) was broken, according to Gregory, the flautist was still an expert musician (that is, the rational soul was still rational), but the flautist's skill could not be made manifest. This metaphor allowed Gregory to explain how brain inflammation might cause the loss of reason, without making the brain the agent of rational thought. Like the flautist and the flute, mind and body were separate. As Nemesius and Augustine also emphasized, injury to the body could not hurt the rational soul, only impede its actions.

Here, Gregory is also referring back to his earlier rejection of both encephalocentrism and cardiocentrism in favor of the theory that the soul permeates the body as a whole.[99] Relevant here is his rebuttal of the medical argument that, since mental illness is associated with injury to the cerebral membranes and drunkenness with heaviness of the head, the mind must have its seat in the brain.[100] Gregory cites the mental illness phrenitis as evidence to the contrary: "I have learned that madness arises not only from heaviness of the head, but also from the membranes that lie alongside the ribs, when they become stretched with sickness; similarly, medical experts define the faculty of thought as becoming sick, calling the affection phrenitis, since the name for these membranes is *phrenes*."[101] Phrenitis was commonly used—and had been used for centuries—to determine the bodily organ of the *hēgemonikon*.[102] Gregory's citation of this disease participates in a long-standing conversation about the role of mental illness in producing knowledge about the organization of the body/soul relationship.

While most used phrenitis to argue that the *hēgemonikon* operated through the brain (if they linked phrenitis to *phronēsis*, "thought") or through the heart (if they linked phrenitis to the *phrenes*), Gregory disputes the localization of the *hēgemonikon* in either location. The language that he uses to describe the theoretical relationship between *hēgemonikon* and bodily organ reveals why, and also gives us some traction in explaining the emphasis of Augustine and Nemesius on calling the ventricles "organs" of the soul. Gregory set out to refute the claims of those who allege that the *hēgemonikon* is "in" the heart, or that the *nous* "dwells in" the brain. What Gregory refutes is not the argument that the brain plays a role in sensory and motor functions, but rather that the soul could be confined spatially within the body.

The scholarly consensus that cell theory transferred the soul and its faculties from the substance of the brain to the empty spaces and *pneuma* within is grounded in an understanding of the model as one of localization: the soul "dwells within" the (ventricles of the) brain, transforming the brain itself into no more than a house or a factory that is divided into rooms. While this does reflect later accounts of the theory, such as that of Theophilus Protospatharius, the earliest accounts of ventricular localization imagined the ventricles not as rooms or containers but as instruments. This was motivated precisely by the concern that Gregory expressed, that the soul should *not* be confined within the brain. When Nemesius and Augustine integrated ventricular localization into their anthropological accounts, they were not interested so much in shifting attention from brain substance to *pneuma,* but rather in emphasizing that the ventricles were instruments in the (figurative) hands of the soul.

THE BRAIN IS A LYRE

Musical instruments were prominent and controversial analogues for the human body in ancient Greek medicine and philosophy. That the body could profitably be imagined as a musical instrument—usually a flute or a lyre—was undisputed; the image went back a long way in Greek philosophy and was influentially deployed by the prominent Neoplatonist philosopher Plotinus.[103] At issue, rather, was the question of whether the soul was to be envisioned as the musician handling the instrument or as the harmony that the instrument produced. The image of the soul as a harmony, attributed to Pythagorean philosophers, was rejected as such by Socrates in Plato's *Phaedo,* by Aristotle in *On the Soul,* and, centuries later, by Plotinus.[104] The central problem with the thesis was that it rendered the condition of the soul dependent upon that of the body and thereby suggested that the soul shared in bodily mortality.[105]

In the early fifth century, the Egyptian monk Isidore of Pelusium wrote a letter to a learned physician, Proeschius.[106] Barred from Pelusium, where he had previously been a priest, Isidore had retired to a monastery on the outskirts of his city and kept up with the world chiefly through his epistolary network. Most of his communicants were priests, bishops, lawyers, and sophists, and many of his letters touch upon aspects of Christian scripture and the Christian life. The letter to Proeschius is not a total outlier in these respects, but it is unusual: its addressee has medical expertise, and its subject—the soul—is discussed in relation to a work of non-Christian literature, Galen's popular work *That the Faculties of the Soul Follow the Mixtures of the Body.*[107] While various late antique Christian authors demonstrate familiarity with the fundamental principles of this text, Isidore offers one of the only extant discussions of it in relation to Christian theories of the soul.[108]

Proeschius has raised a question or made a provocative claim regarding the authority of Galen in matters of the soul. It is difficult to know exactly what this question or claim was because Isidore does not respond directly to anything that Proeschius has said. Instead, he uses the letter as a platform for refuting the central thesis of Galen's text, which is that the condition of psychic faculties such as thought and memory is dependent upon the body's temperament—that is, the balance of bodily qualities (hot, cold, wet, and dry)—with the consequence that an independent (and immortal) entity "soul" might be considered logically unnecessary.[109] "If, then, the reasoning faculty is a form of the soul, it must be mortal: for it too will be a mixture, namely a mixture within the brain."[110]

Isidore situates Galen's theory of bodily temperament in a long history of describing the body as a musical instrument. First, there are the philosophers, such as Pythagoras (seventh century B.C.E.) and Plato (fifth to fourth centuries B.C.E.), who hold that the body is an "instrument" (ὄργανον) in "three dimensions," whilst the soul is incorporeal, immortal, and indestructible.[111] In opposition to the philosophers, there is Galen (second century C.E.), who holds that the body is like a "harmonious lyre" (ἁρμόνιον . . . λύραν) and pronounces the soul to be necessarily mortal.[112] For Galen has argued that "the faculties of the soul follow the mixtures of the body," such that soul is somehow to be defined (Isidore knows not how) as "mixture."[113] We understand by implication that Galen's "mixture," according to Isidore, is the *harmonia*, the music of the lyre.[114] The difference between the theories of Pythagoras and Galen lies in the relationship in each case between instrument and soul. According to Pythagoras, the soul skillfully uses its instrument to produce certain effects. For Galen, meanwhile, the soul is the effect that the instrument produces, skilled user unknown.

Isidore's critique of Galen's model focuses on its implication that injury to the body might damage or destroy the soul. A harmony, he points out, must be lost with the instrument that produces it.[115] At the same time, harmony and disharmony do not correspond so much to life and death as to virtue and vice: thus, the loosening of strings might cause sinful behavior, such that the individual soul cannot be held responsible for the quality of its own actions.[116] Within Galen's theory of bodily temperament the soul loses both immortality and morality, two characteristics which are fundamental to Isidore's Christian conception of the soul.

Even though Galen's temperament-based paradigm and the harmony metaphor alike invoke the balance of the body as the condition of psychic health, Galen's evidence that the soul is dependent upon bodily qualities focuses on a single part—that is, the brain. If the soul were, as Plato claims, immortal (Galen argues), then it ought not to separate from the body upon the brain becoming too cold, too dry, or too wet.[117] Galen's argument here synthesizes his two most famous models for the body/soul relationship: the temperament thesis (*That the faculties of the soul follow the mixtures of the body*) and the local or instrumental model, in which a single part is identified as the "seat" or "instrument" of the ruling part of the soul.[118] Isidore's response is scathing: Galen, for all his knowledge about temperament and the brain, does not understand the ineffable bond between body and soul; what the doctor calls "soul" is not the same thing that philosophers are talking about; he should stick to what he is good at—strictly bodily healing.[119] Notably, however, Isidore does not contest Galen's theory of localization, that is, that damage to the brain results in the separation of the soul. This reflects the extent to which Galen's arguments for the brain as the organ of the *hēgemonikon* had become deeply embedded in both learned and popular culture by the fifth century.[120] Despite the contradiction posed by scriptural emphasis upon the heart as the locus of the mind, most theologians accepted the association between the brain, sensation, voluntary motion, and rational thought.[121]

Precisely how the (corporeal) brain might be related to the faculties of the (incorporeal) soul was another question, the answer to which Isidore touches upon through a striking blend of two popular metaphors. A preferable model for the body/soul relationship, he asserts, would be that of a captain in a ship on a stormy ocean.[122] The captain is the soul, the ship represents the bodily structure, and the ocean is the bodily temperament, which we might visualize as the flux and flow of humors and vapors that affect but do not constitute the soul. Realizing that if the ship of the body were to wreck in the swell of its humors, then the captain must drown, Isidore transforms the ship into a lyre and the soul into a musician. Even if the lyre is broken, the musician is not harmed. Indeed, he goes on, even if the musician holding the lyre falls into the sea, the only reason why the harmony ends is that the lyre does not admit the musician's expertise, and not that the musician is dead.[123] Isidore laces his rebuttal of Galen's theory of temperament with acknowledgement of Galen's medical expertise. For Galen to talk about the soul, he argued, was like an athlete trying to discourse on musical technique.[124] In this way, Isidore redeployed Galen's musical metaphor to represent not only the soul making use of the body, but also the differentiation of authority. The musician was the soul, expert in using its own bodily instrument, and the musician was also the theologian, expert in talking about the music of the rational soul.

Galen was, in fact, a central source for the image of the brain as a lyre. We have already seen how Galen compared the mouthparts (that is, the instruments of rational speech) to a musical instrument. Elsewhere in *On the Useful-*

ness of the Parts, Galen addresses the argument that, since there are acephalous animals (such as crabs) that nonetheless manifest sensory and motor functions, the *hēgemonikon* cannot possibly be located in the brain (the *en-kephalos,* "in-the-head").[125] The tactic that he employs is philological: etymology, Galen argues, is an unreliable indicator of function; the *enkephalos* ought to be defined not as the organ in the head, but rather as the organ that is the source of the sensory and motor nerves.[126] By this reasoning, even acephalous animals could have "brains." It is a simple shift from local to functional definition. In order to facilitate this redefinition, Galen proposed calling the *enkephalos* by its Latin name (*cerebrum*), which did not carry the same local connotation—or by a random word, such as *skindapsos:*

> Well now, instead of *cerebrum* [κέρεβρον], let us call it *skindapsos* [σκινδαψὸς], and just as we call any instrument of vision [ὀπτικὸν ὄργανον] the eye not only when it is in the head but also when it is situated on the breast, so any part of an animal that controls sensation and voluntary motion for the other parts will be called *skindapsos.* Now, if the *enkephalos* is the source of will and motion, and if animals having no head but having an *enkephalos* or something analogous have will and motion of a sort, it is clear that this did not happen through the presence of a head.[127]

Commentators on this passage have emphasized that *skindapsos* was a nonsense word (a "thing-a-ma-bob"), and perhaps Galen intended it as such, but it was also the name of a four-stringed musical instrument: an apt nonsense word, then, for a bodily "instrument" that was supposed to produce rational speech through the movement of *pneuma* and nerves.[128]

The image of the brain as a lyre was useful theologically, so long as the soul could be imagined as the musician, rather than the song; it was anatomically and physiologically appropriate, especially since the word for nerves in both Greek (νεῦρα) and Latin (*nervi*) could also refer to the strings of a lyre.[129] Ambrose of Milan states this clearly in his final hexameral sermon, which gives an account of human anatomy: "The nerves are like an instrument of each of the senses. They descend from the brain like cords and musical strings [*uelut cordae et fides*]."[130] The *pneuma* passed through the hollow cavities within the brain and affected the *neura* that were strung between the brain or spine and the other parts of the body. Through the movement of the *pneuma* over the strings, the bodily instrument as a whole sang with rational thought that manifested in speech most obviously, but also in voluntary motion.

CONCLUSION

The theory of ventricular localization was founded upon a metaphor not of containment but of instrumentalization: in the terms of conceptual metaphor theory, not THE BRAIN IS A CONTAINER but THE BRAIN IS A TOOL. As I have sought to demonstrate in this chapter, the adoption of the ventricles as "instruments" of the psychic faculties was part of a wider project to reject the notion that the soul might be identified with or contained within the brain. Far from imagining that their models displaced the soul from the brain substance to the hollow spaces within, late antique theologians envisioned the soul as a musician, moving air into the instrument from without.

Whether the brain was a flute or a lyre, this metaphor played upon the resonant qualities of hollow bodies and their capacity to make music with the passage of *pneuma* (breath, air). If I am correct, then the metaphor of the brain as a musical instrument—in which the hollow structures, air, and strings collaborated to produce harmonious tunes (the strains of reason)—provided the conceptual apparatus through which the theory of ventricular localization took hold in late antique theological texts. Its appeal was not the deemphasis of brain matter, but the explanatory potential of the lyre as model for understanding how the soul could use the brain to produce rational speech.

Late antique theorists of ventricular localization did not consider different parts of the brain matter to be responsible for different functions in the manner that neuroscience describes. Yet, the dichotomies drawn in modern histories between brain matter and the hollow ventricles or spirit do not adequately represent the late antique imagination regarding the mode in which the brain mediated between body and soul—and, further, they misunderstand the role that theological concerns played in the early development of ventricular localization. If there was a shift to erase the participation of brain matter itself in the activities of the rational soul, then it must be located in subsequent, medieval writers. The earliest, most influential accounts of ventricular localization taught that the ventricles were the instruments that the soul made to sing.

CHAPTER 4

The Governing Brain

While images of the anatomical brain as a lyre elaborated the underlying conceptual metaphor THE BRAIN IS A TOOL, late antique theologians were simultaneously elaborating through a more psychological and spiritual lens a different conceptual metaphor, albeit one that shared its deep philosophical and medical roots: THE BRAIN GOVERNS. These two metaphors highlight different aspects of the relationship between the soul, body, and brain as it was conceptualized in late antiquity. The first, which focuses on the brain/soul relationship, treats the brain as more of an object than an agent. The second focuses on the brain/body relationship and positions the brain as an agent akin to a human being. In keeping with conceptual metaphor theory (see the introduction), we can understand both conceptual metaphors as revealing core ideas about the brain and what it does. It is possible, further, to see how authors sought to reconcile these ideas with one another and with other core theories and beliefs through the ways that they adapted the basic conceptual metaphors in specific images.

Neither metaphor offers a comprehensive map of underlying conceptual structures; instead, each functions as a strategy for negotiating complex and contradictory ideas. The image of the governing brain had seeped into late antique popular culture and become a habit of thought; in addition to meshing well with current medical ideas about the brain, it also offered a neat model for human leadership in a world ultimately governed by God. In anthropological terms, however, THE BRAIN GOVERNS was a troubling image, since it potentially replaced the soul as the source of mental and moral agency.

THE BRAIN IS A TOOL, as we saw in the previous chapter, could resolve this concern but offered limited scope for exploring the implication of the body in action, holiness, and sin. The rising prominence of THE BRAIN GOVERNS in Christian texts suggests the growing importance of this question in the fourth and fifth centuries.

This chapter proceeds in three steps. First, I trace the history of THE BRAIN GOVERNS back to Plato's metaphor of the body as a city. By unpacking the development of the conceptual metaphor, I show how specific elaborations gradually shift from envisioning the civic ruler as soul to the civic ruler as brain. The history of the metaphor also reveals its philosophical underpinnings: when we come across metaphors of the brain as a king, for example, we are not examining mere literary ornament; instead, what we have is a statement (in a strong interpretation) or a trace (in a weak interpretation) of a philosophical position about the relationship between the brain, the body, and the soul.

Second, I turn to metaphors of the brain as a governing figure in theological texts. What is striking in these metaphors is the extent to which they are concerned with honor and self-control. The brain, insofar as it is the "source" or the "governing principle" of the nerves, is responsible for self-control; at the same time, failures of self-control hurt and dishonor the brain, just as disorder within the city dishonors the king. The attraction of THE BRAIN GOVERNS lies partly in the way that it connects the mechanisms and motivations of self-governance.

In the third and final section, I step beyond human governance to examine metaphors of the brain as Christ (as in, Christ the king). Here, I am interested especially in how the Pauline metaphor of the church as Christ's body contributed to reshaping the Platonist metaphor of the governing soul into THE BRAIN GOVERNS. In addition, the metaphor of the brain as Christ opens up new space for imagining the brain as a kind of mediator, participating in two realms of being (body and soul) and transferring knowledge and instructions between them.

What I will argue overall is that late antique Christian texts exhibit a novel interest in THE BRAIN GOVERNS, despite the problems that this metaphor posed for theories of the rational soul. This transition from the soul to the brain as the imagined "king" plays an important role in articulating the hierarchy of governance within a Christian cosmos and offers a model in particular for a hierarchy of governing powers that includes both corporeal and incorporeal (and, further, immaterial) ruling agents. A necessary part of such a hierarchy is that the rulers at each level are exposed to different degrees and types of risk. The conclusion to this chapter will touch upon the vulnerability of the brain as a governing agent and point toward the subsequent chapter, where I explore early Christian rhetoric of the "vulnerable brain" in further detail.

PLATONIST METAPHORS: THE HEAD IS AN ACROPOLIS, AND THE MIND RULES WITHIN

THE BRAIN GOVERNS has philosophical and medical roots. It derives from the claim that the brain is the organ of the *hēgemonikon*, the "governing part" of the soul.[1] In particular, it builds on Plato's *Timaeus*, which compares the body to a city and the head to an acropolis (home to the rational part of the soul), the heart to a guardhouse (τὴν δορυφορικὴν οἴκησιν, home to the irascible or sensitive part of the soul), and the liver as a trough where the common people feed (home to the appetitive part of the soul).[2] The irascible part of the soul is positioned between the head and the liver, "so that it might listen to reason and, together with it, coerce the appetitive part, should the latter at any time refuse to obey the dictates of reason (τῷ τ'ἐπιτάγματι καὶ λόγῳ) from the acropolis (ἀκροπόλεως)."[3] The metaphor of the body as the city with the mind ruling from the head is repeated in *Laws* 12, where Plato writes as follows:

> It is clear that the city itself is the torso, and that the younger guards, as if on the topmost summit [ἐν ἄκρᾳ κορυφῇ] . . . keep watch over the whole city in a circle [κύκλῳ], being on guard, and hand over perceptions to memory, serving as messengers to the elders of all the things that happen in the city; and these [elders] are like the mind [νῷ], in that they have many different wise thoughts.[4]

In neither of these metaphors does Plato allocate any portion of responsibility to the brain. To the contrary, Plato envisions the brain later in the *Timaeus* as a "field" (ἄρουραν) into which the "divine seed" (τὸ θεῖον σπέρμα) of the immortal (and therefore the rational) soul might be planted and take root.[5] That is to say, Plato introduced or popularized the metaphor of the head as the site of civic governance, but his central metaphor of the brain was organic rather than hegemonic, connecting to a distinct figurative tradition, wherein the marrow was envisioned as a nutritive substance that manifested sometimes (as in the *Timaeus*) as the soil, and at other times as the water in a river or the pith within a tree.

Plato's metaphor of the head as an acropolis proved popular among Middle Platonists, who synthesized the passages from *Timaeus* and *Laws* into a single image. This blended metaphor appears first in *Homeric Questions* by Heraclitus (first century), in a comment on Athena's epiphany when Achilles draws his sword on Agamemnon.[6] In order to provide a psychological interpretation for this divine interruption of Achilles' anger, Heraclitus turns to Plato. He summarizes Plato's division of the soul into part 1 (rational) and parts 2a (irrational, spirit) and 2b (irrational, desires), each of which occupies a different space, as if within a single house. This domestic division of labor quickly shifts—as in the *Timaeus*—to the civic scale:

> He thinks that the rational element of the soul has been assigned the top of the head, as a citadel [ἀκρόπολίν], surrounded all around [ἐν κύκλῳ] by a protective guard [δορυφορούμενον] of sense-organs. As for the irrational part, its "spirit" dwells around the heart, while the urges of desire are in the liver.[7]

The protective function that Plato assigns to the irascible part of the soul, which dwells within the "guardhouse" (τὴν δορυφορικὴν οἴκησιν) of the heart in *Timaeus*, has been transferred to the sensory organs, which surround the head/acropolis "all around" (ἐν κύκλῳ), as in *Laws*. This synthesis shifts the focus of governance from controlling the irrational parts of the soul to absorbing, storing, and acting upon information from the external environment.

Shortly after Heraclitus, a second-century philosophical author named in the manuscript as Alcinous but widely identified in modern scholarship as Galen's teacher Albinus repeats the metaphor in his *Handbook of Platonism*.[8] Alcinous/Albinus incorporates key developments from Hellenistic medical and philosophical theory into the metaphor:

> But the gods, having created the human being and bound into its body the soul to govern it, reasonably established the seat of the *hēgemonikon* of the soul in the region of the head, and from there the beginnings of marrow and the nerves and deliriums in the form of affections, with the senses situated around the head, as if guarding [δορυφορουσῶν] the *hēgemonikon*.[9]

Alcinous incorporates both the Stoic term *hēgemonikon* and Hellenistic anatomical discoveries, in particular the notion of the brain as the origin of the marrow-filled nerves. In this way, he shifts the emphasis of the metaphor from the governance of reason over the irrational parts of the soul to the governance of the *hēgemonikon* over the body. Only subsequently does Alcinous name the rational, affective, and irascible parts of the soul: "In this place also is the rational part of the soul, and the faculty of discernment, and the faculty of contemplation. They made the affective part of the soul lower down, the irascible part around the heart, and the appetitive part around the lower abdomen and the places around the navel."[10] Note also that Alcinous makes no mention here of the acropolis. What he seeks to emphasize is not the political metaphor of the human body as a city inhabited by the soul, but the governance of the body via the marrow, the senses, and the nerves.

Perhaps the most important source of this metaphor in late antiquity was the Jewish author Philo of Alexandria (c. 20 B.C.E.–40 C.E). Philo's exegetical works were a central source and inspiration for early Christian theologians.[11] Across his corpus, Philo refers to parts of the metaphor at least thirteen times: three of these references invoke only the head/acropolis metaphor, eight focus on the senses as bodyguards of the mind, and two blend both metaphors together.[12] This last pair are summaries of philosophical accounts of the soul/body relationship. The first is securely Platonist:

> Then they have allotted to the rational part [τῷ μὲν λογιστικῷ] the region about the head, saying that wherever the king [βασιλεύς] is, there his bodyguards [δορυφόροι] are also, and the bodyguards [δορυφόροι] are the mind's [τοῦ νοῦ] senses, being [stationed] around the head, such that the king also might be there, as if allotted the citadel [ἄκραν ἐν πόλει] to live in.[13]

The second incorporates the Stoic and Aristotelian theory that the mind governed from within the heart: "Where does this mind lurk? . . . Some have consecrated [ἀνιέρωσαν] the head to it as the citadel within us, surrounding which the senses lie in ambush; for they consider it to be reasonable for them to be stationed close by, just like the bodyguards of a great king. Others dispute this, believing that it is carried like a statue in the heart."[14]

Neither Philo nor Alcinous nor Heraclitus assigned any governing function to the brain itself. In this, they followed Plato's *Timaeus*. The final passage from Philo above, which summarizes what would now be called "encephalocentric" and "cardiocentric" positions (the theory that the organ of the *hēgemonikon* is the brain or the heart), does not mention the brain at all, but rather contrasts the heart and the head. Even though Hellenistic medical scientists had used dissection to identify the brain as the source of the sensory and motor nerves, the brain nonetheless remained outside the Platonist metaphor of psychic governance.

Consider, in contrast, the following passage from the theologian Gregory of Nyssa, who was certainly familiar with Philo's account.[15]

> Let there be an end to all the speculative and empty talk of those who enclose intellectual activity within bodily parts: both those who argue that the *hēgemonikon* is in the heart, and those who say that the mind dwells within the brain, supporting such claims with superficial but plausible statements. . . . Those who consecrate [ἀφιεροῦντες] the brain to reason say that the head has been constructed by nature just like the acropolis of the whole body; for the mind dwells within like some monarch, guarded all around [ἐν κύκλῳ δορυφορούμενον] by the sensory organs like messengers and bodyguards.[16]

Gregory begins by refuting both encephalocentrists and cardiocentrists. Unlike most ancient philosophers and physicians—but in keeping with a number of other theologians—he insists that the mind (*nous*) or *hēgemonikon* (Gregory uses the terms interchangeably) cannot be located within any bodily part. When he comes to the head/acropolis metaphor, he incorporates all the possible Platonist features, but adds one additional element: the brain. Whereas Philo describes those who consecrate (ἀνιέρωσαν) the head to the mind, Gregory says that these same people consecrate (ἀφιεροῦντες) the brain to reason.

Gregory does not assign the brain a governing role; rather, he draws a connection between the encephalocentric theory of the soul/body relationship and the Platonist metaphor of the head as the acropolis and the center of rule. Nonetheless, a more explicit personification of the governing brain was available, and Gregory may have been responding to it.

We can glimpse this stronger version of the metaphor in a different kind of rebuttal issued by Galen some two centuries before Gregory's lifetime. In his treatise *On the Opinions of Hippocrates and Plato*, Galen seeks to dismiss metaphorical or symbolic proofs for the localization of the *hēgemonikon*. Instead, he insists upon using anatomical evidence. To this end, he refutes even those metaphorical proofs that support his own position, that is encephalocentrism: "Nor is it necessary that because the brain, like the Great King, dwells in the head as in an acropolis, for that reason the ruling part of the soul is in the brain, or because the brain has the senses stationed around it like bodyguards."[17] While it is, once again, the soul that does the governing, this time it is the brain that is compared to a king (specifically the Great King, that is, probably, the King of Persia), surrounded by the senses as bodyguards.

Gregory and Galen were participating in a tradition of reading and applying the metaphors in *Timaeus* and *Laws* to contemporary theories of the mind (or rational soul) and its operations within the body. Within this tradition, which developed within Middle Platonism, the brain was most often passed over as a participant in the key Platonist metaphor of the head as an acropolis with the mind as ruler within; only in later medical and theological contexts did the brain begin to play a significant role.

THE GOVERNING BRAIN IN THEOLOGICAL TEXTS

By the late fourth century, it became imaginable for Christian preachers and theologians to envision the brain not only as the site of governance but as the governing agent itself. This agent was not always the Great King, although it could be. More often, it was some kind of intermediary governing power. These metaphors are not as stable and frequent as the Middle Platonist synthesis examined in the previous section; what they attest to, rather, is the negotiation and expansion of the conceptual metaphor THE BRAIN GOVERNS to explore the nature of the body/soul relationship, especially in relation to self-control. Where we see this most clearly is in pastoral texts, such as sermons, where THE BRAIN GOVERNS is used to motivate appropriate behaviors (such as the avoidance of excess alcohol) by arguing that the neglect of the brain impacts the health of the soul.

A striking example of this elaboration of THE BRAIN GOVERNS for pastoral purposes appears in John Chrysostom's *Commentary on the First Letter to Timothy* 13, in a warning about drunkenness.[18] First, Chrysostom establishes that the vapors of alcohol hurt the brains of bystanders and of drunken individuals themselves. Then he turns to the effects of alcohol on the architecture of the body, describing the blood vessels as "pipes," the internal organs as "reservoirs," and the intestines as sewage pipes ("channels for feces"). Just as his audience members demonstrate civic responsibility in relation to their sewers, he declares, so they ought to act responsibly with regard to their bodies: "and when the excrement rises up to where the king himself sits—I am talking about the brain—we do not consider it worth any forethought. Therefore, indeed, we don't treat it a worthy king, doing all the things [we would for a king], but rather as an impure dog."[19]

Chrysostom also emphasizes this metaphor because it is a fundamental piece of his argument that an individual is to honor the parts of their body and that drunkenness is a source of dishonor. It is striking that, as a clear manifestation of THE BRAIN GOVERNS, this metaphor represents the brain as being *out* of control, subject to damage not only by the other parts of the body, but also by the addressee, that is, by the human individual, the self. This metaphor establishes the brain as a governing power not simply over the other members of the body but over the individual, who is the citizen subject to the king; at the same time, the individual can harm their brain/king by making choices that fail to take care of their body/city. Who is the individual in this image? Not the brain, certainly, but also not exactly the soul.

Chrysostom concludes his metaphor with another link to Plato: "God settled those body parts [sc. the excretory organs] far away [from the brain], so that it might receive no corruption from them."[20] This directly echoes Plato's account of the organization of the human body in *Timaeus*, where the gods divide the head (the locus of the divine part of the soul) from the chest (home to the mortal part of the soul) by the neck, as a kind of isthmus or boundary, in order to avoid upward contamination.[21] Chrysostom's allusion to the *Timaeus* grounds his metaphor in the Platonist tradition and lends his comparison authority: the royal qualities of the brain—and, most importantly for Chrysostom's lesson, the importance of giving it honor—are Platonist, and they are proved through analysis of anatomical design. Chrysostom's figurative arguments for avoiding drunkenness are backed up through reference to philosophical and theological tradition.

Chrysostom's metaphor relies upon ancient medical theory in ways that are simple—and therefore, presumably, recognizable even to the nonexpert—but significant, given the absence of engagement with medical theory in traditional renditions of the head/acropolis metaphor. The opening gambit, that even bystanders' brains are hurt by the "foul smells" emitted from the body of a drunk person, echoes the ancient medical theory that, alone among the senses, smell takes the brain as its organ of sensation. Rather than receiving information or transformed *pneuma* from the eyes, the ears, the tongue, or the sensory nerves, the brain is itself altered through its absorption of *pneuma* that enters through the nose. In this respect, smell is structurally similar to the effects of drunkenness, which causes vapors to rise through the body and enter the skull, causing pain. This was a consistent explanation of hangover in ancient medical texts.[22] To this, Chrysostom adds the idea of pollution: the internal vapors are, according to Chrysostom's metaphor, a kind of waste matter akin to feces. The rhetorical punch of the image lies in this picture of drunkenness as a process that forces abject matter back into the body.

In his *Exameron*, delivered during the Lent of 387, Ambrose of Milan similarly adapted the Platonist metaphor to his own purposes. The *Exameron* is a series of hexameral sermons, that is, sermons explicating the six days (*hex-āmera*) of creation as described in Genesis. Ambrose was inspired and influenced by the hexameral exegesis of Philo of Alexandria (*On the Creation of the World*) and Basil of Caesarea (*Hexameron*, delivered in 378), but he included a more detailed account of the creation of the human being than either of his models.[23] His discussion relies upon the same notion of providential design that we glimpsed above in Plato and Chrysostom. It is worth outlining the basis of this idea before analyzing Ambrose's text.

The basic premise of providential design, as a version of teleology, is that the cosmos—and the human body in particular—was constructed with the human good in mind.[24] Within this framework, it is possible to analyze anatomical details in order to discern the principles and intentions behind the design. This method was developed most explicitly in medical texts (such as Galen's *On the Usefulness of the Parts*), but it was nascent in Plato's *Timaeus* and familiar in subsequent philosophical and theological texts.[25] One prominent example was the idea that the hard and bony skull that encircles and so protects the vulnerable brain is proof that the human body was purposively constructed, since the form of the skull supports its function. Whereas Galen took the agent of this construction to be "Nature," late antique Christian authors used the same arguments as proof of a benevolent God.[26]

Late antique Latin theologians often relied on Cicero for their accounts of anatomical design, and it is no doubt the case that Ambrose was familiar with, and in some respects dependent on, his Roman predecessor.[27] In certain details, however, Ambrose reveals a familiarity with anatomical theories that do not show up in Cicero and that suggest a medical source.[28] In his description of the head, for example, Ambrose introduces the Galenic concept of the brain as the center and source of the sensory and motor nerves:

> Those skilled in the art of medicine maintain, in fact, that the brain is placed in a man's head for the sake of the eyes and that the other senses of our bodies are housed close together on account of the brain. The brain is the source of our nervous system and of all the sensations of voluntary movement. From it emanates the cause of all that we have discussed. . . . Hence, the brain, because it is the gathering point of all the senses, is softer than the other organs. From it emanate the nerves, which report everything.[29]

Here, Ambrose condenses the medical concept of the brain: as the source of the sensory and motor nerves, it is also the source and cause of bodily animation; the brain must be close to all of the sensory organs, since the sensory nerves are soft and bruise easily. As Ambrose has earlier indicated, drawing on the Platonist metaphor of the head/acropolis, the eyes must be in the head, since, like sentries, they require a high vantage point.

Ambrose casts neither the soul nor the brain in the governing role, but, unusually, the head: "Not without reason, therefore, do the other members wait upon the head as to their director [*consultatori suo*]. They surround it like slaves [*seruili*] bearing a litter and carry it aloft as something divine."[30] This focus on the head rather than the brain is unusual among late Platonist renditions of the metaphor, but it does closely echo Plato's own account in the *Timaeus*. Unlike Plato, however, Ambrose clearly personifies the governing member—he does not present the head as the seat or house or instrument of the king (that is, the soul), but as the person who governs. At the same time, this governing member is not king, but *consultator*. Ambrose has personified the governing part of the body, but he does not give it highest powers. Its bodily limitations are signified by its reduced status within the hierarchy of governance. Indeed, the powers of governance that Ambrose describes for the *consultator* are local, rather than imperial: the *consultator* is carried aloft on a litter. Even insofar as it "has censorial power [*censorial potestate*]," this manifests as "directions and orders [that] are given to the slaves and special instructions [that] are relayed to each individual . . . They obey his orders as a *princeps* and serve him as a master."[31]

The choice to render the head, rather than either brain or soul, as governor introduces internal ambiguity: sometimes the head is the acropolis; at other times, it is the "director." Ambrose has already established the head as an architectural structure, writing, at the very opening of his account of the human body, "In this citadel [*arce*] [sc. the head] dwells what might be called regal Wisdom."[32] In Ambrose's account, the head is both the architectural structure (a palace for royal governors) and the agent of power (a bureaucrat). This reflects the difference between psychic and corporeal governance: the soul (although unmentioned) rules as king; the brain (also unmentioned) issues local commands and is carried aloft.

The emphasis that Ambrose places on the orders that the head issues to the other members of the body, combined with his demonstration of medical knowledge regarding the nervous system, further suggests that the "head" in his body/city metaphor also functions metonymically as a signifier for the brain. Actively giving orders to the members of the body, the head's honor is not merely symbolic. It is clear that by "head," Ambrose means not only or not specifically the skull but the brain within.

Both Ambrose and John Chrysostom use basic medical theories of the brain's functions and vulnerabilities to develop their own variations of the Platonist metaphor of the head as the (seat of the) king. Their metaphors personify the brain as a governing agent but do not collapse this governing agent with the person or animal as a whole. To the contrary, it is the responsibility of the individual to look after and honor their brain, suggesting that the individual might be imagined as a subject ranking lower than their brain within the political hierarchy.

Elsewhere, Chrysostom introduces another metaphor of the brain to warn his congregants of the dangers of luxurious consumption, and this time he aligns the brain even more closely with the human subject, lowering its status in the hierarchy of governance by several rungs. Concerned here with the effects of gluttony, Chrysostom asserts the medical axiom that food, like wine, produces vapors that rise into the brain.[33] According to Aristotle, this is part of a necessary cycle that results in the cooling of the body, and in sleep.[34] According to Chrysostom, if food is taken in excess, then the vapors that rise from it will trouble and cause pain to the brain: "And just as a slave [οἰκέτης], when ordered to do something beyond what he is able, is often driven to desperation and insults the one who gave the order [τὸν ἐπιτάξαντα], so too, the [stomach], when under compulsion, often ruins and destroys the brain itself, together with the other organs."[35] We are far from the acropolis here; yet, the brain (like the *logistikon* in Plato's original metaphor) is clearly imagined as "the one who gave the order." As Chris de Wet has pointed out, this metaphor exemplifies a rhetoric of slavery that Chrysostom used frequently to articulate the relationship between different parts of the body.[36] According to de Wet, this rhetoric establishes the brain as a source of governance and the stomach/slave as a source of desire: if the brain fails to control the rapacious stomach, then the stomach masters the brain. As such, the metaphor depends upon the common philosophical motif of the soul as a master and the body as a slave. De Wet's analysis assumes that the brain represents the soul (and so for rational governance), while the stomach stands in for the body (that is, desire). Within this philosophical framework, the soul rules over the body; if the body rules over the soul, then the individual becomes a slave to desire.

Yet, Chrysostom does not—at least, not in this passage—locate desire within the stomach. Rather, desire springs from the one who gives the commands, that is, from the brain. The stomach takes in food under compulsion. To the extent that the stomach reverses the master/slave relationship, it is to attack the brain on the grounds that the brain itself has desired too much. The brain is destroyed not by the desires of the stomach but by the consequences of its own commands. The governing soul, embodied in the brain, is responsible for, not beleaguered by, the desires that it enacts through the bodily parts. Chrysostom suggests in this metaphor that desire cannot be displaced onto the body as onto an entity over which the individual (brain, soul) does not exert control. The brain represents the fallibility of the embodied rational being: the brain might be an instrument of rational thought and even of governance, but it can, through its bodily nature, misthink and, indeed, misgovern. This is, as chapter 5 explores more fully, why cerebral hygiene was so important, both for one's own spiritual health and for the health of the community as a whole.

The images examined in this section reveal how the Platonist head/acropolis metaphor could be elaborated to make the brain the governing agent. The extensive detail of these metaphors further illuminates the complexities and dissonances within the notion of the governing brain at a conceptual level. If the brain governed within the body, then what powers were left to the soul? If the brain were to be identified with the rational soul, then in what manner could desire motivate actions? And if the brain were capable of being compromised by its material conditions, then (how) could the human individual be held accountable for their actions and ignorance? The answer, according to Chrysostom, is that individuals have the responsibility to care for the health of their brain as if for that of their king.

Once the head/acropolis metaphor had been elaborated to include the image of the brain as king, other metaphors of the brain as a ruling figure followed. Gregory of Nyssa, as we have seen, denied that the brain was the "seat" of the governing part of the soul, but in the final chapter of his *On the Constitution of the Human Being* he offered two metaphors for the manner in which the brain controls voluntary movement. First, he compared the power in the cerebral membranes to a mechanism (μηχανῆς) that renders "our earthen statue" (γήϊνον . . . ἀνδριάντα) active and mobile (ἐνεργόν τε καὶ κινούμενον).[37] Next, he described how the brain, "just like a charioteer, bestows impulse and faculty for the movement and rest of every part upon all the meeting-points of bones and joints, as well as upon the sources of the muscles."[38] The first image suggests a humanoid automaton controlled by cords (i.e., the nerves) that are attached to a central point of operation, a metaphor borrowed from the Aristotelian image of the human body as a puppet and the *neura* as puppet strings that loosen and contract through the movement of the *pneuma* within the heart.[39] According to this image, the brain endows earth (the dominant element in the body) with psychic activities, among which the first is movement.

The second image, as noted in chapter 1, is a direct and startling reference to the *Phaedrus*, where Plato describes the relationship between the parts of a soul as follows: The charioteer (representing reason) attempts to control two horses, one obedient (rational or moral impulse) and the other disobedient (irrational appetites and passions).[40] If the charioteer allows the good horse to lead, then the soul will attain heavenly knowledge and virtue; if the bad horse gets the upper hand, the charioteer will fall. Gregory's metaphor aligns the brain with the rational and governing soul. The nerves serve as reins, by means of which the brain controls the parts of the body like a team of horses. Galen had made a similar leap in a discussion of voluntary and involuntary motion: "Choice is like a charioteer who moves the reins and the horses; the nerves are like the reins, and the muscles are like the horses; similarly, the use is the desired end of breathing, as victory is of chariot racing."[41] Whereas Galen cleaves closer to Plato, making the charioteer a faculty of the soul, Gregory introduces a material subject, the brain. In so doing, he draws a clear parallel between the relationship of the brain to the other parts of the body and the relationship of reason to the other faculties of the soul.

Gregory's identification of the Platonic rational soul with the brain sits uneasily alongside his rejection of the localization of the soul in the brain earlier in his treatise.[42] According to Gregory, the *nous* must be immaterial, and therefore cannot be contained by any part of the body; rather, it must permeate the whole.[43] His identification of the brain as charioteer seems to modify his earlier position, attributing to the brain a function that Plato associated with the rational soul. Yet, it can also be read as a limiting strategy: if the mind were to retain its position as charioteer, then the brain would become the chariot, leaving Gregory with a localizationist argument. Instead, he distinguishes the intellectual governance of the mind from the corporeal governance of the brain.[44] The brain governs the body just as the mind governs the irrational parts of the soul. The middle term shared by Plato's soul and

Gregory's brain—the salient function of their charioteer—is not the property of reason, but the act of governance over a lower being. This, according to Gregory of Nyssa, is the hegemonic function of the brain.

Late antique Christian authors mined the Platonist head/acropolis metaphor for new rhetorical resources to negotiate the complexity of the relationship between body and soul. These metaphors were not unthinking reiterations of Plato; nor did they reflect a straightforward assumption of the brain's governing power. While they clearly represent the conceptual metaphor THE BRAIN GOVERNS, they also tease apart that concept, situating the governing brain at shifting points within the body/soul hierarchy and refusing to allow it a stable position.

BRAIN AS CHRIST

In this final section, I examine a different kind of iteration of THE BRAIN GOVERNS, one that seeks not to explicate the brain through reference to political or domestic governance, but rather to represent cosmic governance through reference to the brain. By late antiquity, "king" did not primarily evoke the "Great King" of Persia: far more salient was the interpretation of "king" as Christ. While Chrysostom warns his congregants that they must honor their brain as they would their king, Ambrose describes in his *Exameron* how God placed *sapientia* ("wisdom," often used in reference to Jesus) within the head.[45] In this final section, we will turn to a handful of metaphors that play out this other strand of the head/acropolis tradition: interpretations of Jesus as the head—that is to say, the "brain"—of the church.

Whereas Plato's comparison of the head to an acropolis illuminated an unfamiliar theory of the body/soul relationship through reference to familiar political relationships, late antique interpretations of Christ as the brain within the ecclesial body explicated an unfamiliar theory of the relationship between the church and Christ through reference to familiar medical concepts. That is to say, medical theories of the brain had become sufficiently integrated into everyday understanding that they could be used to clarify theological arguments. Three explicit iterations of this metaphor demonstrate how it served to illustrate claims regarding how the relationship between the church and Christ ought to play out at the level of the ecclesial community. Two of these metaphorical expressions come from the works of John Chrysostom and one from the work of Theodoret of Cyrrhus (c. 393–457). Here, I will focus on the writings of Chrysostom.[46]

In the first case, Chrysostom's homily *On the Beginning of Acts* 3, the brain appears as a representative of governance that is not personified. In this text, Chrysostom explicates 1 Corinthians 12, in which Paul explains that, as members of the body of Christ, each member of the church manifests different gifts: "And God has placed in the church first of all apostles, second prophets, third teachers, then miracles, then gifts of healing, of helping, of guidance, and of different kinds of tongues."[47] In order to explain this hierarchy of gifts, Chrysostom invokes the organization of the body:

> And just as the head, being established in the highest place of all, is not only the beginning and origin of the body, but also the root (for the nerves which manage the body are born from it, and, sprouting from the brain itself and receiving a share of *pneuma*, so administrate the whole creature), so also the apostleship is established not only as beginning and origin for the rest of the gifts, but also contains and comprehends the roots of all things in itself.[48]

The apostleship is the head of the church not only in symbolic terms (it is the highest part of the body), but also according to its function: it contains and is the brain, which is the "root of all things," and it therefore distributes *pneuma* within the body of the church.[49] The transmission of the Holy Spirit through the apostles to the prophets and teachers (Chrysostom adds καὶ ποιμένας, "and the pastors") is aligned to the transmission of *pneuma* through the nerves. The brain and nervous system function as a model for centralized governance through organic integrity. As both the organ from which the nerves "sprout" and are "born" (metaphors familiar within medical texts), and also the organ through which the soul extends control over the body, the brain represents communal wholeness that depends upon natural hierarchy.

In the second case, Chrysostom is more specific about the identity of the brain. He is once again exegeting the Pauline metaphor of the church as the body of Christ. The passage in question is Ephesians 4:15–16:

> Instead, speaking the truth in love, we will grow to become in every respect the mature body of him who is the head, that is, Christ. From him the whole body, joined and held together by every supporting ligament, grows and builds itself up in love, as each part does its work.[50]

Chrysostom begins by remarking that Paul expresses himself with great obscurity. In order to understand the apostle's meaning more clearly, he suggests, it is necessary to interpret "head" as "brain." Christ is like the brain, he explains, insofar as spiritual gifts descend like *pneuma* through the sensory nerves, bringing the power of perception and the nourishment of the *pneuma* to each part in accordance with its capacity.[51] Whereas the previous passage leaves the identity of the brain vague (it is the "root of all things"), Chrysostom makes it clear in this metaphor that the brain is Christ, "contained and comprehended" by the head.

Chrysostom is particularly keen to pin down the significance of the phrase "in love." What does it mean for "love" to be the mode of "the body's growth"? The answer, he explains, is corporate unification:

> For just as if a hand happens to have been torn off from the body, the *pneuma* from the brain seeks out the connection, and, not finding it, does not leap out from the body and, flying through the air, go out to the hand, but, if it does not find it lying there, it does not touch it; thus also here, if we are not bound together by love.[52]

Corporate integrity, while founded upon anatomical connection, is predicated upon the action of the nerves. Chrysostom maps out in precise terms the passage of *pneuma* (whether the psychic *pneuma* of the nervous system or the Holy Spirit) through designated channels and into each part, as determined not only by the spiritual capacity of the part itself but also by its connection to the whole. Separation from the ecclesial body meant disconnection from God and the absence of spiritual gifts. No member could participate in the nourishment provided by the brain without remaining connected to the nervous system through which the brain distributed the *pneuma* to the members. Christianity might be a religion of personal salvation, but one could not obtain that salvation, Chrysostom argued, if one did not participate appropriately in Christian community.

The idea of nervous connectivity was about six hundred years old by the time Chrysostom was writing, but it had become central to medical doctrine chiefly through the writings of Galen in the late second century.[53] Galen had staked his authority as a medical practitioner on his ability to diagnose the source of bodily malfunction (for example, paralysis) in nervous damage across distant regions of the body.[54] He also used anatomical experiments to demonstrate that the brain, rather than the heart, was the hegemonic organ, since damage to the brain affected perception and voluntary motion elsewhere in the body. Nervous connection through the circulation and mediation of *pneuma* was fundamental to ancient medical understandings of the brain/body relationship. Chrysostom's interpolation of the nervous system into the metaphor of Christ as the head of the church was a strategy calculated to establish his political claims about what it means to participate in the communal body through the naturalizing logic of medical discourse.

The medical model of the nervous system provided Chrysostom with a language for talking about not only material but also functional connectedness. This becomes clearer when Chrysostom considers the broader implications of the body metaphor:

> It is necessary that the body be arranged not arbitrarily, but with forethought and skill, since, if it is disarranged, then it no longer exists. . . . One must therefore not only be unified with the body, but also maintain one's own proper place, since if you overstep your position, you do not remain in communion, and will not receive the *pneuma*.[55]

Chrysostom polices the boundaries of the communal body not only in terms of membership (are you in or are you out?) but also in terms of the quality of one's participation.[56] Overstepping one's position within the social and ecclesial order might also cut one off from the Holy Spirit. In the same way that Chrysostom warns his congregants that drinking too much might hurt and dishonor their brain, so here he spells out the negative consequences of undesirable behavior for spiritual health. Again, Chrysostom reinforces this lesson through a medical analogy: "Or do you not see in the dislocation of bones . . . how, whenever one moves from its proper place and occupies that of another, it pollutes the body and often brings about death . . . and is found unworthy of being preserved? For many will frequently cut off that part, leaving its place void."[57] The hand that has been cut off will not receive the *pneuma*. But why should the hand be cut off? Because, according to Chrysostom, it has shifted out of place and poses a danger to the collective.[58] Overstepping the boundaries of one's own position is more dangerous than being cut off from the church, both for oneself and for the body as a whole. The pollution that displacement causes might justify the act of excision or excommunication. Conversely, being cut off from the church implies not only social exclusion, but also alienation from God. After all, one requires connection through the bonds of love in order to receive the *pneuma* distributed by the brain. Through the model of the nervous system, Chrysostom imbues excommunication with theological power, borrowing from the authority of medical science to establish his claim about how bodies "naturally" work.

What kind of "king" is Christ in this metaphor? There is no acropolis in this image, and the brain is imagined not as issuing commands but as controlling the flow of *pneuma*—a nourishing and enabling substance and a source of gifts—to each member of the body. Ecclesial governance is by control and distribution of resources, rather than by direct command. It is clear, further, that while it is Christ who is imagined as the brain, the authority that the metaphor establishes is that of the bishop or priest. The conceptual metaphor THE BRAIN GOVERNS (together with its cousin A GROUP OF PEOPLE IS A BODY) is invoked by Chrysostom ostensibly to explicate the obscure relationship between Christ and the church, but functionally to naturalize the authority of church administrators such as Chrysostom in determining who belongs in the church and who does not.

CONCLUSION

Despite the hesitancy of late antique Christian preachers and theologians to reduce the mind or rational soul to the brain, the anthropomorphization of the brain as governing agent was a distinct trope in late antique Christian rhetoric, repeated by different authors and elaborated with perhaps the greatest sophistication by John Chrysostom. The dissonance between the concepts of the governing brain and the governing soul was smoothed over by making the brain the governor over the members of the body rather than over the human being as a whole. Each of the metaphorical expressions examined in this chapter elaborates the metaphorical concept of THE BRAIN GOVERNS, which has its touchstone in Plato's *Timaeus*. It is on the basis of this core metaphor that late antique Christian preachers and theologians derive the analogies between the body, the city, and the cosmos on which they depend in order to explicate the brain through the city and the church through the brain.

What these metaphors show is a shift toward a concept of the brain as a governing organ, rather than simply a site or instrument in the hands of the governing soul. The anthropomorphization of the brain in these metaphors also hints at a shift toward the elision of the brain with the human being, a conceptual change that we will explore in more detail in chapter 7. Further, they reveal a current of tension underlying these metaphors of the brain, specifically regarding the conceptualization of the brain/soul relationship within medical and theological frames. Late antique Christian authors were insistent that the brain could not be confined within or confused with the rational agent or soul, but they nonetheless found metaphors of the brain as a governing agent to be productive in talking about human governance (and failures in governance) over the self, animals, and one another.

Human reason was—then, as now—a fundamental justification for dominance over the earth and other animals. As such, the brain was a central material symbol of human rulership. Its integration into metaphors exploring different relationships of domination suggests a shared understanding of the basic medical concept of the brain as the source of the sensory and motor nerves, and therefore the bodily instrument of reason and self-governance. These elaborations of THE BRAIN GOVERNS also generated a new set of conceptual tools for talking about aspects of governance not covered by the initial, Platonist metaphor—above all, drunkenness, gluttony, and failure. It is to these aspects of the brain that we turn more fully in the next chapter. How did Christian engagement with the medical concept of the brain as a governing agent shape anthropological and pastoral discourse? As I will argue, two aspects of the brain emerged as central: its role in self-governance, but also, and most prominently, its vulnerability. This physical vulnerability, I suggest, provided the materials for giving an account of the physical and psychological precarity of the (rational, governing) human being.

CHAPTER 5

The Rhetoric of Cerebral Vulnerability

In the third book of the *Iliad,* the Greeks and Trojans swear the following oath of peace: "O Zeus, greatest and most glorious, and the other immortal gods: Whoever first does injury in transgression of this oath, may their brain [ἐγκέφαλος] pour out onto the ground like this wine, and the brains of their children likewise, and may their wives be enslaved to others."[1] The Trojans famously break the oath, launching the conflict that leads to the death of Patroclus and Hector. Of the subsequent six references to the brain in the *Iliad,* one describes the death of Nestor's horse, while the remaining five mark the destruction of Trojan warriors. Amid the variety of fatal injuries that Greeks and Trojans inflict upon one another, the poet cleaves strictly to the terms of the oath. In a quiet but persistent way, the vulnerable brain represents the destruction of the defensive army and the fall of Troy.

The brain is soft and weak, easily injured by sharp objects and blunt trauma. The functions assigned to it by ancient medical authors (sensation, cognition, voluntary motion) are regularly impaired during fevers, drunkenness, and even sleep. Its softness and its implication in mental disorders were commonly recognized in ancient medicine. Lay audiences would have been familiar with its ease of injury from witnessing accidents, experience of combat, sacrificial or culinary contexts (boiled animal brains appear several times in the famous recipe book of Apicius), and, as we see above, epic poetry.

When late antique Christian authors emphasized the vulnerability of the brain, then, they were positioning themselves within a long tradition and in relation to familiar frames of reference. Yet, their interest in the vulnerable brain was more pointed and direct. They were concerned with the softness of the brain not just because of its own susceptibility to damage or the implications that this has for its various functions; according to early Christian authors, damage to the brain represents a threat to the governing soul. At the same time—and in a paradox that neatly captures the Christian ideal of spiritual strength in bodily weakness—the vulnerability of the brain simultaneously confirms both the perfection of human design and human dependence on God.

Insofar as the brain served as a symbol and agent of governance, its vulnerability could represent the fallibility and fragility of human rule both over the self and over others. As the organ positioned on the boundary between body and soul and a participant in both spheres, the brain could cause harm to the body (through the soul's poor command) or to the soul (via bodily damage that causes, for example, delusions). Damage to the brain could impact the individual's capacity for reason and self-control—and therefore for goodness and even, to some extent, salvation. For these reasons, the care of brain became a site of concern for preachers explaining the importance of practices of self-discipline to their congregations.

Yet, it was important also that the brain should not serve as a tool with which humans might control in absolute terms their own spiritual health. In order to ensure continued dependence on God, it was necessary to establish the limitations of ascetic practice. This was a more general problem, but we find it articulated with striking clarity in relation to the brain, which was both the governing organ and representative of human and divine governing figures. Early Christian rhetoric of cerebral vulnerability raised questions about the limits of human reason, the reasons for human weakness, how much control humans have—and should take responsibility for—over their own bodies, and what bearing bodily discipline has on the health of the soul.

By the "rhetoric of cerebral vulnerability," I mean the dual emphasis upon (1) the fragility of the brain and (2) the importance of the brain as instrument of the rational and governing soul. This rhetoric was employed in various ways. First, it helped to explain how care of the body could affect the health of the soul. Second, the physical vulnerability of the brain embodied a necessary weakness in the construction of the human as a rational and autonomous being: the anatomical and physiological conditions necessary for reason make the human being physically vulnerable. Third, the political resonances of the brain enabled preachers to insert themselves not only as physicians of the individual body, but also as physicians attending to the social "body" as a whole. Individual spiritual health, as we shall see, was dependent not only upon one's own cerebral hygiene, but also upon the self-care practiced by others. In this way, preachers used the medical idea of the "brain," together with its attendant characteristics and weaknesses, to forge a vision of a communal Christian body bound by practices of bodily and psychic self-care.

The early Christian rhetoric of cerebral vulnerability was influential. As late as 1869, the Calvinist Baptist minister Archibald G. Brown referred to John Chrysostom as his authority for the claim that pride is "nothing less than a spiritual drunkenness," which "flies as wine to the brain."[2] Brown reflects a motif that was common in late antique medical and theological literature: the fumes of alcohol rise from the stomach into the brain, disturbing reason and the senses. This motif is developed at length in one of Chrysostom's homilies and is mentioned in a homily spuriously attributed to him.[3] As we shall see, it appears also in the works of preachers such as Basil of Caesarea, Asterius of Amasea, and Augustine of Hippo. Chrysostom's more extensive account reflects assumptions in circulation across medical, philosophical, epistolary, and homiletic contexts.

This chapter and the following form a pair in relation to these themes. In this chapter, I argue that early Christian preachers highlighted the vulnerability of the brain in order to motivate moderate ascetic practices, such as avoidance of alcohol, perfumes, and banquets. In the chapter following, I will examine the ways in which ascetic practice itself was thought to hurt the brain when performed in excess and with a view to independent spiritual power. Together, these analyses chart the rhetorical use of cerebral vulnerability to guide and limit ascetic practice and to negotiate the power it could convey.

I begin with a brief summary of the different kinds of cerebral vulnerability that show up in early Christian texts. Following this, there are four sections: the first two examine different kinds of cerebral vulnerability (a delicate temperament; softness) in relation to human design; the final two explore cerebral vulnerability in relation to the consequences of ascetic practices and indulgence in luxury or vice, specifically through the impact of external and internal vapors. The central thread will be the examination of how early Christian rhetoricians used medical ideas about the vulnerability of the brain to craft arguments that were intended to motivate bodily practices and to shape congregants' understandings of their own positionality as human beings in relation to God.

THE WEAKNESSES OF THE BRAIN

> The consequences of the opposite condition [to normal] makes it clear that the brain contributes most to life. For if the membrane around it suffers any wound or lesion, death follows the injury immediately, and nature does not endure the wound for a millisecond. It is just like when a foundation is sunk and the whole building collapses with the part.[4]

Despite his explicit denial of the traditional encephalocentrist position earlier in *On the Constitution of the Human Being*, Gregory of Nyssa did in fact consider the brain to be the center of sensation, the orchestrator of voluntary motion, and the sine qua non of animal survival. His claim that the vulnerability of the brain made the entire body vulnerable is representative of late antique Christian discussions, although his architectural metaphor is a distinctive spin on Plato's comparison of the head to an acropolis. Gregory's metaphor indicates not only the danger associated with wounds to the head but also the structural importance of the brain within late ancient anthropologies.[5] The brain was—for Gregory and for others—the foundation of the human being. Its safety and protection were equivalent to the safety and protection of the human being as a whole.

The brain was subject to various kinds of vulnerability. First, it depended for its functioning on an appropriate balance of temperature and humidity. Second, it was soft, requiring fortresses or helmets of bone for its protection, and being vulnerable to injury by sharp implements, such as swords and spears.[6] Finally, the brain was the receptacle of vapors, both those that rose from within the body and those that were inhaled through the nose; these substances mingled with the psychic *pneuma*, affecting the quality of perception, thought, and self-governance; they could also make the brain heavy and cause it pain, as in drunkenness or the disease of lethargy. These different sources of vulnerability were interrelated. The balance of qualities was the foundation of the softness that enabled the brain to receive sensation, but that also made it vulnerable to blows. Sensation required a soft organ to receive the impressions delivered by the psychic *pneuma*, but this susceptibility to transformation by the air passing through also made the brain peculiarly vulnerable to vapors and fumes rising from the stomach. In the sections that follow, we will examine each distinct source of vulnerability in turn, with an eye constantly toward this overlap and connection.

BALANCING THE BRAIN

John Chrysostom's *Homily on the Statues* 11, delivered in Antioch in 387, sought to demonstrate the providential care of the creator with regard to human beings. Chrysostom drew upon a theme familiar in ancient philosophy: the human body, designed peculiarly as an instrument for reason, is weaker than that of any other animal; yet, through reason, humans have developed tools to surpass and conquer all other animals, and so to rule over the earth.[7] A key piece of the reasoning for this was that sensitivity, which enabled and enhanced rational thought, required soft and impressionable instruments. Insofar as the brain and sensory nerves were considered the instruments of sensation, these were also considered to be soft. By extension, and insofar as it was considered to be an instrument of reason and therefore reliant upon sensation, the human body as a whole was also soft.

Chrysostom relied upon the familiar teleological principle that all characteristics of the human body are designed to support the distinctively human capacity of reason.[8] The upshot of this was that reason was not to be thought of so much as compensation for physical weakness but rather as its purpose.[9] That is, a body designed for reason was necessarily weak in physical strength. In Chrysostom's text, this rationalization of weakness is represented by the vulnerability of the brain to temperamental change:

> Nor did he create the body [without strength] for its own sake, but so that it might participate in the rational soul; for if it were not [created] in such a way, the activities of soul would certainly be impeded; and this is clear from diseases. For if the temperament of the flesh [τῆς σαρκὸς ἡ διακόσμησις] deviates from its accustomed constitution [τῆς οἰκείας καταστάσεως] even trivially, many activities of the soul are in fact impeded—for example, if the brain becomes hotter or colder.[10]

Vulnerability is part of human design in two respects: not only were humans created without natural body armor (the most common example), but, in addition, reason requires a precise bodily constitution.[11] The effect of deviation from this constitution was that one's faculties of reason, perception, and self-control might be lost.

Chrysostom drew upon two medico-philosophical models to make this argument. First, his reference to the "temperament" of the flesh echoes the notion of health as constituted by a balance of qualities, which in Galenic doctrine were the hot, the cold, the wet, and the dry.[12] Second, Chrysostom's identification of the brain as the part whose imbalance might obstruct the activities of soul, presumably those of reason, implies the prominent medical and philosophical argument that the brain is the instrument of the *hēgemonikon*. At the convergence of these two models is the implication that the health or balance of the brain is the fundamental requirement for psychic health.

We encountered in the previous chapter another late antique Christian text that engaged closely with medical theories of temperament in order to negotiate the implications of cerebral vulnerability for the governance of the soul. This was the letter by Isidore of Pelusium to the "learned physician" Proeschius. As we saw, Isidore uses his letter to refute the central thesis of Galen's treatise *That the Faculties of the Soul Follow the Mixtures of the Body*, by aligning this theory with the "harmony" thesis familiar from ancient philosophy (the soul is the harmony produced by the bodily instrument). Whereas John Chrysostom takes the vulnerability of the soul to the imbalance of the brain as an index of divine providence, insofar as the brain is perfectly designed to support reason, Isidore rejects Galen's suggestion that the powers of the soul depend upon the condition of the body and the brain in particular as a variant of the harmony thesis, which renders the soul ephemeral and passive, an effect rather than an agent. A harmony, he points out, must be lost with the instrument that produces it.[13] In support of this, he quotes Galen: "'If the soul is immortal,' he says, 'as Plato wishes, then why is it separated when the brain becomes violently cold or overheated, or excessively wet?'"[14] Within Galen's "temperamental" paradigm, according to Isidore, the soul loses both its function as a moral agent and its immortality. For Chrysostom, meanwhile, the temperamental paradigm was an opportunity to guide and govern bodily care.

Chrysostom's emphasis on the impediment of psychic powers suggests that he and Isidore were in agreement on a fundamental point: imbalance within the brain does not destroy the soul per se. This is a tenet repeated across late antique Christian accounts of the brain. Where Isidore rejects Galen's thesis outright, Chrysostom—ever the rhetorician—finds a way to adapt it to his own persuasive program. The vulnerability of the brain and the psychic faculties it enables signify the precision of God's design of the human being and therefore the importance of human beings to God; it also—although Chrysostom does not go into this here—suggests the potential of the brain as a site for pastoral intervention in the interests of psychic health.

The vulnerability of the brain to the imbalance of qualities or humors might impede the faculties of the soul and as such could serve useful rhetorical purposes for late antique Christian preachers. At the same time, it was a source of anxiety: for early Christian authors, it was important to emphasize that the vulnerability of the brain in no way spelled the destruction of the soul—a point that was sufficiently contested that they reinforced it over and over again.

THE SOFT BRAIN

Human vulnerability was concentrated within the brain not only insofar as the rational faculties were linked to that part and were dependent upon its temperament, but also insofar as the brain itself was soft. Earlier in *Homily on the Statues* 11, Chrysostom celebrates divine providence through a classic anatomical set-piece, that is, the protection that the skull affords the brain: "But who might be able to trace out all the wisdom indicated by the brain? For, first of all, he made it soft, since he gave it the task of being the fountain of all the senses; then, so that it might not be damaged by its own nature, he walled [ἐπετείχισε] it around on every side with bones."[15]

Plato's *Timaeus*, which is the obvious source for the architectural metaphor in Chrysostom's sermon, had also commented influentially on the vulnerability of the brain in relation to the skull. At issue for Plato was not the brain substance itself, but rather the slenderness of the bone that surrounded it. Arguing that the human skull was thin and only lightly covered by hair in order to allow perceptions to travel through, and assuming furthermore that sense perception is the foundation of human reason, Plato proposed a relationship between cerebral vulnerability (a thin skull means a short life) and human intelligence (a dense skull stifles sensation):

> For there is no way that anything whose generation and composition are a consequence of Necessity can accommodate the combination of thick bone and massive flesh with keen and responsive sensation. If these two characteristics did not refuse to cooperate, our heads above all would have been so constituted as to possess this combination, and humankind, crowned with a head fortified with flesh and sinews, would have a life twice or many more times as long, a healthier and less painful life than the one we have now.[16]

The gods therefore made a decision to keep human life brief and vulnerable in order to maximize human potential for sensitivity and therefore reason: "As it was, however, our makers calculated the pros and cons of giving our race greater longevity but making it inferior, versus making it better though less long-lived, and decided that the superior though shorter life span was in every way preferable for everyone to the longer but inferior one."[17] When Chrysostom describes the brain as soft for the sake of sensitivity, yet walled all around by bone, he evokes both the metaphor of the head as acropolis and Plato's compromise between intelligence and vulnerability. Notice, however, a subtle difference between their accounts: for Plato, the skull is the site of vulnerability, since sensations must pass through the skull in order to reach the brain; for Chrysostom, it is the brain itself that is marked as vulnerable. This is presumably because Chrysostom has integrated into his account two fundamental lessons of postclassical medicine: sensation reaches the brain via the nerves, rather than through the skull; and the organs of sensation must be soft—a point to which we will return shortly.

The shift in the locus of vulnerability from skull to brain is particularly clear in the work of Theodoret of Cyrrhus, who writes that the liver and brain are covered by more closely confining bones, "but nonetheless obtain greater security from the creator."[18] With a nod to Plato, Theodoret allows that the bones may appear to be weak, while in fact—through divine protection—they are strong. This notion that human nature requires strength in weakness was a central paradox in early Christian thought, as expressed most famously in 2 Corinthians:

> But he said to me, "My grace is sufficient for you, for my power is made perfect in weakness." Therefore I will boast all the more gladly about my weaknesses, so that Christ's power may rest on me. That is why, for Christ's sake, I delight in weaknesses, in insults, in hardships, in persecutions, in difficulties. For when I am weak, then I am strong.[19]

Like Paul's good Christian, the skull appears weak but is strong because it has been created as a special protection for the brain. This is the upshot of late antique arguments about providence and anatomical design: human beings are weak, but through the assistance of God, they are made strong. The brain, cerebral membranes, and skull represent not only divine providence in creation and the special care that God has for human beings, but also the importance of acknowledging human weakness. The very thing that makes human beings rational also makes them vulnerable. Reason does not give human beings the strength to be independent of God. Quite the reverse: the vulnerability of the brain illustrates the theological imperative to admit dependency on God, rather than seek independence as rational creatures.

Following his introduction of the brain as a soft and sensitive organ protected by the firm skull, Chrysostom discusses how the particular construction of the skull and the two membranes that line it contribute to the protection of the brain:

> Again, so that [the brain] might not become irritated, being grazed by the bones, [God] stretched out a membrane between [the brain and the skull], and not only one, but also a second, one being stretched underneath the bone, and the other being cast around the flesh of the brain, and the first being tougher than the second. He did this for the reason mentioned above, and also so that the brain might not directly receive blows endured by the head, but that the meninges, catching impacts in advance, might dissipate all harm, and preserve [the brain] uninjured. Furthermore, the covering itself is not one continuous bone, but has many sutures all over, so that, again, it might have a secure foundation.[20]

Chrysostom closely echoes Galen in this description of membranes, sutures, and skull, in terms of both the anatomical details and the teleological frame.[21] Medical texts provide the kind of bolster that Chrysostom needs to establish his argument that the human body—especially in its capacity for reason—is dependent upon the design and protection of God. Here, we might recall the social capital attached to expertise in human anatomy that we explored in chapter 1. Chrysostom offers his congregants an abundance of anatomical detail perhaps in the manner of a iatrosophist in order to establish the legitimacy of his claim that human weakness is part of God's providential design.

Galen, both through his own texts and through intermediaries such as Oribasius, underpins much discussion of the vulnerable brain in early Christian texts, not only in anatomical detail, but also in core imagery. His account of the double membranes that protect the soft brain from the hard skull weaves in a metaphor of military defense that draws from the Platonist metaphor of the skull as an acropolis and that lays the foundation for Christian imagery representing the skull as an instrument of divine protection. Galen writes: "The thick membrane is also a covering for the brain: or rather, it should be called not simply a covering but a defensive bulwark [ἀμυντήριόν τι πρόβλημα], so to speak, exposed to the cranium's embrace [or: impacts, attacks] [προσβολαῖς]."[22] This metaphor of military defense became fundamental to early Christian conceptions of the anatomy of the head. Whereas Galen here focuses on the role of the membranes in protecting the brain from the skull, however, most Christian imagery, like that of Chrysostom, identifies the skull as the defensive structure. This was motivated in part by the homophony between τὸ κρανίον (skull) and τὸ κράνος (helmet), a pun that was pointed out by Galen himself.[23] This verbal connection was so strong in Greek medical terminology that the late antique North African physician Vindicianus, writing in Latin, called the cranium *galea* ("helmet") in his anatomical treatise *Gynecia*, despite the fact that *galea* did not ordinarily carry this anatomical meaning.

The pun is most pronounced in texts by Theodoret and John Chrysostom. In his homily *On Providence* 3, Theodoret describes the body as a city, with the head as the acropolis and the brain protected as a treasure within.[24] He then goes on to compare the skull to a helmet, writing that the word "cranium" (κρανίον) gets its name from *kranos* (κράνος, "helmet").[25] In this way, he intertwines Galenic and Platonist metaphors to produce an image of the skull as the ultimate defensive architecture, protecting both the individual and the city from external attack.

The same analogy, albeit not the etymological connection, is echoed in Chrysostom's homily *On the Letter to the Hebrews* 5, where the "helmet of salvation" of Ephesians 6:17 is identified as the skull.

> And it is necessary for us to have a helmet [περικεφαλαίας] also, since the rational part of the soul [τὸ λογιστικόν] happens to be there [sc. in the head], and by this it is possible either to be saved, if what is necessary comes about, or to be destroyed, if that which ought not be the case [is done]. Because of this, he says, "And the helmet of salvation" [Καὶ τὴν περικεφαλαίαν σωτηρίου]. For the brain is soft by nature, and so is concealed from above by the bregma, as if by a shell; and it is the cause for us of all that is good and all that is bad, knowing the things that are necessary, or the things that ought not be.[26]

The "rational part of the soul" is the source of salvation, through its control of "necessary" or "obligatory" actions (τὰ δέοντα). The brain, meanwhile, is the cause of good and bad, providing the material conditions for knowledge of the necessary actions that the soul enacts. Since the brain is "soft" (ἁπαλός), the skull protects it like a helmet or a shell (belonging to shellfish, rather than to eggs). The location of both the soul and brain within the head is more than a coincidence, and the skull, in protecting the brain, preserves the integrity of both.

Chrysostom's connection between reason, virtue, and the brain is striking. The brain was to be protected because it was weak (as instrument of sensation) and also because it was important (as instrument of reason). While most of Chrysostom's contemporaries were willing to accept that the brain played some part in cognition, the idea that the rational aspect of soul that was responsible for virtue could be confined within any bodily part was strongly contested, as we saw in chapter 3, since it risked making the soul subject to the body, rather than transcendent of it. Chrysostom's identification of the cranium with the "helmet of salvation" and his explanation of this association in terms of brain function—that is, one must "know" the things that are necessary—suggests, to the contrary, that the integrity of the brain might be a precondition for salvation. One's ability to discern the good from the bad and that which should be from that which should not was the "helmet" that protected the soul.

Chrysostom does not in this passage connect the softness of the brain to its faculty of sensation, but it is clear from the passages already discussed that this connection was fundamental to his understanding of the brain. It was axiomatic in late antiquity that the softness of the brain enabled sensitivity, and thereby contributed to reason. In his treatise *On the Usefulness of the Parts,* Galen had explained that both the brain and the sensory nerves need to be soft in order to receive sensory impressions, "for a substance easily altered is most suitable for such actions and affections, and a soft substance is always more easily altered than one that is harder."[27] Indeed, the brain, being the common instrument of sensation, needed to be softer even than the sensory nerves.[28]

The theory that the sensory organs must be soft was based on the belief that sensation is a matter of *tupōsis* ("impression") or *alloiōsis* ("alteration") of the sensory organ or the *pneuma* within.[29] This understanding of the sensory process remained influential until the early modern period.[30] As Ambrose wrote in his *Exameron,* "the brain, because it is the gathering point of all the senses, is softer than the other organs."[31]

This theory is presented in condensed form in a homily *On Holy Easter* by Gregory of Nyssa. Addressing the question of how the resurrection of bodies will take place at the end of days, Gregory invites his congregation to think about human genesis—not the original creation of humankind, but the daily creation of individual human beings in the womb. Through the model sphere of the astronomer, Gregory argues, one can understand the whole, invisible cosmos. In the same way, gestation provides a model for resurrection. Gregory's account of embryological development is formulated as a condensed rhetorical question:

> For how is the seed—being a kind of being [οὐσία οὖσα] that is wet and unshaped and formless—congealed in the head and solidified in the shin-bones and the ribs, and [how does] he make the brain soft and loose [ἁπαλὸν καὶ μανὸν] and the bone surrounding it correspondingly hard [σκληρὸν] and resistant [ἀντιτυπὲς], and the elaborate construction of the living creature, so that I might speak concisely, without dragging out these things one by one in minute detail?[32]

This is a Platonist account of human creation, framed explicitly in cosmological terms. The seed of human life is planted in the head and in the bones, and it is this seed—Gregory goes on to say—that will ripen to pregnancy once again at the end of days. At the center of Gregory's account is the brain. Indeed, whereas Plato planted the immortal seed of human life in the cerebral marrow as in a fertile field, Gregory seems to identify the seed—wet, unshaped, and formless—with the congealed bodily fluid that is the brain itself. His contrast of the "soft and loose" brain to the "hard and resistant" skull is fundamental to his conception of "the elaborate construction of the living creature."

It was commonplace to contrast the brain, being "soft" (ἁπαλὸν)—or even "loose" or "porous" (μανὸν)—to the skull, which was "hard" (σκληρὸν). Gregory's choice of the additional adjective "resistant" (ἀντιτυπὲς) reveals the underlying resonances that he attaches to this polarization: ἀντιτυπὲς contains within it the verb τυπόω ("to impress, stamp, mold"), which Gregory uses to describe the formation of the previously shapeless "seed" in the process of resurrection: "the seed, being shapeless in the beginning is molded [τυποῦται] to a model."[33]

The word ἀντιτυπὲς also contains the stem of τύπωσις, a common word, as noted above, for the imprinting process necessary for sensation. The brain is not only the site for the implantation of the divine soul, but also the organ of sensation—in contrast to the skull, which, as Plato had claimed, dulls human sensory powers. In his juxtaposition between brain and skull, Gregory builds on Plato's account. It is not only that the skull obstructs the sensory powers of the brain, but that the material constitution of skull and brain determine their relation to perceptual activities: the soft brain receives sensation, while the resistant (ἀντιτυπὲς) skull resists sensory impression (τύπωσις). The physical quality of the skull describes its obstructionist role in the sensory process.

The softness of the brain signified the vulnerability of the human being and the necessity of relying upon divine protection. It was also necessary for the faculty of sensation, and therefore provided a starting point for embodied human reason. As the following section explores in further detail, this association between sensation and vulnerability was no accident; sense perception was precisely the source of the vulnerability of the human soul. By making the brain both soft and responsible for sensation, early Christian authors explored the conjunction of physical and psychic weakness.

EXTERNAL VAPORS: SMELL

Despite the importance of sense perception for making rational and moral judgements about the world, softness and sensitivity carried negative connotations. "Softness" was traditionally a feminine quality, signifying dissolution, dissipation, and a lack of critical rigor or self-control.[34] Thus, one word for "ascetic discipline" was σκληραγωγία ("training in hardness").[35] Sensitivity was similarly gendered: in his exegesis of Genesis, Philo wrote that the senses were to reason as Eve was to Adam, luring the masculine intellect away from devotion to God.[36] The "soft" quality of the brain therefore refers both to its material texture and to luxury and love of pleasure. The attribution of the sensitive faculty to the brain endowed it with "feminine" characteristics that threatened its security and the security of "masculine" reason.

Late antique Christian authors were ambivalent about whether the senses were to be celebrated as points of access to the divine—through, for example, perception of the created world—or to be feared as conduits through which sensory impressions might warp and damage the soul.[37] While this metaphor might be understood in psychological terms as an "entryway" for "temptation," Gregory Smith has shown that it must also be interpreted physiologically: the openings of the sensory organs allowed external impressions, carried upon the air, to alter the substance of the *pneuma* within the brain in a manner akin to the invasion of demons.[38] Sensation could be understood along the lines of an "invasion model" of disease, polluting the spirit within through contact with sensory objects.[39]

Illustration of this can be found in another of Chrysostom's sermons, *On Vainglory and on Raising Children*. Here, Chrysostom argues that vainglory is one of the most dangerous passions, affecting even and especially those who lead otherwise upright lives.[40] Avoidance of vainglory must therefore be taught from early childhood, and Chrysostom lays out a method for doing so. His central strategy is to control sensory input, in order to avoid encouraging the impressionable child to seek out sensuous experiences.[41] Just as a lawgiver establishes regulations regarding traffic in and out of the city gates, so a parent guards the sensory organs of his child from undesirable visitors:

> If not blocked up, this gate [sc. the nose] also permits great mischief to enter, such as spices and the fumes of incense. For nothing so loosens, nothing so slackens the tension of the soul, as to take pleasure in fragrant smells. "What, then," one might say, "must we rejoice rather in filth?" This is not what I am saying: I mean that we must enjoy neither one nor the other. Let nobody introduce perfume, for the brain, upon receiving this, immediately and entirely slackens [or: "slackens the whole"]. From that point on, pleasures are kindled, together with a great desire for fulfilment.[42]

Chrysostom encourages stuffing up the nostrils in order to prevent the invasion of "great mischief," which will affect both the physical quality of the brain and the child's susceptibility to pleasures.

In Chrysostom's account of the senses, it is only with regard to smell that he mentions the brain.[43] This is in keeping with late antique medical doctrine, which taught that smell, of all the senses, acts most directly upon the brain. In his treatise *On the Usefulness of the Parts*, Galen writes that "the perceived material proper to this sensation must, in fact, alter [ἀλλοιῶσαι] a portion of the brain."[44] Indeed, the organ of smell was not the nose but the front ventricles of the brain itself, on the grounds that only these contain the vaporous substances that must be altered by vaporous smells from outside.[45] Galen elaborated this precept, assumed in *On the Usefulness of the Parts*, in his *On the Olfactory Instrument*.[46] This work was summarized by Oribasius in his fifth-century medical encyclopedia, and also by Nemesius in his treatise *On the Nature of the Human Being*.[47] Chrysostom's particular source is unknown, but the general derivation of his concerns about odors is clear: according to contemporary Galenic doctrine, smell was the sense that acted most directly upon the brain.

The intimate relationship between smell and the brain provoked anxiety more broadly, rendering smell both the most acute and the most unstable of senses.[48] Smell was, quite literally, transformative: in theological metaphors, it represented divine epiphany; in ascetic discourse it more commonly signified intractable temptation to indulge in sensual pleasure.[49] Laurence Totelin explains this tension in terms of the juxtaposition of reason and perception within the brain:

> Although smell was probably the most animal sense, Galen felt able to locate its organ in the brain, which he considered the seat of the rational soul. It is little surprise to find, then, that the complex and controversial status of olfaction was also a subject of considerable debate among contemporary philosophers, for whom the connections between body and smell, and the relationship between perception, knowledge and understanding, were likewise subjected to intensive scrutiny and analysis.[50]

The localization of both smell and reason within the brain offered a material counterpart to philosophical discussions about the relationship between bodily perception and the incorporeal mind.[51]

This relationship was not only symbolic but also mechanical: the proximity of the organs of smell and thought does more than represent their juxtaposition in philosophical questions; through the intrusion of odors into the front ventricles of the brain, the "vaporous" substance within—that is, the psychic *pneuma*—must be altered. Since this is the same *pneuma* that works through the middle and rear ventricles of the brain also, to bring about thought, memory, and voluntary motion, the odors that enter through the nose and alter the vapors affect the substrate of thought itself.[52] The instruments of the rational soul (both *pneuma* and the brain substance) are materially transformed by smell.[53]

This puts into a new light the association in late antiquity between smell and demons. According to Evagrius of Pontus, demons "reportedly enter their victims through the nose."[54] Evagrius writes in his *Praktikos*, "Given the overpowering stench in demons, the soul typically is enflamed toward thoughts [λογισμοὺς] whenever it senses them drawing near."[55] Demons affected the brain directly by entering like (or as) smells through the nose.[56] Discussions of cerebral vulnerability in relation to bad smells had clear implications for the vulnerability of the soul to more than luxurious perfumes.

Chrysostom represents the entanglement of physiological and psychological causalities within the brain through his repetition of the verb "slackens" (χαλᾷ/ἐχάλασεν), first in relation to the soul and then in relation to the brain and body: "For nothing so loosens, nothing so slackens [χαλᾷ] the tension of the soul, as to take pleasure in fragrant smells. . . . Let nobody introduce perfume, for the brain, upon receiving this, immediately and entirely slackens [τὸ πᾶν ἐχάλασεν]."[57] The dissolution of the child upon exposure to pleasant odors is overdetermined, as the temptation of pleasure operates with an attractive and a loosening force at the levels of both brain and soul. A further meaning of slackens emerges if we take the phrase τὸ πᾶν ἐχάλασεν not intransitively (the brain "entirely slackens") but transitively (the brain "slackens the whole"). In the first reading, "slackens" describes the alteration of brain substance by the entering odor; in the second, "slackens" describes how the brain loosens the rest of the body when affected by perfume, via the slackened nerves that branch out from the brain and spine. It is possible that Chrysostom intended both meanings, and it is certain that both meanings could be heard. Perfume slackens both the brain and the "tension" (*tonos*) of the soul, and in so doing it slackens the control that the brain and soul hold over the body via the nerves.

In his commentary on Aristotle's *Categories*, the late antique philosophical commentator Simplicius of Cilicia (c. 490–560) reveals that Chrysostom's term χαλᾶν ("to slacken") was also used by Stoic philosophers to articulate the impact of bodily practices on the health of the soul: "Further, even the Stoics," writes Simplicius, "concede that in cases of torpor, melancholy, and lethargy, and in cases of drug-taking, a loss of virtue itself along with the entire rational state comes about; vice does not supersede it, but the firmness is slackened [χαλωμένης] and slips into a state that the ancients called intermediate."[58] Chrysostom's warning that pleasant smells "slacken" the tension, or *tonos*, of the soul (and also the brain or body as a whole) was grounded in Stoic teachings about how the condition of one's body could inform one's psychic health.

By late antiquity, the concept of *tonos* had accumulated rich layers of meaning that emphasized the interpenetration of body and soul in affective events: (1) In physics and engineering, *tonos* referred to "the peculiar property of elasticity," as exploited, for example, in spring catapults.[59] (2) In anatomical texts, *tonos* was a term for the nondifferentiated category of "tendons, sinews, muscles."[60] (3) Within Stoic physics, *tonos* was a quality of the *pneuma*, enabling a continuum of unified bodies, with differentiation between inanimate, animate, irrational, and rational beings, with the souls of rational animals displaying an extremely high level of pneumatic tension, irrational animals slightly less, and plants and inanimate objects such as rocks the least tension of all.[61] (4) In Stoic psychology, meanwhile, the *tonos* of the soul referred both to the *tonos* of the *pneuma* (that is, the material substance of soul) and also to the strength of what we might call the "will."[62] In her discussion of "Stoic Tonics," Martha Nussbaum writes that philosophy's "medical function is understood as, above all, that of *toning up* the soul—developing its muscles, assisting it to use its own capabilities more effectively."[63] The "toning" of the soul "is not just a metaphor but a literal physical idea."[64] The *tonos* of the soul is the *tonos* of the psychic *pneuma*.[65] (5) According to Galenic medical theory, *tonos* works both physiologically and psychologically: a loosening of the *tonos* of psychic *pneuma* within the cerebral ventricles, for example, may lead to stupor.[66] Elsewhere, Galen associates *tonos* with the *thumos* (the spirited part of the soul), which Plato located in the heart and made responsible for enforcing the commands of reason over the body: understanding the *tonos* of the soul to be a function of the *thumos* akin to the boiling of innate heat within the heart, Galen explained the importance of this *tonos* as enabling the *thumos* to manage the relationships between the other two parts of the soul, protecting reason from desire and enforcing the commands of reason when desire gets in the way.[67]

In his warning that perfume will "slacken" the *tonos* of the soul, Chrysostom situates himself firmly within Stoic psychology. Yet, by paralleling this slackening to the slackening of the brain, Chrysostom flags his awareness that psychic *pneuma* is located not in the heart, as Stoic philosophers had claimed, but within the brain and the cerebral ventricles. The slackening of soul, the slackening of the whole brain, and the brain's slackening of the whole body are versions of the same psychophysiological event.[68] When perfumed *pneuma* slackens brain matter, according to Chrysostom, it slackens the *tonos* of the soul also.

We have already encountered a similar overdeterminism at work in Gregory of Nyssa's *On the Constitution of the Human Being*, where, after denying medical arguments for the brain as the seat of the mind, Gregory likens the power in the cerebral membranes to the force and mechanism (μηχανῆς) that might bring a humanoid puppet (ἀνδριάντα) to life and to the guidance that a charioteer (ἡνίοχος) gives to horses, imparting to the muscles both impulse and power.[69] Gregory appears to borrow not only the charioteer from Plato's *Phaedrus*, but also the "puppets" described by Aristotle and by Marcus Aurelius (although both these philosophers identified the "mechanism" of the puppets with the heart, rather than with the brain).[70] While Gregory's comparison of cerebral power to a "mechanism" suggests a separation between the autonomous soul and the instrumental body that reflects his overall perspective on the soul/body relationship, his allusion to Plato's charioteer metaphor introduces an element of ambiguity. Is the brain the mechanism (by which soul acts) or the operating agent? More bluntly, does the brain make the governing soul superfluous?[71]

Chrysostom's repetition of the verb "slackens" in his discussion of the effects of perfume on the *tonos* of the soul and on the brain suggests a similar ambiguity. Upon exposure to perfume, the child becomes softer and more susceptible to the temptations of sensuous pleasures. The locus of this attraction lies in both in the brain and soul.[72] The concern which Chrysostom demonstrates for the health of the brain is tied to the human capacity for rational self-governance. In this way, the preacher justifies his intervention into bodily practices as conducive to the health of the soul: alteration of the brain influenced its control of the rest of the body. The brain could serve as a marker of human vulnerability, since the health of the soul—that is, its resistance to temptation—was determined in part by the health of the brain. That the slackening of the brain could stand in parallel to the slackening of the *tonos* of the soul suggests a kind of psychophysiological causality that we do not find in Plato, in Galen, or even in the Stoics. For Chrysostom, the brain seems to represent the necessary vulnerability of the soul as interpenetrated with the human body, such that one's care of the soul is mediated physiologically through one's care of the brain.

Ancient Christian authors were not entirely against the use of scented ointments and perfumes, which were regularly used in religious rituals. Clement of Alexandria (c. 150–215) offers a contrast to Chrysostom's text in his *Paedagogus*, where—despite his argument against the use of ointments and perfumes on the grounds that they are feminizing and lead to sensual temptation—he outlines ways in which these products can serve therapeutic purposes, especially in their effects upon the brain. Their key functions are to soften and to alter the temperament of the body.[73] Oil, which Clement considers preferable to ointment, "is sufficient to lubricate the surface and to loosen the sinewy part [τὸ νευρῶδες]."[74] As a younger contemporary of Galen, it is likely that Clement was familiar with the interpretation of *neura* as nerves; here, however, he is almost certainly referring to the oiling down that was associated with massage and athletic activity in antiquity.[75] When it comes to the effects of fragrance, however, he focuses in on the brain and stomach: "For there are fragrances that are neither soporific nor aphrodisiac, that do not smell of sexual intercourse and indecent friendship, but are healthy in moderation, nourishing the brain when it is in a bad condition, and strengthening the stomach."[76] The "bad condition" (καχεκτῇ) of the brain is a reference to the concept of *hexis*, a technical term with a range of meanings that include (1) a stable arrangement or disposition (for example, the health of the body) and (2) the stability or cohesion that *pneuma* provides for the cosmos within Stoic physics.[77] The *hexis* of the brain is both its general condition or health and the condition of the *pneuma* that (within Stoicism) organizes all things, and (within medicine) permeates and animates the brain and nerves. Fragrant smells affect the brain through their impact upon the *pneuma*.

Clement goes on to indicate the therapeutic utility of ointment in relation to bodily weakness, flux, chills, and dissatisfaction. He cites as his authority on this an anonymous "comic poet," who has been identified by editors as Alexis (375–275 B.C.E.): "The nostrils are anointed with myrrh; the greatest part of health is to render excellent odors to the brain."[78] Clement emphasizes the effects of fragrance on the brain not only by including a quotation to back up precisely this point, but by choosing a quotation that claims this as holding principal importance in human health. Alexis, although active some fifty years before Hellenistic medical scientists began to investigate the features and functions of the brain, here anticipates the medical encephalocentrism that was to take hold in the Hellenistic period and after, as well as the much later claim by John Chrysostom, examined above, that the activities of the soul depend upon the temperament of the brain. The conception of cerebral health as central to human well-being had early roots that were readily incorporated into Christian texts.

Clement subsequently clarifies how fragrance affects the brain: "In this way, physicians—explaining in scientific fashion that the brain is cold—consider it appropriate to anoint the breast and the tip of the nostrils with myrrh, so that the fiery inhalation might strongly warm the chill, passing gently through."[79] In general, the brain was considered a cold organ; it is not clear here whether the physicians are talking about the medicinal use of myrrh to warm a brain that is abnormally chilled or if, rather, they consider regular application of myrrh useful in maintaining the overall balance of the brain. What does seem likely is that the healing properties of myrrh (warming) overlap with the dangerous properties of myrrh (softening, slackening) as described by Chrysostom, since warmth typically softens cold substances—a suspicion confirmed by Clement's own lengthy discussion of how perfumes soften and slacken the person who wears them. Clement and Chrysostom were working with shared assumptions about the effects of myrrh on the brain but turned these assumptions to different effects.

Perfume was a site of tension in ancient understandings of how the body was implicated in ethical responsibilities and regimes. Central to its ambiguous status was the expectation that it softened the body and altered bodily temperament. To take one influential example, the late classical author Theophrastus of Eresos (c. 371–287 B.C.E.) described perfume as having warming, drying, and dilating effects upon internal bodily vessels, but also as having an effect, if used in excess, similar to that of drunkenness and stupor.[80] The weakness of the soft brain lay not only in its vulnerability to physical trauma, but also in the very function of this softness in enabling sensation, which could transform both brain and soul, above all in the form of pleasant smells. Christian and ascetic management of the sensory environment was as much a manipulation of the brain as of the soul.

INTERNAL VAPORS: ALCOHOL

Just like external vapors and fragrances, internal vapors—particularly those that rose out of the stomach—could damage the brain and affect the cognitive faculties. These vapors might be the product of alcohol or of the regular digestion of food.[81] Late antique preachers used this medical knowledge to discipline their audiences into the moderate ascetic practice that was supposed to characterize the Christian congregation. In this closing section, I examine the role of medical theories about cerebral vulnerability in warnings against excess consumption of alcohol. Through close attention to the metaphorical and technical details that preachers employed, we can see the rhetoric of cerebral vulnerability at work in late antique Christian pedagogies of the body.

The medical theory of hangovers crops up frequently in late antique Christian texts. In his homily *Against Drunks,* Basil of Caesarea writes that "whenever the cerebral membranes become full of soot, which wine carries aloft in evaporation, the head is struck by unbearable pains."[82] In his angry letter "to the notables of Neocaesarea," Basil instructs his addressees to bid farewell to "heads heavy with wine, which are made to see fantasies by the vapor which is carried upward in the swell of intoxication."[83] Augustine, in his treatise *On Catholic Morals,* defends the regular use of old wine by arguing that it is not so potent as new wine, which more quickly destroys the sensitive faculty: "so that if [the wine] has remained in the vat for a little time and has fermented a little bit, it drags down headlong those looking in from above, striking their brains."[84] In his *Homily on the Holy Fast,* Asterius of Amasea describes how fasting lessens pulsation within the brain, which was typically caused by an "influx of vapors" thought to "darken" the brain.[85] A sermon *On Prayer* (spuriously attributed to John Chrysostom) informs the congregation that alcohol does not help in prayer, since the "evaporation" (ἀναθυμίασις) from excessive nutriment enters into the ventricles of the brain and makes reason turbid.[86]

These references reflect the medical teaching that, following consumption of wine, warm vapors filled the head, causing heaviness and pain.[87] We see this outlined clearly in *Problems*, a collection of philosophical questions and answers that likely dates to the late second or early third century, the lifetime of the Peripatetic philosopher Alexander of Aphrodisias, under whose name it circulated: "Wine, being upward-rising, burns the brain with fever and forces the first organ of the soul (that is, ethereal pneuma), being excessively damaged, to enact its thoughts."[88] The vapors of wine, rising through the body, disturb the *pneuma* within the cerebral ventricles, strike the brain, and clog up the cerebral membranes, leading to headache, fuzzy reason, and uncontrolled behavior. When preachers drew on this theory, they sought to enforce a standard of behavior (sobriety) that was motivated by its connection to the health of the soul. Whereas most such discussions focused on how wine could increase susceptibility to temptation by loosening inhibitions and encouraging sensuality, the use of a medical theory introduced the idea that wine affected the soul and its capacity for restraint by damaging the brain and the *pneuma* within. By blending physiological and moral explanations for how wine affects human behavior, preachers sought to motivate their audiences to conform to specific behavioral expectations.

In his homily *On the First Letter to Timothy* 13, John Chrysostom offers an elaborate illustration of how this appropriation of medical knowledge about the brain could work within a pastoral context. The homily explicates 1 Timothy 4:11–18 and 5:1–7; by far the majority of the text, however, focuses upon 1 Timothy 5:6, which condemns widows who choose to live in pleasure: "But the widow who lives for pleasure is dead even while she lives."[89] What does it mean to be dead while still alive? Chrysostom's answer is that it is to be drunk. The core of his argument against drunkenness is the theory of vapors just discussed. He begins, however, not with medical doctrine, but with dramatic imagery:

> Just as a sky that is fully and continuously overcast does not allow the brightness to shine through, in the same way the vapors of luxury and wine—obscuring the brain like some rock [σκόπελον] and settling a dense cloud [νέφος . . . πυκνὸν] there—do not then allow reason to reach through, keeping the drunken man within a deep and moonless dark.[90]

Tropes of reason as light and mental disturbance or drunkenness as a fog were common in antiquity.[91] More unexpected is the rock (σκόπελος) that stands in for the brain, which itself stands in for the subject, that is, the "drunken man." The drunken man stands in darkness, just as the rock/brain stands shrouded from the light of reason. As the bodily organ of the rational soul, the brain here substitutes for the entire rational organ, that is, the human being.[92]

But how is a rock (σκόπελος) like a brain? There are two core meanings of σκόπελος: a rock or cliff, typically in the ocean, or a lookout point (a usage that highlights the echo of σκόπ-, "see").[93] Since, within city/body analogies, the eyes were often designated the "scouts" or "look-outs" of the soul, we might interpret the σκόπελος as a central site for perception of and engagement with the outside world.[94] While the eyes perform the activity of "looking out," the brain supports the analogous activity of reason, which is, in common metaphor, the "eye" of the soul.[95] If the brain is shrouded in mist, then the lookout (the soul) on the lookout point (the brain) can see nothing.

The most famous "cloud-covered" σκόπελοι in antiquity were, however, the "Clashing Rocks" through which Jason passed on his way to Colchis, and which Circe describes to Odysseus in the twelfth book of the *Odyssey:* "There are two rocks [σκόπελοι]; one reaches the expanse of heaven with its sharp peaks, and a dark blue cloud [νεφέλη] envelops it."[96] Chrysostom's congregation, immersed in Homeric poetry through elementary education and popular culture, may have heard the echo of these lines in Chrysostom's evocation of a single "rock" (σκόπελον), shrouded in a "thick cloud" (νέφος . . . πυκνὸν).[97] That the echo is intentional is suggested by a more explicitly marked use of the Homeric image in a letter by another famous rhetorician of Antioch, Libanius, who may have been Chrysostom's teacher.[98] In this letter, which describes the difficulty of achieving calm during the school vacation, Libanius compares his mental distractions to the "continuous cloud" (διηνεκεῖ νεφέλη) that covers the peaks of the two rocks (τοῖν σκοπέλοιν), as "Homer called to mind" (Ὅμηρος ἐμνήσθη).[99] Was Chrysostom familiar with this letter, had he heard Libanius allude to the line, or was the echo an accident of the saturation of late antique culture in Homeric poetry? Suggestive of Chrysostom's familiarity with Libanius' letter is the fact that Chrysostom's description of the "sky that is fully and continually [διηνεκὴς] overcast [συννέφεια]" contains another echo, this time not of the Homeric passage itself, but of the "continuous cloud" (διηνεκεῖ νεφέλη) in Libanius' letter. For Chrysostom and Libanius alike, whether through accident or design, a thick cloud covering rocky peaks represented the interminable fog of mental distraction.

There are further echoes of the cloud-covered rocks in Chrysostom's second homily *On John*, where worldly concerns are said to cloud the soul. He writes as follows:

> For, just as the eye, whenever it is pure and translucent, is also sharp of vision and does not easily tire out, even when observing the slightest bodies, but whenever, with some evil humor pouring into it from the head or murky smoke having been borne up from below, a dense cloud [πυκνή . . . νεφέλη] forms in front of the pupil and does not allow it to see clearly even grosser [bodies]; thus it is also with regard to the soul.[100]

According to Galen, *pneuma* flowed between the front two ventricles of the brain and the eyes through the optic nerves, thereby enabling vision.[101] Humors and vapors, especially digestive vapors, could also enter through these nerves, thereby damaging vision.[102] The common association of the eye with the rational soul, and of sight with the activity of thought, made this physiological event a suitable analogue for the passage of disruptive thoughts (for example, concern for one's business affairs) into the soul, obscuring contemplation of God.[103] Yet, this analogy lacked a key term: corrupt humors travel from the brain into the eye. What was the source of the disruptive thoughts (φροντίδα βιωτικὴν) that entered the soul? As the instrument of discursive thought, the brain is, again, the most obvious candidate. Worldly thoughts travel from the brain into the soul in the manner of vapors and corrupt humors.

For the audience to Chrysostom's homily *On the First Letter to Timothy* 13, then, the fog settling over the rock/brain/drunken man obscures clarity of vision in the same manner as the "dense cloud" of worldly thoughts (humors) in one's eye or the "continuous cloud" that envelops Libanius during the school holiday. This diverges from the image in its Homeric context, where the risk posed by the cloud-covered rocks depends upon the viewer being located in a ship at sea and the rocks themselves being hidden from view. Chrysostom's initial metaphor presumably would have evoked this direction of vision, together with the threat posed by invisible rocks. We are not, I think, supposed to lose this taste of danger when the rock is transformed first into a brain and then into a drunken man, although it is now the rock/brain/man that is at risk, rather than the Odyssean sailor looking on. Through these transfigurations, Chrysostom distances his audience from the drunken man, situating those who listen to him on the side of reason. The audience is offered a split perspective: drinking is dangerous because it prevents you from seeing out (seeing reason), but also because it transforms the brain into a rock upon which one might destroy one's craft. Failure to take care of one's brain increases the danger that the body poses to the health of the soul.

A common metaphor for the human person was a ship at sea, piloted by a soul.[104] Chrysostom splices this image with the canonical analogy of the human person and the city, shifting from his image the brain as a rock to a scene of urban confusion, as the storm of alcohol washes into the city:

> For just as, when a flood has come about and water has risen over the entrances to the workshops, we see the inhabitants in constant panic [ἀεὶ θορυβουμένους], contriving to use urns and jars and sponges and many other things to bail out the water, so that it might not rot through the foundations and render all of the equipment useless. Thus it is with regard to the soul also, that whenever it becomes flooded with excessive luxury, the internal thoughts begin to panic [θορυβοῦνται μὲν ἔνδον οἱ λογισμοὶ], being no longer strong enough to empty out that which has already gathered.[105]

Where previously the wine was imagined as the fog hanging over the sea, it now becomes the water itself which breaks into urban spaces, threatening to flood the buildings within, and sending the inhabitants into panic as they bail the water out of their workshops. Most strikingly, however, this is the first mention of the soul in this account of drunkenness.

While one might initially imagine the site of the storm as the body with its various internal organs, Chrysostom reveals at the culmination of his analogy that it is in fact the soul that "has become flooded" (ὑπέραντλος γένηται) and the "thoughts," rather than the members within the body, that are stirred up in panic (θορυβοῦνται μὲν ἔνδον οἱ λογισμοὶ).[106] This does not mean that the flooding is immaterial: as we have seen, the manifestation of soul within the body required (or perhaps was identical with) the material substrate of *pneuma*. The flooding of the soul with luxury refers to the effect of alcoholic vapors upon the *pneuma* within the brain, an interpretation supported by a comparable metaphor in a letter from the same period by the Roman theologian Jerome to his one-time friend but now despised enemy, Vigilantius. Accusing Vigilantius of forgetting how much he approved of Jerome's preaching, Jerome suggests that a recent sea voyage has damage his opponent's brain:

> Recall, if you will, that day when you leapt up beside me as I preached on the resurrection and truth of the body, stamping your feet and acclaiming my orthodoxy. After you set out on your sea voyage, however, and the rot of bilge water [*sentinae putredo*] reached your innermost brain [*ad intimum cerebrum*], you remembered us as heretics.[107]

The word translated as "flooded, saturated" in Chrysostom's description of the drunken storm is ὑπέραντλος, which can be broken down into two parts: ὑπέρ-, "over, super, excess," and -αντλος, "bilge-water, flood." While ὑπέραντλος extended beyond its literal meaning, -αντλος evokes a nautical context.[108] For both Chrysostom and Jerome, the effect of bilge-water is to rot and to corrupt.[109] Jerome locates that corruption in the brain but assumes its effects on the soul. Chrysostom, on the other hand, identifies the soul as the locus of water damage, but charts a similar process of moisture (bilge-water or vapors) entering the brain.[110]

Following his description of the flooded city, Chrysostom turns swiftly to focus once again on the body itself. This time, the body is likened both to the city as a whole and to a single workshop, from the furnace of which smoke belches forth. This extended metaphor, which we encountered briefly in chapter 3, elaborates upon connections between cerebral, psychological, and political vulnerability that the other texts we have examined merely hint at. Here, it is worth examining the passage in full:

> When we indulge ourselves further, the more we fill ourselves with foul smells, leaking like a wineskin from all over the body. Someone belches such that even bystanders' brains are hurt. As if from a furnace, smoky vapors are emitted from all over the body, through the heat of corruption within. Now, if bystanders are pained, what do you think the brain within is suffering, continually assailed by these vapors? What of the pipes of heated and obstructed blood? What of those reservoirs, the liver and the spleen? What of the channels for feces? It's ridiculous that we tend to sewers, so they do not get blocked and spew up their filth, and do everything possible on account of this, thrusting through them with poles and dragging them with mattocks but in no way clean the drains of our own stomachs, but rather block them up and choke them. And when the excrement rises up to where the king himself sits—I am talking about the brain—we do not consider it worth any forethought. Doing all these things, we don't treat it a worthy king, but rather as an impure dog.[111]

The consumption of wine produces fumes and smells that, like perfume, can alter the brains of others, as well as that of oneself. As in Chrysostom's previous metaphor, wine is envisioned a civic problem, although here the source of harm is located within the individual, rather than as a storm overcoming the city from outside. That is to say, the individuals are required, in considering their own ascetic practice, to see themselves not only as responsible for the care of their own souls, but also as members of a community, producing the environmental conditions (and the external vapors) by which the brains and souls of their fellow humans are formed.

The drunken belch is also envisioned within a civic and an architectural frame. "As if from some furnace," Chrysostom writes, the fumes of wine are released "from all over the body"—that is, from the major orifices and also through the *poroi*, what we might think of as pores, in the skin. The individual body is part of the urban landscape, a furnace that is necessary to the maintenance of civic life but that is also a source of danger and discomfort to the populace. The blood vessels, meanwhile, rather than perform their proper task of circulating nourishment within the body, are overcome by wine. The liver and spleen, which act as reservoirs upon which the blood vessels might draw, are similarly affected.[112] The stomach drains like a cesspit into the sewage system of the intestines.[113] Within the body of the drunken individual, physiological and civic disorder converge. The architectural details connect Chrysostom's extended metaphor back to the Platonist image of the head as an acropolis and the body as a city.[114] The reader is primed to expect the appearance of the king as the rational, governing part.

Unlike the Platonist head/acropolis metaphor, Chrysostom is more interested in the management of waste products than in the operations of governance. In this, he echoes medical sources. Plumbing was a structuring metaphor in ancient medical conceptions of the flow of blood, humors, and other substances within the body. In *On the Opinions of Hippocrates and Plato*, Galen explicitly figures the liver and veins as an aqueduct: "If you wished to describe the distribution of water brought into a city, you would not pass over its first entrance and find some other point from which to begin the account," that is, the source of blood within the body.[115] Urban plumbing that connects the various parts of the body to the brain/king specifically evokes Galen's simultaneous presentation of the brain as the organ of the *hēgemonikon* (a theory that, as he acknowledges, is associated with the metaphor of the brain/*hēgemonikon* as king) and the brain as an architectural structure oriented around the accumulation and distribution of fluids (that is, the plumbing beneath the citadel, necessary for the maintenance of the city, but rarely seen), especially in *On the Usefulness of the Parts*. As Julius Rocca has observed in his analysis of Galen's anatomy of the brain ventricles: "Galen draws his analogies from structures and systems that deal with the containment or distribution of fluids."[116]

Blockage, moreover, was a key medical concern. Different kinds of wine, as Galen described in *On Hygiene*, were known to "block up" (ἐμφράττεται, cf. Chrysostom's ἐμφραγῶσι) the liver, kidneys, and spleen, especially in the elderly.[117] In general, medical authors describe blockage (ἔμφραξις) in these organs, typically caused through the ingestion of certain foods, and remedies for it.[118] By drawing upon architectural imagery and terminology common within medical texts, Chrysostom lends his sermon a technical tone, enhancing the authority of his instructions in the care of the body.

Blake Leyerle has argued that Chrysostom's fondness for scatological imagery was a technique for shaming his wealthier congregants into giving up their luxury and excess.[119] In the passage considered here, Chryosostom is talking about more than the personal bodily pollution of diarrhea. The enmeshment of bodily and civic architecture invokes the obligation of the citizen to maintain civic hygiene as a support for the obligation of the individual congregant to care for the health of their individual body. Just as one must clean the gutters and prevent the blockage of the sewers in order to create a pleasant environment for all citizens, so one must purify one's stomach and bowels in order to participate healthfully in the larger community.

The individual has, in particular, a responsibility to provide clean lodging for their king. Chrysostom writes, as we have seen: "And when the excrement rises to where the king himself sits—I am talking about the brain—we do not consider it worth any forethought." The rising sewage represents the alcoholic fumes that rise into the head from the stomach. The image is striking insofar as it elides the governing soul into the brain, such that the effects of drunkenness upon the soul might be understood in entirely material terms. As bodily representation of the soul, the brain deserves the honor of a king, but instead, within the polity of a drunken body, experiences pollution and pain. Chrysostom's scatological account turns on its head the traditional image of the monarchical soul ruling from the acropolis of the skull. Rather than focusing upon the distribution of political function across the parts of the body, he highlights failure in sociopolitical duty through the breakdown in urban sanitation. Healthcare is, Chrysostom insists, no longer a private concern. How one takes care of one's body constitutes a sociopolitical and a spiritual responsibility.

The brain was a fragile organ, susceptible to physical trauma, to pleasant smells, and to the vapors of digestion and strong wine. At the same time, it was the internal source of reason, virtue, and self-governance. Chrysostom's emphasis upon the brain as the bodily source of these qualities, which are fundamental components of the health of the soul in the philosophical tradition, reveals the high stakes of cerebral self-care, as he taught it to his congregation. Damage to the brain compromises the ability to govern one's own actions, affects, and thoughts in a manner conducive to the health of the eternal soul.

CONCLUSION

In late antique Christian rhetoric, the brain could be described as the foundation of the human being. Its protection was considered vital to the well-being of the human being as a whole. Its vulnerability was a matter of concern. Further, as I have argued in this chapter, it was not simply the case that preachers and theologians worried about the vulnerability of the brain—more significantly, they emphasized its vulnerability in order to establish theological arguments about providential design, encourage political compliance, and motivate moderate ascetic behaviors. This was a central contribution that late antique Christian authors made to subsequent conceptualizations of the brain.

Key modes of vulnerability included temperamental imbalance, softness (and, by extension, sensation), and susceptibility to external and internal vapors. Late antique Christian authors drew upon medical terminology, theories, and imagery to develop the existing understanding of the brain as vulnerable into a powerful rhetorical tool that was also an object of anxiety and control, insofar as the vulnerability of the brain could threaten the health of the soul. Cerebral vulnerability served useful rhetorical purposes for late antique Christian preachers: it encouraged habits of self-care considered proper to Christian communities as spiritual, sociopolitical, and medical responsibilities. It also provided material for articulating the necessary weakness of the rational human being, as a creature able to choose salvation or destruction, capable of divine contemplation, but enmeshed in material form. Not only as the instrument of the governing soul, but also as a soft, vulnerable organ, the brain became the ideal metonymic representative for the human being.

As we have seen, Christian preachers elaborated upon medical concepts, theories, and images, integrating them fully into their arguments and making new connections between the vulnerability of the brain and that of the soul. The medical metaphors that structured early Christianity (sin as disease, salvation as healing, preachers as physicians of the soul) provided a context in which this close engagement with medical expertise not only made sense but could be generative at both figurative and literal levels. Early Christian preachers considered the care of the brain to be a useful rhetorical tool for talking about the care of the soul, but they also actively encouraged specific ascetic practices precisely to ensure the health of the brain. In the next chapter, I turn to a related set of rhetorical practices that sit similarly at the boundary between metaphorical and literal speech: that is, the use of brain-based mental illness to describe religious "deviance," in particular, excessive ascetic practice. Just as in the emphasis on cerebral vulnerability in this chapter, the instrumentalization of "crazy" as a tool for disciplining congregants and opponents operated in both metaphoric and literal terms.

CHAPTER 6

Insanity, Vainglory, and Phrenitis

The previous chapter examined how late antique Christian authors deployed a rhetoric of cerebral vulnerability in support of moderate ascetic practices, such as avoidance of wine and perfume. We found that preachers drew upon medical ideas about the vulnerability of the brain to support their claim that sensual pleasures could compromise the health of the soul. In this chapter, we turn to the opposite problem: the damaging effects of excessive ascetic practice on the brain. On the one hand, flooding the brain with alcoholic fumes could threaten rational thought through damage to the cerebral membranes, the ventricles, and the *pneuma* within; on the other hand, total abstinence from food and other necessities could dry out or otherwise damage the brain, while at the same time encouraging ascetic practitioners toward self-righteousness and vainglory. As I will argue, the medical concept of the brain was not simply a tool for motivating certain modes of self-care (for example, sobriety), but also served to demarcate the limits of human behavior, since both luxury and abstinence could destroy it and, in doing so, could impair the faculties of the soul.[1] In this way, the rhetoric of cerebral vulnerability was deployed to guide audiences along a middle course: neither form of bodily autonomy (luxurious living, outstanding asceticism) was safe for the health of the brain and soul. Conformity with pastoral guidelines on the care of the body and trust in the grace of Christ were fundamental to salvation. The vulnerable brain was the site where these tensions between different paths to psychic health and salvation played out.

At the heart of my discussion is the ancient disease phrenitis, which was considered to be among the most dangerous of mental illnesses. In late antiquity, phrenitis was defined as a strong but short-term fever accompanied by delirium.[2] Its etiology varied among medical authors, but by late antiquity it was most commonly associated with the brain. Thus, the poet Prudentius could write without clarification: "This is your grave and rational speech, Marcion—or, rather, this is obviously the phrenitis [*frenesis*] of a thunder-struck brain [*attoniti . . . cerebri*]."[3] As Prudentius illustrates, phrenitis was a medical term, but its meaning was regularly extended. In popular speech, it commonly denoted deviance from a social norm.[4] In Christian texts, phrenitis was often invoked to denounce one's religious opponents—pagans, Jews, Manichaeans, as well as any Christian, such as Marcion, considered heretical in doctrine or practice.[5] Used in this sense, it was similar to the modern English words "crazy" and "mad," generic terms that cover the whole gamut of alien phenomena, from fashion choices and weather events to religious extremism and random acts of violence.

The metaphorical application of "phrenitis" to forms of deviance operates on a continuum with more obviously physical disorders, such as gangrene and ulcers, which regularly served in this capacity. Yet, mental disorders bridge the physical and the moral—and the literal and the metaphorical—in ways that gangrene and ulcers do not. Just as perpetrators of mass violence are not merely called "crazy," but are often (whether or not correctly) assumed to suffer from mental illnesses, so phrenitis continued to carry—in sermons, in polemical pamphlets, in letters, in poems—the baggage of its medical definition.[6] When Christians called their enemies "phrenetic," they did not only intend the generic insult "crazy," but were also invoking the structuring metaphor of early Christianity, that is, salvation as the healing of the soul.[7] The traffic between literal and metaphorical interpretations of phrenitis is crucial to understanding the complex role of the brain in early Christian understandings of sin.

Exploring the medical character of phrenitis gives us access to a discourse of "crazy" that was riven by tensions peculiar to late ancient Christianity but resonant up to the present day: if deviance is a product of the brain, then in what cases and to what extent can a person be held responsible for actions deemed inappropriate or destructive? Should disease or malfunction of the brain mitigate the punitive consequences of "bad" behavior?[8] Is deviant action or thought always to be assigned to a malfunction of the body?[9] Where is there room, in this model, for responsibility and the notion of the will?[10] These questions were as prominent in early Christian literature about orthodoxy, sin, and salvation as they are in contemporary discussions of criminality, social justice, and neuroscience.

The first part of this chapter presents phrenitis from the perspective of ancient medicine. Here I make the argument that in late antiquity phrenitis signified above all the loss of self-governance through bodily damage. More precisely, illnesses of the brain undermined one's ability to control one's own thoughts or actions, and so challenged the generally accepted notion that self-responsibility belongs to the soul. Second, I focus upon ascetic practice and the role of the brain in setting limits to human feats of endurance. Here, I focus on the story of Macarius of Alexandria, an Egyptian monk who compromised ascetic discipline to ensure the health of his brain, which he seems to have considered a fundamental condition of human reason. I argue that phrenitis is to be interpreted as a bodily correlate to vainglory, the affect that endangers every perfected monk. Through the discourses of phrenitis and vainglory in combination, late antique Christian authors sought to discipline ascetic practitioners to respect the limitations that bound them to the community of their fellow human beings. Finally, I turn to the polemical application of "phrenitis" as a diagnosis of religious difference in the sermons of perhaps the most influential Christian teacher in late antiquity, Augustine. For Augustine, I argue, the loss of self-governance represented by phrenitis offered a model for understanding how a person might be sick but refuse treatment and so for justifying nonconsensual therapy.

PHRENITIS IN ANCIENT MEDICINE

Phrenitis was a disease of hot and dry swellings. An anonymous doxographic work *On Chronic and Acute Diseases* (generally dated to the first century C.E.) records the opinions of the late classical physicians Praxagoras and Diocles that phrenitis was, respectively, a "swelling of the heart" (φλεγμονὴν τῆς καρδίας) or a "swelling of the diaphragm" (φλεγμονὴν τοῦ διαφράγματός).[11] Galen, meanwhile, insisted upon the localization of phrenitis in the region around the brain. In his work *On Symptoms and Causes,* he explains that "phrenitis does not simply arise through hot humors [θερμοῖς . . . χυμοῖς] but also is brought about after inflammation in the brain and cerebral membranes [τοῦ φλεγμονὴν . . . κατά τε τὸν ἐγκέφαλον καὶ τὰς μήνιγγας]."[12] Another of his works, *On Trembling, Palpitation, Convulsion, and Rigor,* describes how phrenitis is triggered by "dryness" of the nerves, and then adds that phrenetic symptoms are caused by "swelling of the source of the nerves" (τὴν φλεγμονὴν τῆς ἀρχῆς τῶν νεύρων), that is, the brain.[13] By late antiquity, hot and dry swellings around the brain were a standard explanation, as we discover in the popular medical handbook by Alexander of Tralles (sixth century C.E.): "Genuine phrenitis comes about, then, from yellow bile, whenever this is produced and creates swelling around the brain or the membrane within it [φλεγμονὴν . . . περὶ τὸν ἐγκέφαλον ἢ τὴν ἐν αὐτῷ μήνιγγα]."[14] Alexander's contemporary, the medical author Aëtius of Amida, reports the view of the physician Posidonius, writing probably in the fourth century C.E., that "phrenitis is the swelling of the membranes around the brain [φλεγμονή . . . τῶν περὶ τὸν ἐγκέφαλον μηνίγγων], together with acute fever, and brings with it derangement and wandering reason."[15]

This brain-centered etiology was complicated by the contested etymology of phrenitis. In ancient literary and medical tradition, phrenitis had two etymologies.[16] According to one, phrenitis was derived from the Greek word *phronēsis*, and meant "disturbance of the intellect or mind." The second explained phrenitis as inflammation of the *phrēn* (pl. *phrenes*), which was an archaic Greek word for a part of the body, often identified as the diaphragm.[17] These two etymologies supported different etiologies, each framed by a different relationship between the body and the governing part of the soul. Encephalocentrist thinkers tended to prefer the derivation of phrenitis from *phronesis*, arguing that, since phrenitis meant "disturbance of the intellect or mind," the localization of phrenitis in the cerebral membranes proved the localization of the mind within the brain. Cardiocentrist thinkers, meanwhile, tended to highlight the root *phrēn/phrenes*, arguing that the inflammation that caused mental disturbance must be located somewhere inside the torso. As Galen wrote in *On the Affected Parts*: "Our forebears all named the boundary below the chest the *phrenes* [φρένας], either because it simply occurred to them, or, as some think, because sick people suffer damage in their intelligence [φρόνησιν] when this part is inflamed [φλεγμαίνοντος]."[18] The cardiocentrist perspective still had some followers in late antiquity, as Gregory of Nyssa demonstrates:

> For we have also learned that insanity comes about not from heaviness of head alone, but also from the membranes underlying the ribs [τῶν τὰς πλευρὰς ὑπεζωκότων ὑμένων] being in a pathological condition, just as the experts in medicine explain the sickness of the rational principle, calling the affection "phrenitis," since *phrenes* [φρένες] is the name of those membranes.[19]

According to Galen, the *phrenes* perhaps get their name from *phronēsis* ("intelligence"), which is lost when they suffer from phrenitis. According to Gregory, meanwhile, phrenitis gets its name not from *phronēsis* at all, but rather from the *phrenes*.

The use of disease etiology to support a persuasive account of the body/soul relationship was acknowledged in antiquity. The late antique North African medical writer Caelius Aurelianus (fourth/fifth century C.E.) explains the many etiologies of phrenitis as corresponding to each author's position regarding the localization of the soul:

> Now some say that the brain is affected, others its foundation or *basis*, which we translate as "seat," others its membranes, others the heart, others the apex of the heart, others the membrane which encloses the heart, others the artery which the Greeks call the *aortē*, others the thick veins, others the diaphragm [*diaphragma*]. But why go on when we can easily clarify the matter by stating what these writers really had in mind? For in every case they hold that the part affected in people suffering from phrenitis [*in phreniticis*] is that in which they suspect the ruling part of the soul [*animae regimen*] is situated.[20]

As Caelius observes, the contested etymology and etiology of phrenitis was leveraged to prove different theories about the localization of the rational and governing soul within the body.[21] It is unsurprising, then, that phrenitis became an attractive model for the sickness of the soul in early Christian discourse. Arguments about the localization of phrenitis function as an index of where any given author believes the ruling part of the soul to be located.[22] Across medical, philosophical, and theological texts, phrenitis evokes the contested relationship between brain, body, and soul.[23]

Historians have noted that excessive ascetic practices were thought to lead to madness.[24] It was in this context that phrenitis became prominent among mental disorders that late antique Christian writers cited when seeking to define the limits of asceticism. In this sense, it played a role similar to vainglory, a passion of the soul thought to threaten the spiritual health of expert ascetic practitioners. Excessive ascetic endurance could provoke both phrenitis and vainglory, which mapped onto one another as inflammation of one's brain and inflammation of one's pride. In order to explore this in more depth, we will begin with the story of a celebrated Egyptian monk, Macarius of Alexandria, who yielded his ascetic discipline for the sake of his brain.

ASCETICISM AND THE HEALTH OF THE BRAIN

Early in the fifth century, Palladius of Galatia, then bishop of Helenopolis, wrote a description of the journey he had undertaken through Egypt as a youth. This text, known as the *Lausiac History*, became one of the most popular ancient accounts of the early Christian monastic movement.[25] It included dialogues with and biographical accounts of the ascetic communities and hermits whom Palladius had visited.[26] Among the stories Palladius tells is that of Macarius of Alexandria, who lived in the monastic community known as Kellia, deep within the Nitrian Desert.[27] Faithful to the hagiographical tradition, Palladius recounts feats of bodily endurance as an index of Macarius' spiritual prowess. "Here is another practice [ἄσκησις] of his," Palladius reports: "He determined to dispense with sleep, and he told us how he did not come inside under a roof for twenty days, that he might conquer sleep, being inflamed [φλεγόμενος] by heat, and shriveled up with cold by night."[28]

Bodily injury was a sign of holiness within the ascetic paradigm.[29] Indeed, cultivating and enduring illness was an ascetic discipline in its own right. It is surprising, therefore, when Macarius sets a limit to his task of endurance, on the grounds that he risks damaging his body and becoming sick. Palladius reports: "He added this: 'Unless I had come inside under a roof and got some sleep rather quickly, my brain would have so dried up [μου ἐξηράνθη ὁ ἐγκέφαλος] as to drive me into delirium [ἔκστασίν] for ever after. But I conquered so far as depended on me, and I gave way so far as depended on my nature, which had need of sleep.'"[30] While Macarius might seek the burning and shriveling up of his body as a whole, he is careful not to permanently injure his brain, in case he should lose control of his mind.

Macarius' concern for the health of his brain represents a tension described by the historian Andrew Crislip in his work on illness in ascetic narratives: "Illness may render bodily self-control impossible and culminate in the annihilation of the body and the self. But this may have a transcendent and salutary effect as well," functioning simultaneously as an opportunity for "mimesis of Christ's suffering" and "the clearest possible signifier of God's wrath."[31] Illness was a form of suffering attractive to late antique Christian ascetics. At the same time, illness of the brain or mind compromised the self-control necessary to ascetic identity.[32] We can see this tension at work in the phenomenon of the "holy fool," that is, the late antique ascetic practice of concealing sanctity with a performance of insanity.[33] This behavior and trope was effective because, on the one hand, it tapped into the idea that holiness could be misunderstood as madness, insofar as it contravened social norms, while on the other it challenged the preconception that "unpredictable, bizarre, and ostensibly anti-social behavior" could not represent holiness.[34]

Macarius' concern that he might dry out his brain echoes ancient medical accounts of phrenitis. The Byzantine medical encyclopedist Paul of Nicaea writes as follows:

> What is phrenitis? It is acute delirium with acute fever because the brain is parched of moisture [ξηραινομένου τοῦ ἐγκεφάλου ὑγροῦ], from which sleeplessness also follows. Such an illness arises from a hot and dry imbalance [ἀπὸ θερμῆς καὶ ξηρᾶς δυσκρασίας] in the case of burning fever when vapors are dispersed from the brain [ἀποπεμπομένου τοῦ ἀτμοῦ τοῦ ἐγκεφάλου]. For the brain is dried out [ξηραίνεται γὰρ ὁ ἐγκέφαλος] by the departure of moisture and excess of dryness. And continual sleeplessness follows these things, together with disturbance of thought; sometimes, becoming angry and wild, they run outside; at other times, being gentle and compliant, they lie down inside.[35]

The qualities of hot, cold, dry, and moist were fundamental to the ancient conception of human health and disease, and the temperament of the brain was considered essential to the work of the rational and governing soul. As John Chrysostom declared to his congregation: "For if the temperament of the flesh deviates from its accustomed constitution even trivially, many activities of the soul are in fact impeded—for example, if the brain becomes hotter or colder [εἰ θερμότερος ἢ ψυχρότερος ὁ ἐγκέφαλος γένοιτο]."[36] Temperament was the foundation and the explanation for one's physical and mental condition. Galen's influential treatise *That the Faculties of the Soul Follow the Mixtures of the Body* called into question the necessity of theorizing an incorporeal soul and instead proposed that individual character supervenes upon the measure of one's temperature and humidity.[37] In his introductory work *The Art of Medicine,* Galen describes the effects of bodily temperament localized within specific organs. Here is how he describes the compound imbalance of a brain that is hot and dry: persons who possess such brains "are lacking in excretions, endowed with acute perceptions, extremely insomniac, and become bald early."[38] A hot and dry brain is conducive to insomnia.[39] Correspondingly, sleep moistens the brain.[40] This is perhaps a hint as to why Macarius goes out into the desert to avoid sleep. The physiological effects that he both seeks out and fears will help him stay awake.

Insomnia is also, as we saw in Paul's account, a symptom of phrenitis.[41] This was already conventional wisdom by the second century, when Galen attributed it to "most physicians."[42] As Galen writes in his distinction between diaphragm-based delirium and brain-based phrenitis: "No few symptoms anticipate the person's condition, all of which are known as phrenetic signs [φρενιτικὰ σημεῖα] and have been written about by all those who came before me. For example: insomnia or dreams that are troubling because of the clarity of the visual images."[43] The same symptoms are described also by Alexander of Tralles, who states that insomnia and vivid dreams signify the onset of phrenitis, a warning that all is not well in the region of the brain.[44] Macarius' fear that lack of sleep and a dried-out brain might push him toward delirium makes sound medical sense.

Yet, the trajectory of causation in Macarius' text should give us pause for thought. Macarius does not discover himself to be sleepless, diagnose himself with impending phrenitis, and withdraw from the desert. Rather, he seeks out insomnia by simulating the conditions of a phrenetic brain, and only then worries that in doing so he might bring on the full-blown illness.[45] This point is worth dwelling on because it highlights an aspect of phrenitis that is salient to our broader question of the relationship between cerebral health, responsibility, and self-care: individual behavior affects the condition of one's brain. While one's mental condition—that is, reason, self-governance, and perhaps even salvation—is dependent upon the health of one's brain, this does not mean that the mind and soul are at the mercy of the body. The consequence is rather that one has, like Macarius, a responsibility to look after one's brain.

Excessive ascetic practice was a problem with which ecclesial leaders of the fourth and fifth centuries were familiar. The religious authority cultivated by ascetic experts challenged the official hierarchy of the church.[46] Among ascetic practitioners, there was concern that individual self-discipline might undermine the very purpose of disciplinary practice.[47] A common response to this was often to suggest that overenthusiastic asceticism was the consequence of demonic attacks or vainglory.[48] Vainglory was the one passion known to target the otherwise perfected monk.[49] In ascetic texts, it functions as a limit upon the individual's self-discipline.[50] One must abstain not only from food, sleep, and other bodily comforts or necessities, but also from ascetic practice itself, when that practice threatens to make one vulnerable to the demon or disease of vainglory. Strikingly, this spiritual disorder could sometimes manifest as a bodily disease. In this case, disease was not an ascetic practice, but a symptom of an illness of the soul. Andrew Crislip expresses the paradox thus:

> Illness, thus, for some or many in the decades following monasticism's rapid rise in popularity pointed to an *askēsis* gone awry. It raised a number of fundamental questions. Did the illness of the ascetic indicate the obverse of Antony's or Paul's health, a failure of asceticism? Did illness come from the devil or from god? How much responsibility should the individual ascetic, or his peers, bear for illness? Should one be allowed to choose such an injurious lifestyle?[51]

This is, precisely, the dilemma faced by Macarius. What are the moral and ethical implications of choosing "an injurious lifestyle" that might result in the loss of his reason and his inability to further pursue ascetic practice? Macarius' identification of his brain as the part of his body that he is afraid to injure suggests that not only bodily illness, but also specific kinds of bodily illness worked to limit the scope of ascetic discipline.

It was the brain's involvement in voluntary motion that made it so central to a lifestyle of self-control. When Macarius claims that he "conquered so far as depended on [himself]," but "gave way so far as depended on [his] nature," he draws a distinction between intentional action (that is, the sphere of psychic *pneuma*, which carries out the activities of the rational part of the soul) and involuntary motion (the province of vital and natural *pneuma*, each of which performs unconscious activities such as digestion and pulsation).[52] While the brain may be the organ of reason and site of the psychic *pneuma*, the healthy functioning of the brain is dependent upon physiological processes not subject to conscious control. Fragile organ of the *hēgemonikon* that it was, the brain set a limit to ascetic discipline.

The threat of cerebral dysfunction, like that of vainglory, could serve as a tool for disciplining the ascetic practitioner. We see this parallelism more clearly if we consider another story that follows shortly after Macarius' withdrawal from desert exposure: "Having ordered my whole way of life as I desired, I then came to another desire, wherein I wished at that time to keep my mind for five days alone undistracted from God."[53] Once again close to perfection, the anchorite tries to surpass the limitations of his human nature. This time he seeks the transcendence not of the human need for sleep, but of human community itself: "After deciding upon this, I closed the cell and the courtyard so that I might not give answer to any human being; and, starting from the second hour, I took my stance. I ordered my mind, then, saying: 'Do not descend from the heavens; there you have angels, archangels, the powers above, the god of the whole; do not descend below heaven.'"[54] Once again, however, Macarius' attempt to discipline himself into superhuman reverie is thwarted—this time by a demon, which appears in fiery form:

> And when I had endured for two days and two nights, I provoked the demon so much that it became a flame of fire and entirely consumed everything of mine in the cell, with the result that even the little rush mat on which I had taken my stance was burned up, and I thought that I myself would go up in flames. At last I was struck by fear and stepped aside on the third day, unable to render my mind undistracted; I descended instead to contemplation of the cosmos, so that delusional vanity [τῦφος] might not be reckoned to my account.[55]

The inflammation that strikes Macarius on this second occasion is an affective rather than a medical disorder. Or is it? The word *tuphos* ("delusional vanity") was a technical term in both medicine and psychology. The Hippocratic text *Internal Affections* describes *tuphos* as a fever causing excessive heat, loss of bodily control, extreme pain, and—when one is at the point of death—confidence in one's own health.[56] It was also used more broadly to refer to "vanity," as in Clarke's widely used translation of the text.[57] Thus, the late antique lexicographer Hesychius explains *tuphos* as "boastfulness, swelling, vainglory [κενοδοξία]."[58]

Tuphos was commonly associated with vainglory across Christian and non-Christian texts alike. The second-century satirist Lucian of Samosata provides an example in his *Dialogue of the Dead.* Entering the underworld, the Cynic philosopher Menippus (c. 300–250 B.C.E.) encounters the Presocratic philosopher Empedocles (c. 495–434 B.C.E.), who is blistered and burned from his death in the fiery crater of Mount Etna. When Menippus asks Empedocles why he jumped into the volcano, Empedocles cites the illness melancholy (μελαγχολία). Menippus rejects this diagnosis: "No, by Zeus! Rather, it was vainglory [κενοδοξία] and vanity [τῦφος] and much drivel."[59]

Macarius dreams of burning up. He becomes scared, consequently, that *tuphos* (vanity; burning fever) might be "reckoned to his account."[60] We can read this as a retelling of his story about the avoidance of sleep: In this instance, feverish delirium and vainglory are explicitly aligned as pathological effects of disciplining one's body and mind to surpass ordinary human limitations. The affective and physiological consequences that Macarius fears are intertwined.

Advice to Ascetic Women on the Care of the Brain

Macarius and Palladius were not alone in these concerns. In 414, their contemporary, the bishop Augustine of Hippo, wrote a treatise *On the Good of Widowhood* for the wealthy widow Juliana, who had fled to North Africa in the wake of the Visigothic sack of Rome in 410.[61] Written a couple of years after Juliana's arrival on his shores, this treatise sought to dissuade Juliana from adopting celibacy as a mode of spiritual purification:

> But as for those who condemn the marriages of women who have been widowed, even if they exercise their own continence marvelously and fervently [*feruenter*], restraining themselves from many things that you yourself enjoy, do not let them lead you astray on this account, such that you think what they think, even if you are not able to do as they do. For no one wants to suffer from phrenitis, even if she should see that the energy of the phrenetic person [*phrenetici*] is stronger than the energy of those who are healthy.[62]

Augustine's opponents are the British theologian Pelagius and his followers, who argued that human beings are born free from sin, such that one might—indeed, must—earn salvation through obedience to Christian discipline.[63] Augustine seeks to impose a different kind of discipline on Juliana: the moderation of her ascetic perfectionism in acknowledgement of her inescapable imperfection, that is, her need for Christ's grace. His strategy for discounting Pelagian views repeats centuries of Christian and Greco-Roman polemic: he undermines the authority of his opponent by diagnosing a mental disorder. Yet, whereas most such polemic invoked "crazy" in the sense merely of difference or deviance in thought and behavior (for example, through the noun *insania*), a more precise diagnosis lies behind Augustine's use of the word *phreneticus*. The Pelagians who condemn marriage do not suffer from merely any kind of crazy, but from the kind associated by Macarius with vainglory, that is, inflammation of the brain.

The triangulation of asceticism, vainglory, and cerebral health is repeated in another letter that Juliana must have read in the years following her relocation to North Africa. In 414, the Roman theologian Jerome, a colleague and opponent of Augustine, wrote to Juliana's teenage daughter Demetrias, who had renounced marriage in favor of dedication as a holy virgin.[64] Jerome is famous for, among other things, mentoring aristocratic women, all of whom he urged to adopt austere ascetic practices and at least one of whom was thought to have died under his instruction.[65] It is surprising, then, that in his letter to Demetrias, Jerome helps himself to a pinch of moderation. In this passage, Jerome makes the argument that, while some people privilege solitary over communal ascetic practice, isolation can make the minds even of men—not to mention women—slide into illusions of self-sustenance and pride.[66] Nor is this all. Jerome writes: "I have seen the health of the brain [*cerebri sanitatem*] damaged through excessive abstinence [*per nimiam abstinentiam*] in certain individuals of both sexes, and especially in those who dwell in cells that are damp and cold, with the result that they do not know what they are doing or in which direction they turn, what they ought to say, what they ought to do."[67] Jerome's warning resonates with the strategies suggested by Augustine and Macarius for limiting ascetic practice through reference to the weakness of the brain. Nonetheless, he does not suggest that isolated ascetic practitioners suffer from phrenitis—quite the reverse, their problems are caused by an excess of moisture and an absence of heat. Within the framework of ancient medical assumptions about the qualities associated with the gendered body, the extremes reached in each text suggest that Macarius and Augustine are concerned about hypermasculinization (excessive dryness and heat), while Jerome is worried about hyperfeminization (excessive damp and cold). Based on ancient medical assumptions about the gendered qualities of the brain, one might say, in fact, that Jerome's solitary ascetics have feminized their brain by making it cold and wet, whereas Augustine's phrenetic ascetics have hypermasculinized their brain by warming it up and drying it out.

Gendering the Brain in Early Christian Asceticism

Ascetic practices reinforced and challenged gender identity and expression in late antiquity. In particular, the bodies of ascetic women were subject to masculinization, just as earlier martyr narratives had regularly represented the bodies of female martyrs as masculinized through their endurance of violence and deprivation.[68] The shift in focus from martyrdom to asceticism carried this masculinizing potential with it. This was understood both in symbolic terms—luxury and sensory pleasure were feminized in ancient Greco-Roman and early Christian culture—and also through a medical lens. In ancient medicine, the male body was typically considered dry, while the female body was wet.[69] Drying out the female body through diet, bodily activities, or disease rendered it masculine, as Helen King has explored in her analysis of the Hippocratic case study relating to the widow Phaethousa, whose body is rendered masculine—a condition that turns out to be deadly.[70] By late antiquity, this foundational assumption of gendered differences in the qualities of flesh had absorbed new significance from the theory of temperaments, which held that health, physical characteristics, and character all depend upon a balance of the four qualities (hot, cold, wet, and dry).[71] This theory of temperaments meant that the difference between "male" (hot, dry) and "female" (cold, wet) bodies could predict other differences also, in the realms, for example, of sense perception, intelligence, and affect.

The difference between "masculine" and "feminine" flesh extended to the qualities of the brain. On the one hand, the brain was generally considered to be a cold and wet organ; on the other hand, female brains were considered wetter than male brains.[72] This had consequences: women were more prone to diseases involving flux from the head, for example, and were also (as we will see momentarily) more likely to keep their hair. The former consequence is visible in the Hippocratic text *Airs, Waters, Places:* "Men with a phlegmatic temperament and women are likely to suffer dysentery, with phlegm flowing down from their brain, through the wetness of their nature."[73] The ordinary humidity of the female body mimics the physiological behavior of phlegmatic male bodies, that is, it causes the accumulation of phlegm within the brain, and so triggers dangerous flux. Female brains are constitutionally endowed with excess phlegm.

As a consequence of their cold bodies, women lacked body hair.[74] Yet, if beards were a defining characteristic of ancient masculinity, it was women who kept hair on the tops of their heads. The connection between the gendered brain and baldness crops up across several ancient medical and philosophical texts. In his commentary on the Hippocratic text *Epidemics* 6, Galen writes as follows:

> For you learned in the treatise *On Mixtures* that hair grows neither in skin that is excessively moist, nor in skin that is excessively dry. Now then, the skin around the head is moist in children and women and eunuchs, but disproportionately dry in bald men. That the brain in newborns, being soft and wet, touches the cranium and takes up all the space within, while in the old it pulls back, drying out and collapsing, you have observed often in the dissection of animals.[75]

In eunuchs, women, and children the scalp is wet, but in bald men it is exceedingly dry. This is a consequence of aging and its effects on the softness and moisture of the brain. It is also—as the association of children, women, and eunuchs suggests—associated with sexual activity. The pseudo-Aristotelian text known as *Problems* poses the question as follows: "Why do eunuchs not go bald? Is it because they have a big brain?" No, he concludes: "This happens to them because they do not have sex with women. For semen derives from the brain through the spine."[76] Male pattern baldness was thought to be caused by sexual intercourse, which drained fluid from the man's brain for the production of semen.

The idea that male and female brains might be different, and that their difference might be manifest in human hair, appears also in Aristotle's *On the Generation of Animals.* Identifying baldness as akin to the shedding of leaves, feathers, and fur, Aristotle explains the cause of all these conditions as the deficiency of hot moisture that occurs in winter for plants and animals, and later in life for humankind: "That is why before the time of sexual intercourse no one becomes bald, and why at that time it is in those of the sort whose nature is more eager for it. For by nature the brain is the coldest part of the body, and sexual intercourse makes one cold. For it is in fact the secretion of pure and natural heat."[77] The brain, being naturally cold, is the first organ to feel the effects of this cooling of innate heat, and thus the hair withers. This effect is not experienced by other animals because the human brain is "much the largest and the wettest."[78] Women, of course, do not go bald, "because their nature is about the same as that of children. For both are sterile of spermatic secretion." The same is true of eunuchs, who (Aristotle goes on to suggest) "change from the male condition to the female."[79] That is to say: men can cool down their brains through sex or, alternatively, retain the heat that characterizes the female brain through castration.

Pseudo-Aristotle builds on the work of Aristotle himself in his connection between the emission of semen and hair loss. Yet, he goes one step further and claims that semen itself comes from the brain. Within this framework, it is not heat that departs from the brain, but moisture. This shift is suggested by Aristotle's own distinction of human brains not as the coolest/hottest among all animals, but as "much the largest and the wettest." The female brain, with its follicular fecundity, was distinguished not by its retention of heat, but by the retention of moisture; correspondingly, the male brain did not so much cool down as dry out. This explains the disjunction between Aristotle's side comment that only human beings go bald because they have the biggest brains and pseudo-Aristotle's initial suggestion that perhaps eunuchs do not go bald because they have big brains. Aristotle argues that the cooling effects of a large brain are greater than of a small brain. Pseudo-Aristotle, meanwhile, rejects the supposition that eunuchs' brains retain moisture for hair growth because their brains are larger in the first place. In fact, as Pseudo-Aristotle explains, the reason eunuchs have wet brains is that they do not drain their brains of moisture through the emission of seed.

By late antiquity, it was popularly understood that semen derived from the brain. As the North African medical author Vindicianus wrote during the fourth century: "Seed is said to originate in the brain and the marrow of the spine. For it is the moisture in food, produced through bodily concoction and disseminated through the blood vessels and the marrow."[80] Some even suggested that this view went back to the archaic medical author Alcmaeon of Croton, who, it was suggested, considered semen to be a "portion of *enkephalos*," that is, a portion of the brain.[81] Men's brains dry out, as evidenced by their loss of hair, because their brain drips down their spine. This was a necessary process in (and became a sign of) their transmission of form to a child. In this way, the brain itself stood in for the man as a whole. We can see this most clearly in the doxographic split described by the pseudo-Galenic author in the textbook *Medical Definitions*: "Semen, according to Plato and Diocles, is secreted from the brain and the spinal marrow but, according to Praxagoras, Democritus, and in addition Hippocrates, from the whole body."[82] According to the latter theory, that sperm originates from every part of the body, the transmission of features is dependent upon seed from each corresponding part. According to the theory of encephalomyelogenesis (derivation of seed from the brain marrow), information about each of these parts (and their formative power) was consolidated within the brain. When a man grew bald, this served as a sign that he had participated in the activities necessary to imprint himself upon an heir.

Self-restraint with regard to sexual activity was regarded as a necessary condition of masculinity across the ancient Mediterranean world. Sex was not a universally masculinizing activity. Excessive indulgence in sexual pleasure was considered both pathological and feminizing.[83] This tension is reflected in brain physiology also: while a wet (feminine) brain might cause flux, an excessively dry (i.e., hypermasculine) brain could lead to the illness phrenitis—this is the fear that drives Macarius back into human community and into shelter. The point was moderation. While women were considered—by nature—to have sex more often than was necessary, without changing the quality of their brains, how men chose to look after their bodies—how they regulated their sexual behavior—was informed by concern about how they might transform their brains, with highly visible results.[84]

Male ascetic practitioners were like eunuchs, on the one hand, insofar as they abstained from sex and so avoided transmuting their brain substance into semen. On the other hand, both male and female ascetics could dry out their brains, through deprivation of food, drink, and sleep. Ascetic practice was a process of masculinization and sex-free maturation for both men and women. As Macarius reveals, however, even masculinization had its limits. Hypermasculinization, like hyperfeminization, could lead just as surely to insanity. Ideal ascetic practice and the avoidance of vainglory or pride were oriented toward a moderate and mature masculinization that stripped the brain of its moist and labile properties but did not inflame it into arrogance. Gendering the brain is not only about the politics of gender but also about the politics of human vulnerability, potential, and salvation.

Vainglory, Asceticism, and the Brain

Sickness of the brain stood in parallel to vainglory as a consequence of excessive ascetic practice because brain injury impaired the ability to achieve spiritual health. At the same time, brain injury or disease could cause affective disorder. As I discussed in chapter 1, Evagrius of Pontus identified the brain as a particular site of vulnerability for the perfected monk: by touching and palpating the brain and its associated blood vessels, the demon associated with vainglory conjures up a sense perception of God, thereby suggesting to the monk that the goal of prayer has been accomplished, that is, they have achieved perfection.[85] The cause is both the passion (vainglory) and the demonic manipulation of the brain.

Vainglory is a distortion of the perceptual faculty, such that the individual seems to (but does not in fact) see a vision of God. This is because the perceptual faculty is distorted by the physical intervention of a demon; in order to distort one's perceptual faculty, the demon must "touch" and "kindle" the brain and palpate the blood vessel in that region.[86] According to Evagrius, the passion known as vainglory occurs through a physiological mechanism that is triggered by a demon working within the brain. The demon's kindling of the brain and bending of light echo Macarius' account of his own incendiary dream vision. The localization of vainglory within the brain further supports the argument I have put forward in this section, that brain damage and vainglory were parallel risks faced by those who sought ascetic perfection. Sometimes they appeared together as equal threats; sometimes they served as metaphors for one another; and sometimes, one was cited as the other's cause.

As a passion linked to hallucinatory perceptions of God and of oneself, it is unsurprising that vainglory was located within the brain. Its association with phrenitis in particular was fostered by the long-standing figurative relationship between vainglory, vanity, and heat. The association was further supported by certain characteristic symptoms of phrenitis, above all the preternatural strength experienced by the phrenetic patient. As Augustine wrote to Juliana, "no one wants to suffer from phrenitis, even if she should see that the energy of the phrenetic person is stronger than the energy of those who are healthy."[87] The next section explores what Augustine means by this remark. The symptom of preternatural strength proves central to the diagnosis of phrenitis in those who seek salvation through virtue alone.

PHRENITIS, SELF-RIGHTEOUSNESS, AND THE BRAIN

The bishop Augustine named phrenitis over forty times in extant letters, sermons, and polemical tracts, chiefly as a diagnosis of religious opposition.[88] In each instance, Augustine uses phrenitis as a model for sickness of the soul, in particular, a sickness that masks itself from the patient, such that the physician or clergyman is obliged to intervene. A central thread that runs throughout Augustine's engagement with phrenitis—and one that ties it to the anxiety exhibited by Macarius and Jerome that ascetic behaviors in excess might damage the health of one's brain—is Augustine's focus on phrenitis as representing the delusion of self-sufficiency and strength. This was a key symptom in Augustine's understanding of the disease, and he weaves it through his diagnosis of Pelagians (who rely on their ascetic practice for their spiritual strength), of Jews (who rely on their obedience to the law), of Manichaeans (who rely on their superior knowledge), of Donatists (who think that they have achieved purity through a clerical lineage free from capitulation during imperial persecutions), and of "pagans" (who simply do not know that they are in need of salvation). In this section, I examine a series of texts in which Augustine issues a diagnosis in order to draw out the ways in which Augustine employs a medical framework to motivate coercive therapies within his religious and political communities.

While much attention has been paid to Augustine's use of a medical framework for conceptualizing sin, salvation, and pastoral responsibilities, there has been no sustained examination of phrenitis as a discrete and embodied diagnosis in Augustine's medicalization of religious difference.[89] This lack of attention is partially explained by the tendency to render the Latin words for "phrenitis" (*phrenitis, phrenesis, frenitis, frenesis*) and "person suffering from phrenitis" (*phreneticus*) in generic terms, such as "insane," "overwrought," and "delirious." What Augustine refers to is not, in fact, a general "crazy," but rather a discrete medical condition with a set of symptoms that Augustine adapts from technical discourse to suit religious difference and its therapies. By paying attention to how Augustine interprets religious difference or deviance as (like) a disease of the brain, we can develop a deeper understanding of how Augustine uses medical discourse to articulate a vision of Christianity not simply as a healing religion, but as a healing religion that sick people, as a consequence of their sickness, reject.

Phrenitis and the Experience of Strength in Disease

According to Augustine, phrenitis was caused by a problem with the nerves that connect the brain to the sensory and motor organs. In the final book of his *Literal Commentary on Genesis*, Augustine describes the hallucinations caused by phrenitis as the consequence of disturbance (*perturbatio*) of the passages (*iter*), that is, the nerves, that the attention (*intentio*) of the soul follows when it departs from the brain.[90] Since the soul could not, in these circumstances, make use of the sensory organs, and since it could not cease from its own activity, it invented its own images, imprinting them upon the spirit that ran through the brain and nerves as agent of soul.[91] While Augustine's account avoids medical terms, it reflects the Galenic doctrine that *pneuma* travels from the brain into the sensory organs in order to actualize the faculty of perception.

In his philosophical treatise *On the Magnitude of the Soul*, Augustine turns specifically to the effects of phrenitis upon the *nerui* responsible for voluntary motion. Addressing the question of how bodily and spiritual strength might be related, he determines that bodily strength is no index of spiritual power. It is clear, he writes, that people suffering from phrenitis can struggle and resist "with greater strength than in full health," even though their body is wasted by the disease; this is because excessive heat "stretches and hardens their *nerui*."[92]

The superhuman strength of the person suffering from inflammation of the brain was not an Augustinian invention. In a text from the popular philosophical genre of questions and answers, an unknown author poses the question of "why those suffering from phrenitis are strong while they are subject to the affliction, but weak when it departs." The answer is that a "dry imbalance" (ξηρὰ δυσκρασία) has taken hold of the brain and the nerves, which gives the nerves (νεῦρα) tension (τόνον) for activity.[93] It is unlikely that Augustine read this text, not least because it is subject to doubt whether Augustine ever fully learned Greek, the language in which it was written.[94] Nonetheless, the physiological mechanism that the author describes has traveled into Latin clearly enough for Augustine to invoke it not merely as an explanation of phrenitis, but also as a model for how the experience of strength might be caused by disease.

We have already seen this strength invoked in Augustine's critique of Pelagian injunctions to celibacy: "No one wants to suffer from phrenitis," he writes to Juliana, "even if they should see that the energy of the phrenetic person is stronger than the energy of those who are healthy."[95] This was to become a motif in Augustine's writings, especially in polemic against Judaism. In a sermon on Psalm 58, which was preached at Carthage at around the same time that he sent his letter to Juliana, Augustine denounced the strength of "people who base their self-assurance" on wealth, on a muscular body, on high rank, on political power, or—most dangerously of all—on the strength of their own righteousness. These individuals are akin to those who suffer from phrenitis. "But such strength, belonging to those who trust [*praesumentium*] in their own justice," he adds, "has prevented the Jews from entering through the eye of the needle. For, since they trust [*praesumunt*] in themselves as righteous and seem to themselves to be healthy, they have refused medicine and even killed the physician."[96] The preternatural strength of the body that is affected by phrenitis provides a model for the reliance of the Jewish people on their commitment to the law as a guide for righteous living.[97]

In an exposition of Psalm 70, Augustine again devotes his attention to the necessity of grace for the salvation of the soul.[98] His argument is "that all our hope is to be in God, and we are to trust nothing to ourselves, as though in our own strength."[99] The verb translated here as "to trust" (*praesumamus*) recurs in the beginning and end of this sermon, each time in connection with medical care. Speaking again of the Jews, Augustine reports the words of Paul: "Glorying as if in deeds, [Paul] said, they shut out grace from themselves, and they spit out the medicine, as if trusting [*praesumentes*] in their own false health."[100] Augustine concludes with clarification of this medical frame, praying that he will not, like the Jewish people, rely on the law rather than on grace: "Let me not take glory in my own strength; let me not linger in texts; let me reject erudition, that is, the people who glory in texts, meanwhile trusting [*praesumentes*] perversely in their own strength, like those suffering from phrenitis [*phreneticos*]."[101]

Augustine's repetition of *praesumentes* frames his sermon and suggests the import of his diagnosis. The bodily strength characteristic of phrenitis not only masks a deeper bodily disorder, but also causes the sick person to rely upon their own strength. This has two consequences: phrenetic patients act in ways dangerous to their own health; and phrenetic patients resist medical care, sometimes with violence.[102] When, in his sermon on Psalm 58, Augustine accuses the Jews of killing their "physician," he evokes not only the Christian narrative of Jesus's death, but also the more widespread trope in ancient medical discourse that the physician must necessarily tolerate the unpleasant and sometimes dangerous task of caring for the sick (especially the mad).[103] In consequence, a central therapeutic strategy that Augustine highlights is to bind down the phrenetic patient in order to prevent them from doing damage either to themselves or to others.[104] The conclusion to Augustine's sermon on Psalm 70 ("trusting perversely in their own strength, like those suffering from phrenitis") echoes not only his opening use of the word *praesumere*, but also his description earlier in the sermon of how the Christian evangelist Stephen criticized the Sanhedrin (Acts 7:51): "He bound with words those who, suffering from phrenitis, were raving savagely."[105]

Following the medical paradigm of phrenitis, Augustine constructs a set of characteristic symptoms (preternatural strength, unfounded confidence in one's own health, resistance to the physician) and a mode of treatment (bondage; but also, as we will see, soothing words and medication) for a theological or a spiritual disease—that of refusing Christian salvation.[106] The invocation of phrenitis establishes a bind wherein declaration of one's own health, indeed, the voicing of opposition to the Christian model, is a symptom of disease.

Augustine's sermons on the Psalms form a cornerstone in his anti-Jewish polemic.[107] This is in large part because he is engaged in a typological project, reading the Jewish Psalms as prophecies foreshadowing the coming of Christ.[108] His goal is to undermine Jewish readings of the Psalms, in order to appropriate them for the Christian context as supporting evidence both for the life of Jesus (through anticipatory signs that could be identified in the texts) and for the broader narrative of salvation that Jesus's death set into motion. Phrenitis appears in ten of Augustine's sermons on the Psalms, where it functions to undermine Judaism as a form of madness characterized by reliance upon the old narratives of salvation (the law) instead of upon the new (that is, grace).[109]

Twenty-four of Augustine's references to phrenitis (that is, roughly half) are oriented polemically against the Jewish people. Throughout these texts, Augustine uses the trope of Christ the physician to construct a narrative wherein Jews suffer from the same illusion of strength as those who strive for ascetic self-salvation.[110] The Jews—in Augustine's eyes—think that they are strong because they follow the law; in fact, they are fatally ill; in their delirium, the Jews resist the physician with violence. While many have commented that Augustine's Jews are affected by frenzy, it has not been pointed out that, for Augustine, this mental disturbance is not a general but a discrete diagnosis—and one with which we are now familiar. The Jews of Augustine's text suffer from phrenitis, that is, from inflammation of the brain.

All but one of the twenty-four texts in which Augustine diagnoses the Jews with phrenitis are sermons. His account of Jewish resistance to medical care was a narrative that congregations throughout his episcopal territory were to hear repeated again and again.[111] Through this narrative, Augustine taught his congregants—and the congregations who heard his sermons repeated by later medieval preachers—to think about the origin narrative of Christianity in terms of a conflict between Christ the doctor and his phrenetic patients, the Jews.

Sometimes Augustine elaborated further upon the treatment appropriate for the phrenetic patient. Those who rejected Christ were not only to be tied down, but were also to be offered a *medicamentum*, that is, the blood of their own physician:

> You recognize the people suffering from phrenitis [that is, in the context of the sermon, the Jews who called for Christ's death]; recognize the doctor also. "Father, forgive them, because they do not know what they are doing." Those men were raving with their minds destroyed, and they poured out the blood of the doctor through their savagery. But he, meanwhile, was making drugs for the sick out of his very own blood.[112]

The Jewish people refuse the physician, but the medicinal compound that will actually bring about healing is produced through this act of rejection. This is grounded not in the naturalistic medical tradition, but rather in theological symbolism. Nonetheless, Augustine's repetition of this theme renders the metaphor tangible, rather than abstract, in perhaps an unexpected way. The medicine for phrenitis is not only the persuasive speech of the preacher or the philosopher, but also the substance of Christ's blood.[113]

The implications of this become clearer when we recognize that it was not only, according to Augustine, the Jewish people who suffered from phrenitis and who could benefit from this medicine. In a sermon on Psalm 77, Augustine again describes the crucifixion in pharmacological terms:

> The doctor understood that the persons suffering from phrenitis killed the doctor because their minds were destroyed, not knowing that by killing the doctor, they were making a medicine for themselves. For we have all been cured by the death of the Lord, redeemed by his blood, and freed from hunger by the bread of his body.[114]

"We have all" been sick with phrenitis, Augustine tells his congregation.[115] The defining moment of Jewish phrenitis—the resistance to medical treatment that ends in the doctor's blood—paradoxically provides the remedy through which Augustine ensures the salvation of himself and his flock. This is how Augustine prepares his congregation for the Eucharist that is to follow: the wine served to members of the church becomes a medicine for the phrenitis of disbelief.[116] The Jews are not the only people to have suffered from phrenitis; yet it is the Christians who take their medicine and enjoy mental health. This has consequences for how Christians interact with their religious opponents. Above all, diagnosis of a mental disorder establishes a kind of epistemological authority that not only undermines an opponent's theological position, but also justifies one's own intervention into their spiritual care.

In the texts we have considered so far—and, indeed, in Augustine's diagnosis of the Jewish people more generally—Augustine does not speak to any sanctions or therapeutic interventions that might be carried out upon the Jews. Their doctor is Christ, and their medical case history lies in the past. Their importance lies in the establishment of a Christian mythology, wherein the Jewish people represent the mentally ill patient whom the Christian strives not to become. In the next subsection, we turn to contexts in which Augustine the preacher and bishop acts as physician to religious opponents of a more local and immediate context—that is, pagans, Pelagians, and Donatist Christians.

Therapy for the Sick

In a long sermon delivered in the small town of Boseth, close to Carthage, Augustine addresses the non-Christians in his audience directly: "If you still mock," he declares, "you are phrenetic. . . . Phrenetic people often knock down even their doctors, and yet they, being sympathetic of heart, not only do not get angry with those who knock them down, but even seek their health."[117] The doctors here, while they are modeled on Christ the physician, do not represent Christ alone. Rather, they stand in for the body of Christ, that is, the members of the church, and above all the bishops and priests. Christians, Augustine asserts, do not get angry when they are mocked, and actually seek the salvation of those who mock them.

This is, perhaps, a rendition of the Christian scriptural teaching to "turn the other cheek."[118] Yet, it carries here the additional edge that the one who turns the other cheek is not a peer but a doctor, carrying the authority of diagnosis. A similar epistemological hierarchy is constructed in Augustine's treatment of Donatist Christians. Donatism was a rival North African Christian group that was characterized by the demand that none tainted by capitulation during the persecutions should be accepted into, much less appointed as clergy within, the church.[119] By the early fifth century, those who had yielded to imperial demands were dead, but those whom they had appointed as their successors were discredited, in Donatist eyes, by association. Meanwhile, Donatist Christians had elected their own clergy, who presided alongside "Catholic" (or "Caecilianist") priests and bishops across North Africa.[120] In this new world, "Catholicism" meant collaboration with the imperial government, while "Donatism" signified resistance.[121] When Augustine became preacher, the Donatists were powerful; during his episcopate, and partly through his own efforts, the Donatists were slowly crushed by imperial legislation.[122]

Like excessive ascetic practitioners and like the Jews, Donatists were condemned by Augustine as purists who assumed a position of self-righteousness in order to deny the righteousness of others.[123] This self-righteousness was identified by Augustine as a symptom of phrenitis, a symptom that in turn evoked a cluster of other symptoms, including resistance to therapeutic care imposed by their physician. In a sermon on Psalm 34, for example, Augustine argues that suffering alone does not a martyr make.[124] If this were the case, he suggests, the mines would be filled with saints.[125] Rather, what feels to some like persecution might in fact be justifiable punishment (in the case of the criminal), commendable correction (in the case of the son), or therapeutic intervention (in the case of the one who is sick). Thus, he declares:

> Isn't the doctor, being summoned for healing, frequently armed with a knife? This is against the wound, however, and not against the human being. He cuts that he might heal. And yet, when he cuts the sick man, the latter is in pain; he shouts out; he resists; and, if he happens to have lost his mind through fever, he even

> strikes the doctor. But the doctor does not desist from healing the sick man; he does what he knows how to do, and he does not care that the other curses and denounces him. . . . The lethargic are roused up, and the phrenetic are tied down; yet, both of them are treated with love.[126]

Medical intervention is a classic philosophical example of pain that is in fact a good, rather than an evil.[127] I endure the insertion of a drill into my mouth only if I anticipate the removal or avoidance of pain; I allow a knife to cut away parts of my body in the belief that the knife is a medical instrument in the hands of a doctor, who is acting to ward off death and disease. The appropriation of this everyday example for philosophical discussions of virtue and vice lends to medical therapy—and its endurance—a virtuous aspect. It is, by implication, morally valuable to endure short-term pain for the sake of long-term health. Yet, as Augustine also suggests, medical treatment is not always a choice. Psychiatric care, in particular, is enforced regardless of the patient's consent.[128]

Historians of early Christianity have emphasized the similar responsibilities pertaining to preacher and philosopher. In part, these responsibilities involve the moral education of communities through rhetoric.[129] "The long-standing tradition of philosophers who attempted to teach morality to the public," writes Jaclyn Maxwell, "helps us to make sense of the Christian preacher's role in late antique society."[130] In part also, the preacher and philosopher share a medical framework for attending to the psychic health of the individual.[131] There is a clear continuity between philosophical and Christian therapeutics.[132] Psychological affections—"passions"—migrate from the therapeutic texts of Seneca and Galen to the sermons and letters of bishops such as John Chrysostom and Augustine.[133] Anger and grief, for example, are accompanied by physiological events, but are at root behavioral and affective orientations that the individual can, through intentional redirection and recommended modes of self-care, transform.[134] Therapy, in the psychic therapeutics of philosophy and Christianity, is grounded in a practice of pedagogy and an assumption of choice.[135] No individual can moderate their emotions and desires without the intention to do so.[136]

The differences between anger and phrenitis as models for Christian healing are, at least on the surface, fairly clear: philosophical therapy relies upon self-diagnosis and treatment, under the guidance of a teacher; physicians dealing with phrenitis, on the other hand, operate on the assumption that treatment should be enforced regardless of the patient's understanding, participation, or desire.[137] Phrenitis provides a model for therapeutic intervention in a context where the patient refuses treatment: "It was not the Donatists' happiness that Augustine desired . . . but their salvation."[138]

This is clarified in a letter of approximately 417, which Augustine sends to the Roman official Boniface, in an effort to enforce the oppression of Donatist leaders.[139] Boniface is new to his position and asks Augustine to clarify the situation.[140] Augustine explains the relationship between Catholic and Donatist Christians through the analogy of phrenitis:

> For the doctor annoys the raving patient who suffers from phrenitis, and the father his undisciplined son—the first by tying him down, the second by beating him, but both by loving care. Indeed, if they neglect them and allow them to be destroyed, this false gentleness is in fact cruel. For if *the horse and the mule, who have no intellect* [Ps. 32:9], resist with biting and kicking the human beings by whom their injuries are to be treated and healed, the human beings, even though they are often in danger and are sometimes injured by teeth and hooves, do not abandon them until they have returned them to health through medicinal pains and torments. How much less is the human being to be abandoned by the human being, the brother by the brother. Otherwise, he might perish for eternity, who, being corrected, would be able to understand what a great kindness was offered to him, when he was complaining that he suffered persecution.[141]

Augustine situates himself as a doctor responsible for healing the Donatists from the self-righteousness he identifies in their doctrine. The chasm of self-knowledge that diagnosis opens up widens such that the individual loses responsibility not only for their actions, but also for their capacity to know whether they are healthy, and what will make them well. The conflict between Catholic and Donatist Christians is transformed into a combination of (1) therapeutic violence perpetrated by the physician upon the patient, and (2) the irrational violence of the patient who resists medical care. Through this medical lens, what feels to the Donatists like "persecution" is reimagined as necessary therapeutic intervention.[142]

The partnership of "persecution" and "therapeutic intervention" crops up elsewhere in Augustine's account of the conflict between Catholic and Donatist Christians. Early in the fifth century, a series of councils at Carthage and delegations to the imperial court provoked multiple edicts condemning Donatism and prescribing punishment for its leaders and adherents. Most notorious is the "Edict of Unity" (405), a document intended "purely and simply to proscribe Donatism."[143] The text of this edict evokes, albeit more loosely, the discourse of "crazy" that we find in Augustine: "No one is to recall the Manichaean to mind, no one the Donatist, who, as we have discovered, does not desist from raving madness [*furere*]."[144]

Either that year or the next, Augustine reinforced this diagnosis in one of his most important anti-Donatist works, *Against Cresconius, the Grammarian of the Donatist Party*.[145] In this work, Augustine is responding to a letter that Cresconius had sent to him sometime around 401–2, defending the Donatist leader Petilianus.[146] Nonetheless, the recent imperial measures cannot but have been forefront in Augustine's mind as he addressed his opponent's argument that the true Christian does not engage in persecution.[147] Catholic treatment of Donatist Christians does not, Augustine asserts, amount to persecution. As in his sermon on Psalm 34, the significance of pain inflicted depends upon the goal: "Accordingly, since the *freneticus* troubles the doctor and the doctor binds the *freneticus*, either each persecutes the other in turn, or, if persecution is only that which is done wickedly, the doctor does not persecute the *freneticus*, but the *freneticus* persecutes the physician."[148] In this polemical work, phrenitis allows Augustine not only to reimagine Catholic treatment of Donatists as a "kindness" rather than as "persecution," but also to transform Donatist resistance itself into a form of persecution, that is, persecution of Catholics.

This is surprising, given that perhaps the most significant characteristic of phrenitis, for Augustine as for Nemesius and other authors of this period, is lack of self-governance and compromised intentionality. Indeed, phrenitis was a touchstone example of pardonable violence, on the grounds that the individual did not know what they were doing.[149] In a sermon titled *On the Lord's Sermon on the Mount*, Augustine explains the command to "turn the other cheek" with regard to the behavior of infants and *frenetici*.[150] John Chrysostom writes similarly that "people who are sick with phrenitis [οἱ τὴν φρενῖτιν νοσοῦντες] say many evil things to those standing around them, but their listeners do not think that they are being insulted."[151] As Jerome had written of solitary ascetics who injure their brains, "they do not know what they are doing or in which direction they turn, what they ought to say, what they ought to do."[152]

Augustine interprets the violence of the *freneticus* as persecution because he wishes to highlight not only Donatist resistance to the Catholic imperative to convert, but also the acts of violence carried out by Donatist clergy and Circumcellions.[153] The Circumcellions were an anti-imperial group affiliated with the Donatists.[154] They were made notorious through Catholic polemic for encouraging martyr-suicides and acts of violence against Catholic Christians.[155] Augustine continues in his treatise against Cresconius as follows: "Therefore, your savagery and most violent audacity, which are made known through your Circumcellions, who are attendants to your clerics, had to be suppressed by all the laws that have been carried against you, and had somehow to be tied down."[156]

Augustine emphasizes a similar theme in a sermon delivered at Hippo Diarrhytus (Bizerte), an old port town between Hippo Regius and Carthage, several months after imperial measures had been laid down against the Donatists at the Council of Carthage in 411.[157] The sermon is framed around the theme of brotherhood and reconciliation, and begins, appropriately enough, with the conflict between Cain and Abel. Donatists and Catholics, Augustine explains, should be reconciled like brothers. The relationship was, of course, as egalitarian in the eyes of Augustine as that between the sons of Adam. The truth was that it was not (according to Augustine) Donatists and Catholics that needed to be reconciled, but the Donatists that had to be brought into agreement with Catholic norms. Augustine frames this disparity in medical terms:

> Troublesome are those who suffer from phrenitis, who have lost their minds, and who wander hither and thither, sick, raving, and armed with weapons, searching for whom they might kill, whom they might blind—for it was recently announced to us that they have cut out the tongue of one of our priests. Those wicked men suffer from phrenitis. Care must be taken for them, and they are to be loved.[158]

The violence that Augustine identifies as characteristic of the Donatists is not aimed at the physician, but at the family members attendant upon the sick. *Phrenetici* attack not only their physician, but also their fellow Christians. They are to be treated forcibly (albeit with loving care), both for their own sakes, and for the protection of their religious brethren.

Phrenetic patients are endangered not only by their fevers, but also through their own irrational behavior. In a letter written to Vincentius, bishop of Cartenna, in 407 or 408, Augustine argues for the imperial measures that Vincentius disputes:[159]

> For if anyone were to see his own enemy, made phrenetic with dangerous fevers, run headlong, surely in that case it would be to return evil for evils to permit him to go on thus, more so than if one took care that the other was seized and tied up? And yet, one would seem most troublesome and hostile to him, at the very time when one was being most useful and most sympathetic.[160]

Invoking a now-familiar theme, Augustine justifies therapeutic intervention that is undesirable to the patient on the grounds that therapeutic violence is an act of love. Indeed, it is an act that even the person suffering from phrenitis (the Donatist) will appreciate upon recovery:

> Clearly, however, when his health was restored, he would give thanks all the more freely the less he felt he had been spared. Ah, if I could exhibit for you just how many from among those Circumcellions we now consider to be sure Catholics, who condemn their own previous way of life and miserable error, because of which they used to think that whatever they did through their own unquiet and brazen folly, they were doing for the Church of God.[161]

There is symmetry to Augustinian healing practices: The more that the patient resents the therapy they are compelled to receive, the greater their gratitude once their sickness has passed. In this passage, perhaps more clearly than in any other, "Circumcellion" signifies "sick," while "Catholic" means "with health restored." The delusion of the Circumcellions—that is, that they act "for the Church of God"—reflects the confidence in one's own health characteristic of phrenetic patients, founded as it is on preternatural physical strength (in the medical disorder) and "restless temerity" (in the disorder which is Augustinian). Augustine concludes by highlighting the key therapeutic action undertaken in this instance: "Yet, these people would not have been brought to health, had they not been bound like phrenetic patients with the chains of those very laws that displease you."[162]

Augustine's emphasis upon the therapeutic necessity of chains (*uinculis*) is startling. It is not, after all, the chains themselves that bring healing, although cords and bonds were regularly used to delay self-injury.[163] One way of understanding the distinction might be to align the chains here with secular or political intervention ("the chains of those very laws"), in contrast to the pharmacological quality of the Eucharist ("he, meanwhile, was making drugs for the sick out of his very own blood"). Yet, this leaves unclear the role of medicinal speech: do Augustine's sermons, polemical pamphlets, and letters work to heal his religious opponents, or merely to bind them, whether for their own protection or in preparation for healing? The philosophical tradition teaches us that words and rhetoric have a medicinal power.[164] Nonetheless, the line is sometimes blurred, as we see in Augustine's treatise *On the Grace of Christ and Original Sin*.

Here, Augustine discusses the punishment of Caelestius, an associate of Pelagius. Caelestius had been brought before Pope Zosimus and condemned for his view that human beings can attain perfection through virtuous behavior, and (therefore) that babies are born free from original sin.[165] His treatment, which was, according to Augustine, more therapeutic than punitive, nonetheless involved being metaphorically bound: Pope Zosimus "tied up [Caelestius] with his own questions and that man's responses" in order to prevent him from "being carried headlong" (*ferri . . . praecipitem*) or falling "off that precipice" (*in illud abruptum*).[166] When Caelestius promised to condemn whatever was condemned by the See of Rome, "he was treated gently, just like someone suffering from phrenitis, so that he might calm down." Nonetheless, "it was believed that he should not yet be released from the chains of excommunication."[167] Caelestius is bound equally by the chains of speech and those of legal intervention. Augustine seeks to emphasize a continuity between theological defeat and political or religious sanction. His solicitation of formal measures against local enemies is no more than a continuation of his daily sermons and occasional debates; it is certainly not a form of persecution. To the contrary, through the medical lens that Augustine constructs, legal suppression of Donatists and Pelagians is therapeutic intervention that turns pain to a beneficial end.

The strength that was characteristic of phrenitis enabled Augustine to explain how another's self-perception as spiritually healthy could be absorbed into a narrative of Christianity as *the* healing religion. The self-masking properties of phrenitis and the propensity of *phrenetici* to resist medical treatment made the disease a valuable model for demonstrating that individuals could be sick while experiencing themselves as healthy. Augustine justified his intervention into the spiritual lives of his religious opponents by asserting their mental incompetence.

As a disease of the brain, phrenitis also inscribed within the body the cognitive, affective, and behavioral deviance that Augustine identified in his opponents. The body was crucial to late antique accounts of sin and salvation, despite the denigration of the body within ascetic discourse and practice.[168] On the one hand, the body was the locus of human mortality, weakness, and sin. At the same time, Christian practices of asceticism and martyrdom relied upon an understanding of "the body as a blank canvas for Christian inscription," such that bodily change could transform the person as a whole.[169] The resurrection that Christians hoped for was precisely a resurrection of the body.[170] While Christianity might share with pagan philosophy an emphasis upon the transcendence of the soul, Christian spiritual practice demanded the body as its raw material, and aimed itself at an embodied end.[171] The invocation of phrenitis as a model for spiritual sickness weakens the already porous boundary between deviance as a product of the body (not within one's control) and deviance as a product of the soul (within one's control).[172] It thus creates space for a vision of psychic deviance—that is, sin—as a product of bodily and psychic disorder, and so both in one's control and not in one's control. Phrenitis exemplifies the condition of being not in control of one's own psychic health. This was, precisely, Augustine's understanding of original sin.[173] "Thus," as Peter Brown writes, "the Christian life, as seen by Augustine, could only be a long process of healing."[174]

One of the biggest theological questions that Augustine faced was how one must be "healed" (that is, saved): by virtue, or by grace. This was, above all, a question provoked by the teachings of Pelagius and Caelestius.[175] Could the individual earn salvation? Augustine argued vehemently to the contrary, but this left him with an awkward proposition: that spiritual discipline contributes nothing to salvation, and furthermore that God has already marked out those who will be saved, in some sense predetermining the damnation of the rest.[176] A version of this problem is illuminated by the Augustinian theologian Ellen Charry:

> The third and last book of *On Free Will* tackles the difficult question of divine foreknowledge and freedom of the human will, asking whether God makes us happy or whether we make ourselves happy. Augustine wants to maintain the force of both positions, and he ultimately argues that even if God knows that one will be happy a year hence, this does not rob one of the will to happiness now. . . . He teeters on a trembling fence, fearing that any concession of power to us would undermine God's power, but also knowing that denying all power to humans would destroy moral responsibility. It is not clear that Augustine ever resolves this tension.[177]

As Charry later points out, we might replace the adjective "happy" here with the word "saved."[178] Human beings have, in Augustine's conception of salvation, a moral responsibility to make themselves happy, that is, to be healed; at the same time, their capacity to attain happiness is dependent upon factors beyond their control—namely, the intervention of God.

Augustine sought a resolution to this problem through his conceptualization of original sin, grace, and free will. Yet, as Charry makes clear, the tension was never definitively settled, and theologians continue to try to resolve it.[179] In Augustinian phrenitis, we might observe not only a spiritual illness that causes the experience of strength in illness, but also a translation of the problem of predetermination from the divine to the bodily realm. Organic mental illness illustrates how embodiment might render one incapable of actions and attitudes conducive to spiritual health.[180] In this respect, it offered a paradigm within which to understand human rejection of God as an action that one might not be able to control, but the effects of which one nonetheless suffered. One might, after all, not intend to run off the edge of a cliff, but one nevertheless strikes the ground with the same force.

CONCLUSION

This chapter has examined late antique Christian metaphors of phrenitis that center upon the idea that excessive ascetic practices (and their psychological equivalent, self-righteousness) might cause, be caused by, or be identical with, inflammation of the brain. Just as the previous chapter demonstrated how luxurious behaviors and indulgence in sensory pleasures might endanger the vulnerable brain by flooding it or softening it, so also excesses of asceticism threatened the soul, by hardening and drying out the brain. The rhetoric of cerebral vulnerability was employed in late antique Christian texts to guide audiences toward a moderate care of the body that might ensure the health of the brain, and therefore the integrity of psychological functions, emotional well-being, and even, by extension, virtue and salvation. As my analysis of Augustine's use of phrenitis to diagnose religious "others" reveals, this rhetoric of cerebral vulnerability was not simply pedagogical, but underwrote a program of political and ecclesial coercion and an ideology of ecclesial community that depended upon assuming an identity as "healed."

Metaphors and models of phrenitis were not simply tools for shoring up one's own authority, or indeed for undermining the salvation and reason of others. They also created a context for working out tensions in the Christian worldview, in particular the question of whether and how an individual might contribute to (or obstruct) their own salvation. The slippage between phrenitis of the brain and phrenitis of the soul that emerges across the different texts examined in this chapter was part of a broader deployment of the brain as a site for negotiating the tensions that arose from the Christian appropriation of a medical paradigm for individual salvation and the resurrection of body and soul. It is this broader deployment of the brain in late antique theological anthropologies that I turn to in the final chapter.

CHAPTER 7

Humanizing the Brain in Early Christianity

Animal brains served as the basic model for brain anatomy and function in human beings within the ancient Mediterranean world. With the exception of a fleeting window of opportunity in Hellenistic Alexandria and the occasional roadside skeleton or body that washed out of its tomb, human vivisection and dissection were strictly taboo. Anatomical demonstrations designed to prove that the rational soul or mind operated through the brain were performed on animal bodies. There was a latent tension in this: human anatomy was thought to enable distinctively human activities, yet these functions could be demonstrated through animal brains. The introduction of Christianity compounded this tension. The difference between humans and animals was not just a question of categorization or even of power but of planes of being and access to immortality. Humans were uniquely intended for corulership with God. Unlike both animals and angels, humans had access to salvation. While these faculties pertained to the soul, they were fundamentally rooted in the body—the ultimate promise of Christianity, after all, was bodily resurrection, and its mechanism was the death of the embodied Christ.

According to early Christian authors, human bodies were peculiarly designed for reason and governance, which were crucial to the capacity for salvation. We see this in the repeated use of anatomical knowledge, borrowed from medical and philosophical texts, to support the claim that human bodies are providentially designed for rational governance over other animals. The brain was considered fundamental for these activities—especially reason, but also moral choice and rulership. This is clear both from direct explanation and from the newly burgeoning personification of the brain as a governing figure. Strikingly, however, we never see any reference to comparison between animal and human brains in early Christian texts: while Christian authors compare hands, stature, mouths, and other parts of the body in order to demonstrate the ways that human anatomy supports rational governance, and even though they claim the brain is the instrument through which this rational governance is enacted, they never compare human brains with their animal counterparts. This absence is challenging to explain, but by exploring it we can begin to unpack the stakes that early Christian authors had in the brain as a conceptual tool for talking about what it meant to be human.

This chapter proceeds in six parts. First, I return to two key texts in which early Christian authors address comparative anatomy: Tertullian's *On the Soul*, which rejects animal models for the human soul, and Hippolytus' *Refutation of All Heresies*, which rejects the brain as a model for the cosmos. Next, I lay out a brief history of the comparative anatomy of the brain in ancient medical and philosophical work, with a focus on the use of a teleological lens to explain anatomical structures in terms of their functions. The third section turns to the incorporation of comparative anatomy into early Christian texts in order to support the legitimacy of human governance over other animals. This section highlights the absence of the brain from these anatomical discussions; part 4 examines possible reasons for its exclusion. In order to further unpack the implications of this absence, I turn in part 5 to Christian discussions of the brain in relation to governance: both the role of the brain in self-governance and metaphors of the brain as a human ruler. I suggest that the absence of the brain from comparative accounts might, somewhat paradoxically, reflect its centrality to the understanding of what it meant to be human. That is to say, perhaps early Christian authors eliminated the brain from their comparative anatomy in order to present the brain as a distinctively human organ. Finally, I explore the implications of this particular association of the brain with the human being qua rational governor in light of the modern concept of cerebral subjectivity, that is, the idea that the human self is identified with the brain.

COMPARATIVE ANATOMY AND THE *HĒGEMONIKON*

In Tertullian's treatise *On the Soul*, a reiteration of a common package of ideas takes an unexpected turn. The chapter titled "On the Governing Part of the Soul" poses the question of whether there is in fact any "governing part," and whether it has a bodily location.[1] Tertullian listed off the usual suspects (Plato, Hippocrates, and so forth), then turned to those authors—above all, Asclepiades—who taught there was no *hēgemonikon* (in Tertullian's Latin, *principale*) at all. According to Asclepiades, the organ of the *hēgemonikon* cannot be the brain because there are some animals that "continue to live and be sentient" even with their heads cut off (the examples that Tertullian provides are flies, wasps, and locusts). On the other hand, the organ of the *hēgemonikon* cannot be the heart, since some animals similarly maintain conscious awareness "if you cut out their heart" (for example, Tertullian adds, goats, tortoises, and eels).[2] Animals that exhibit the functions of the *hēgemonikon* without either hearts or brains serve as evidence that there is no *hēgemonikon* at all, that is, no entity that is exclusively responsible for sensation, voluntary movement, and other mental activities.

Asclepiades' argument relies on the assumption that (1) the *hēgemonikon* is coextensive with its bodily organ and (2) this bodily organ must be the same in all creatures.[3] For Asclepiades, animal anatomy provides a basic and non-negotiable template for theorizing how the human body functions, since all bodies are formed according to shared structures and logics. We catch a glimpse of the intellectual background to this argument in Galen's *On the Usefulness of the Parts*, which reports a debate about the observation that crustaceans do not have heads.[4] The focus of the debate seems to be the question of whether the *hēgemonikon* takes the brain or the heart as its instrument. Within the cardiocentrist position, the head and the brain appear to have no function, if we (as Galen does, at some length) discount Aristotle's theory of the brain as a kind of refrigerator.[5] For the encephalocentrists, meanwhile, the organ of the *hēgemonikon* is typically in the head, except where a head is lacking, in which case it is in the chest. Crucially, for Galen, this organ is the *enkephalos*, wherever it is located. This is because, despite its name (*enkephalos*, "in the head"), the proper definition of any bodily part must refer to its function rather than its placement within the body: just as "eyes" are called "eyes" no matter their form and position, "so likewise, then, the instrument in control of sensation and motion is one and the same in all animals, even though it is found in different locations."[6]

For Galen, the crucial point is that the lack of a head in some animals should neither compromise his argument for encephalocentrism nor imply that the *enkephalos* is functionally useless, since some animals do not appear to require it. The important point for our purposes is that Asclepiades' assumption that the organ of the *hēgemonikon* must be the same across all animals was rooted in medical and philosophical debates and may have emerged (as in Galen's account) out of conflict between different paradigms and opinions. Tertullian is clearly tapping into a conversation of which only fragments remain. Whereas Galen resolves the problem of the missing heads by reinterpreting the *enkephalos* as the instrument of the *hēgemonikon* (specifically, "the instrument in control of sensation and motion") rather than as the "organ in the head," Asclepiades explains the question of why some animals maintain sensation and motion without heads or without hearts by suggesting that there is no *hēgemonikon* (and therefore no instrument of the *hēgemonikon*) at all.

Tertullian was having none of this. In his view, it is necessary for the activities of human reason to be embodied. "Flesh is the thinking-room of the soul [*animae cogitatorium*]," as he argued elsewhere.[7] Given his Stoic influences, Tertullian unsurprisingly favored the heart as the instrument of the *hēgemonikon*; however, he reserved his harshest criticism for Asclepiades and his ilk. He does not draw on medical knowledge in his refutation. Instead, he cites scriptural references to the heart as the site of the soul and the source of moral knowledge in order to make his first point; when it comes to his second point, he turns to brute insult: "Besides, everyone knows that he who judges the nature of the human soul from the condition of animals is himself without either heart or brain."[8]

In Latin literature, "brainless" was a surefire synonym for "stupid." This was true even among those who held to a cardiocentrist position: Jerome, for example, interpreted the Hebrew word *raca* as "κενός, that is, 'void' or 'empty.' We can express this by the popular insult 'brainless' [*absque cerebro*]."[9] Tertullian stretches this insult to include the heart and makes both quasi-representatives for reason. Those who lack either are lower than animals, which, within the argument as framed here, have one or the other. There's also a kind of etymological argument embedded in this insult: if neither the heart nor the brain were the organ of the *hēgemonikon*, the reader is supposed to understand, then "heartless" and "brainless" would not be popular insults.

The absence of medical arguments here—either for the identification of the heart as the organ of the *hēgemonikon*, or for the existence of a *hēgemonikon* and associated organ in the first place—perhaps speaks to the fact that by the second century C.E., medical encephalocentrism clashed with the cardiocentrism of Stoic and Christian texts. It may also reflect a lack of familiarity with anatomical handbooks or public dissections of the kind that we saw, back in chapter 3, mirrored in the detailed ekphrasis of brain anatomy offered by the contemporaneous theologian Hippolytus of Rome. Yet, while there is a clear distinction between Hippolytus' explicit familiarity with medical perspectives on the brain and Tertullian's use of scripture and insult, the two have in common two key strategies: denying the possibility of using the (animal) brain as a model for higher orders of intelligence and ensoulment. Tertullian could have said that those who think there is no *hēgemonikon* are heartless and brainless; instead, he chose to dismiss comparative anatomy wholesale as a source for understanding human anatomy.

Hippolytus, similarly, rejected the use of the brain as a cosmological and theological model. Recall how Hippolytus describes the anatomy of the brain in order to refute the idea attributed to hebdomadal theologians that the brain might itself be interpreted as a physical model for "the substance and the power and the paternal godhead of the universe."[10] As I discussed in chapter 3, Hippolytus' account of how the *pneuma* is propelled through the ventricles and channels of the brain offers the reader an ekphrasis of a vivisection, very possibly an event that Hippolytus had witnessed or at least heard about in Rome. I argued further that this ekphrasis, which does not contribute obviously to Hippolytus' argument, might be interpreted as an assertion of rhetorical and perhaps even medical authority. What I want to suggest here is that implicit within his account is a demystification of the brain by summoning in the reader's mind the image of a brain that belongs to an animal.

While Hippolytus does not specify whether the brain that he is describing is human or animal, the implied context of his description suggests the latter. Apart from a very brief window of opportunity in Hellenistic Alexandria and some rare cases of head injury, there was no way for ancient audiences to witness the vivisection (or even, with some rare exceptions, dissection) of a human brain. In his representation of a working brain visible to the human eye, Hippolytus calls to mind performances and descriptions of the vivisection of animals familiar from the writing of Galen.

Hippolytus' reason for doing so is perhaps to neutralize the potency of the brain as a model for the organization of the cosmos and divine power. The image of an animal brain—exposed on the dissection table, operating through the movement of material parts and the flow of *pneuma*—is his entire argument against the use of the brain as an analogy within hebdomadal theories. Whereas the human brain epitomized the inexplicable manifestation of immaterial intellect through material bodies that hebdomadal theorists saw writ large in the universe, the animal brain merely functioned to enable sensation, voluntary motion, and consciousness, each of which could be explained in material terms and without reference to reason. The animal brain was a kind of boundary object that gestured to the inexplicable animation of the rational human being, while itself remaining solidly in the world of natural and irrational functions, without the capacity either to organize and govern or to serve as a useful analogy for the organization and governance of the cosmos. By representing the brain as subject to vivisection, Hippolytus implicitly evoked the animal brain, and so limited its symbolic potential.

In Tertullian and Hippolytus, we find two distinct refutations of the comparative anatomy of the brain (animal/human, brain/cosmos) that reflect existing debates about how the brain might model the invisible and inexplicable activities of reason as it operates in and through material bodies. Tertullian's rejection of animal models for the embodiment of the human soul represents a critical moment in Christian engagement with the tools and texts of comparative anatomy that were available within the medical and philosophical traditions. By asserting that animal models were worse than useless as models for the exceptional rationality of the human being, Tertullian indicated the need for a specifically human anatomy. What was it about the human body that enabled the activities of the mind? In a way, although he would thoroughly have resented this, Tertullian's rejection of animal models and his inclusion of the insult "brainless" pointed the way toward the erasure of animal bodies from accounts of the brain, such that it could become, at least in symbolic terms, a distinctively human organ, responsible for such human activities as kingship and self-control.

Hippolytus' rejection of the brain as a model for the cosmos seems to have held sway. We rarely witness subsequent Christian authors employing brain anatomy to illustrate or prove the relationships between different levels and kinds of spiritual and material beings—with the important exception of the relationship between God and humans. Within these analogies, the brain sometimes represents the divine ruler over other parts of the body (i.e., Christ as the "head" of the church, as we saw in chapter 4) and at other times represents the embodied intelligence unique to human beings. Following upon the interventions that Tertullian and Hippolytus performed into the ways that brain anatomy was used to model deeper mysteries, the brain seems to have narrowed to a model for humans and their place within the cosmic hierarchy.

While Tertullian and subsequent Christian authors were clearly aware that most animals had organs inside their head (the generic meaning of *enkephalos*) and organs responsible for sensory and motor functions (Galen's definition of *enkephalos*), comparative discussion of animal and human brains was no longer on the table. Animals ceased to serve as suitable models for understanding how the rational soul operated through the human brain, and the concept of the brain itself became increasingly associated with human identity, agency, and judgment.

If the functions of the human brain were learned through experimentation on animals, then what was it that made the brain itself responsible for human activities, such as governance and reason?[11] We find no answers to this question in late antique texts, only silences: subsequent authors followed Tertullian in excluding comparative anatomy from their accounts of the human brain and its functions. In their metaphors and descriptions of the brain, animals are absent; in their comparisons between animals and humans, the absence is the brain.

COMPARATIVE ANATOMY AND THE BRAIN

In most ancient Greek philosophical and medical frameworks, anatomical knowledge was organized around the principle of teleology, that is, each bodily structure or material perfectly serves its proper end or function. Examples of this range from the obvious (the stomach is constructed to digest food) to the obscure (according to Aristotle, the brain is as a cooling system whose function is to counterbalance the innate heat of the heart) and from the very broad (the human body is the instrument of the rational soul) to the minute and specific (the spongy quality of the skull is designed to lighten the head as a whole and prevent the animal from collapsing under its weight, according to Galen).

Teleological anatomy could be presented in terms of a creator's act of design (as in the work of Plato and in Christian texts) or in terms of a more or less personified nature/Nature and theoretical principles about how things in nature ought to be (especially Aristotle and Galen). While teleology was a very common principle, its application was varied, and it raised a number of philosophical questions: Did each anatomical part have only one function or several? If the latter, then was one function primary? Were there parts of the body that had no function at all? What were the boundaries that defined an individual part? We have already seen this last question, for example, in the debate regarding whether the brain is to be defined by its location or by its function; when defined in terms of function, the further question arose of whether the *enkephalos* was the organ in the head (or equivalent) alone or if it extended to include the spinal cord and nerves.

For early Christian authors, the medical and philosophical tradition of teleological anatomy became central to arguments about the providential design of human bodies as exceptional among created beings. That is to say, theologians and preachers borrowed arguments about how anatomy supported the functions of the parts to support their claim that God specifically designed human bodies to be uniquely capable of intelligence and suitable to rule over creation. As we will explore in the subsequent section, they focused specifically on comparative anatomy of specific parts of the body thought to support reason; while they were aware of the central importance of the brain, it is absent from their comparisons. Here, I focus on places where the brain appears in ancient comparative anatomy in order to identify possible texts and traditions that early Christians chose not to incorporate into their own accounts.

Aristotle: Human Brains Are Bigger and Wetter

Aristotle was a central source for teleological explanations of the parts of the body and, especially in *Parts of Animals* and *History of Animals*, for comparative anatomy also. Subsequent discussions of the features of the human body that made it peculiarly designed for reason and governance tended to draw on Aristotle's work, especially in relation to stature, mouth parts, and hands.[12] When it came to the brain, Aristotle's comparative observations were less relevant. Since Aristotle was a cardiocentrist, the differences between human and animal brains did not, for him, have any direct bearing on the differences between human and animal intelligence. Instead, he focused on the function of the brain as a cooling device: according to Aristotle, human brains were the biggest and wettest among all animals. The reason for this was the need to counteract the intense heat produced by the human heart.[13] This comparison does not show up at all in the teleological anatomy that late antique Christian authors incorporate into their accounts of human superiority.

Erasistratus of Ceos: Human Brains Have More Convolutions

The Hellenistic anatomist Erasistratus of Ceos, born shortly after the death of Aristotle, argued that there was one key anatomical difference between human and animal brains—a difference that contributed specifically to cognitive capacity: "Just as in other animals—deer, hare, and any others that far surpass the rest in running, being well provided with the muscles and sinews useful for this activity—so too in humans, since they are far superior to other animals in thinking, the cerebellum is large and has many folds."[14] That is to say, the human brain is larger in its rear portion and is more convoluted than that of the animal. Erasistratus builds on Aristotle's claim that the human brain is the largest among all the animals but explains its distinctive size in terms of cognitive capacity. According to Erasistratus, the brain can be conceptualized like a muscle.

If cognitive capacity correlates to the size and convolution of the cerebellum, then the difference between human and animal brains—and between human and animal cognition—is one of quality or degree. The act of "thinking" is the same kind of thing among all embrained creatures. It is perhaps predictable, then, that this view does not show up at all in early Christian accounts of comparative anatomy. Yet, it seems to have been popular or prominent enough for Galen to feel the need to explicitly reject it, using as his evidence the observation that donkey brains are bigger and more convoluted than those of humans.[15]

We might ask ourselves whether Galen's motivation in rejecting Erasistratus' theory reflected the urgency of reporting his own anatomical observations (here, of donkey brains), the need to assert a theory of brain function that focused on the movement of *pneuma* through the ventricles, or qualms about the notion that the difference between brains and their capacities might be quantified. As we see in the next section, Galen did think that animal and human brains did the same kind of thing, but he did not comment at all on how or why they did it differently.

Galen's Experimental Design

Galen sought to prove through experiments upon living animals that the brain was responsible for reason and self-governance.[16] Since he understood rational thought to be a distinctively human quality, Galen designed experiments that measured something other than the manifestation of rational thought. The relevance of his experiments to human bodies derived from the assumption that the difference between human and animal capacities was again one of degree rather than kind, such that an examination of the structures and functions of the animal brain might prove the attribution of similar (but more advanced) functions to similar or identical structures within the human brain. Two of Galen's most infamous experiments provide ample illustration.

The first involved an ox. Galen performed this demonstration for students and in public; he also wrote about it in his anatomical handbook *On Anatomical Demonstrations* and in his philosophical treatise *On the Opinions of Hippocrates and Plato.*[17] It was supposed to prove that the brain was the seat of sensation, voluntary motion, and consciousness. The experiment focused on the ventricles within the brain. The basic point that Galen sought to demonstrate was that sensation, voluntary motion, and consciousness were dependent upon the presence of *pneuma* within the ventricles, rather than upon the integrity of the substance of the brain itself.

Galen first sliced through the skin and the pericranium, then cut away the bone and peeled back the outer cerebral membrane.[18] In his discussion *On the Opinions of Hippocrates and Plato,* he offers a detailed description of what follows:

> After the bone of the head has been removed—the animal being still alive—and once the outermost membrane has been laid bare, when you have pulled it back with hooks on each side of the middle line at which it is doubled and descends into the brain, if you merely cut it or if you remove it entirely, the animal does not lose sensation or motion. Nor does it lose them if you cut or remove that portion of it which covers all the back part of the brain. And even if you cut away the brain itself in any manner, even then the animal does not lose motion and sensation, until the incision reaches one of the ventricles.[19]

Galen offers us a slow reveal that draws in the reader's attention. Sensation and motion are *not* lost if the outermost membrane is "merely cut" or removed, *nor* if the part that covers the back part of the brain is removed, *nor* even if the brain itself is cut away in any manner, but only once "the incision reaches one of the ventricles." He draws out the suspense to add weight to his big reveal (the answer to the question, *What part of the brain is responsible for motion and sensation?*), which itself indicates the answer to an even bigger question (*What part of the brain is responsible for self-governance?*).

Like Hippolytus, Galen uses ekphrastic techniques to mimic the experience of watching a vivisection of a functioning brain in order to demonstrate a point beyond that which the vivisection itself exhibits. By revealing the operations of the bovine brain, Galen seeks to prove how the soul gives rise to consciousness and reason within the human body. Whereas Hippolytus rejected the use of the brain as a model for the materialization of intellect in the cosmos,

Galen had no such qualms. Probing or cutting each ventricle of the brain in turn, he showed his audience that each ventricle played a vital role in animal consciousness:

> Should the brain be compressed on both the two anterior ventricles, then the degree of stupor which overcomes the animal is slight. Should it be compressed on the middle ventricle, then the stupor of the animal is heavier. And when one presses down upon that ventricle which is found in the part of the brain lying at the nape of the neck, then the animal falls into a very heavy and pronounced stupor. This is what happens also when you cut into the cerebral ventricles, except that if you cut into these ventricles, the animal does not revert to its natural condition.[20]

Galen thought that cutting into the cerebral ventricles sent the animal into a stupor because it allowed the escape of psychic *pneuma*, the gaseous substance that traveled from the brain through the nerves to enable sensory and motor functions. The same mechanism, Galen asserted, explains the loss of sensation and voluntary motor activity in human beings. In oxen, the sign of reduced sensory and motor functions was simply "stupor," an apparent loss of consciousness that stands in for self-report (*Can you see my hand moving? Can you move your hand?*). Despite the presumed innate stupidity of the ox, Galen assumed that bovine and human brains perform the same basic sensory and motor functions.

Galen's second experiment involved a squealing pig.[21] This experiment was a response to the following Stoic argument: the voice is an indubitable function of the governing power of the soul; the physical source of the voice is the lungs; the lungs are closer to the heart than to the brain; therefore, the heart must be the command center from which the words—given force by the lungs—are dispatched.[22] Galen dismissed this "argument by proximity" as incidental and insisted that anatomical connection was essential for demonstrating functional association.[23] Identifying the nerve that runs between the larynx and the brain as the anatomical connection necessary for speech, he designed an experiment to prove his case. Taking a live (and squealing) pig, he opened the animal up and tied its laryngeal nerve with a strip of wool. Immediately, the animal stopped squealing. Once Galen released the ligation, the animal resumed its cries. Clearly, so Galen argued, the laryngeal nerve carries the chief impulse for speech from the brain into the voice box.

Galen's animal experiments served as the foundation of medical knowledge in late antiquity.[24] Yet, what they demonstrated was not how physiological processes produced reason and self-control, since animals were not thought to possess these qualities, but rather the activities on which they depended—sensation, voluntary motion, vocal expression, and consciousness. The assumption that underlay Galen's experiments was that if you could identify the bodily origin of some faculties associated with governance (vocalization), then you could identify the bodily source of them all (verbalization).[25] He was careful, however, not to call these animal functions "reason" or "self-control." The connection remained implicit.

For practical reasons, the animal brain was the standard model for the anatomy and functions of the human brain in the ancient world. Comparisons between human and animal brains were limited by the taboos around dissecting or vivisecting human bodies: the chief points of comparison were of magnitude, humidity, and complexity, rather than of the presence or absence of specific structures. Erasistratus and Galen, whose dissections of the brain (together with those of Herophilus) established the framework for all subsequent knowledge of brain anatomy within the Greek and Roman medical traditions, treated human brains as doing the same kind of thing as animal brains, albeit at a different level of sophistication. The knowledge that they produced served as the foundation for Christian accounts of the brain as central to self-governance and reason; the absence of animal comparisons from Christian discussions might reflect the desire to draw a clearer distinction between human and animal cognition as fundamentally different kinds of activities.

ANATOMICAL ARGUMENTS IN SUPPORT OF HUMAN HEGEMONY

Early Christian authors borrowed medical and philosophical arguments about comparative anatomy to support the claim that humans were intended as rulers over creation. This strategy was part of what animal studies scholars have identified as the early Christian consolidation of earlier philosophical tendencies to privilege the human being over other animals, establishing theological foundations for speciesism.[26] While Aristotle and the Stoics denied animals the faculty of reason and so justified practices of sacrifice and consumption, early Christians used the concept of an exclusively human reason to explain why human beings alone should enjoy communion with God and access to salvation. It was only insofar as they were rational that human beings could be said to be made in the "image of God," who was the ultimate rational being.[27] As a consequence, humans were the only legitimate rulers over the created order, mirroring God's governance over the cosmos.

This section will outline in detail the ways in which early Christian authors used anatomical knowledge to construct this argument. My purpose is to establish the textual and theological framework within which the absence of the animal brain carried meaning. First, I will examine the use of comparative anatomy to argue for human governance and exceptionalism. I will then turn to noncomparative discussions of brain anatomy to argue that the absence of the brain does not reflect lack of relevance or knowledge but an active choice to avoid comparison.

Sharing a material body with animals but immaterial reason with God, the human being was, in the words of Nemesius, "assigned a place on the boundary between the non-rational and the rational nature."[28] So he explains: "That is why they also define man as a rational animal, mortal and receptive of intellect and knowledge. An animal, because man too is an animate, sensitive being: for this is the definition of an animal. 'Rational,' in order to separate him from non-rational animals. 'Mortal,' in order to separate him from rational immortals."[29] Humans who indulge in the pleasures or concerns of the body, Nemesius continues, sink into the condition of nonrational animals, while those who dedicate themselves to reason become like heavenly creatures, assimilating themselves to God. Distinct from animals, humans were thought to have rational souls. Distinct from angels, humans were thought to have material bodies. Alone among all created beings, humans could move from mortality to immortality, through the process of salvation—a product both of divine grace and also of human virtue and self-control: one way of thinking about it, Nemesius writes, is that the human being "was created mortal, but capable of being immortal if perfected by progress: in other words, potentially immortal."[30]

The exceptionality of human reason was the foundation not only of Christian salvation, but also for the assumption of human dominance over the rest of creation.[31] The human being, wrote Nemesius, was "established as ruler" over the animals, just as the rational soul is ruler over the body: "If the rational part in us rules the nonrational part in us, how is it not reasonable that it should also have mastery over the nonrational things external [to us] and that they should have been given to serve its needs? For it is the natural role of the nonrational to serve the rational, as was shown with regard to ourselves."[32] The rational soul governs the nonrational "part" of the human being *and also* all other nonrational things, such as plants and animals. Self-governance was both the premise and model for dominance over the environment. This was not only a matter of degrees of power (that is, reason makes humans more powerful than animals), but of the role of the human being as a link in the chain between animal (nonrational, material) and divine (rational, immaterial) beings: it was the rational soul at work in the human body that enabled the human to rule the material world. Human exceptionality as a rational, self-governing, embodied species was the premise for understanding the position of the human being within the cosmos: not only near the top of the chain-of-being familiar in ancient philosophy, but a mediatory being, joining "things intelligible and things visible" in the organization of the cosmos.[33]

The human participated in both body and soul, earth and heaven, animal and god. Within the body, the brain played a similar role. It was a material governor over material parts, and it gained its governing power through its communion with the immaterial, rational soul.[34] Within the ecclesial community, the brain could be used also as a figure for Christ.[35] Such imagery tapped into the metaphor THE BRAIN GOVERNS in order to cast political, ecclesial, and sometimes domestic dramas within the microcosm of the individual body, but the role of the brain was not restricted to analogy. The brain was directly responsible for the human activities that enabled governance over one another and over creation: reason; moral choice; self-governance.

According to early Christian doctrine, this was no accident. Each individual part of creation was designed for its own proper function. Since the human body was the instrument of the rational soul, individual parts of the body could be understood to have been tailored to enable rational and governing activities.[36] These parts were necessarily different from the parts of animal bodies. Not only this, but the human body was thought to surpass "all things in grace and beauty."[37] Through comparative anatomy, theologians charted the exceptionality of the human soul. Strikingly, however, their accounts systematically excluded the brain.

The central argument of early Christian comparative anatomy was that the human body is physically weaker than the body of many animals, but that human reason—effected through the careful design of the human body—enables domination of animals, nonetheless. This claim was grounded in philosophical and medical tradition. Aristotle, in *On the Parts of Animals*, rejects the claim that "the human being has been constructed not better but worse than [other] animals," given its lack of innate bodily protection or weaponry.[38] Aristotle's rejection of this claim depends upon the hand, which is uniquely adaptable, enabling humans to employ multiple kinds of weapons, and thereby manifesting human intelligence. While hands may seem weak, they are in fact the perfect tool. "Nature," Aristotle goes on, "invariably gives each tool to the [creature] that is able to use it."[39] That is to say, hands indicate human rationality. Galen echoes Aristotle in the opening to *On the Usefulness of the Parts:* "Now to the human being—for this is an intelligent animal and, alone of all creatures on earth, godlike—in place of any and every defensive weapon, [nature] gave hands, instruments necessary for every art and useful in peace no less than war."[40] Concluding his elaboration of Aristotle's point, Galen adds one more thing: "Now just as the human body is bare of weapons, so the soul is destitute of skills. Therefore, to compensate for the nakedness of the body, [the human being] received hands, and for his soul's lack of skill, reason. . . . For if he had been born with a natural weapon, he would have that one alone for all time, and just so, if he had one natural skill, he would lack others."[41] Physical weakness and a lack of instinctual skills are necessary to reason, since any creature that has sufficient innate tools and methods for survival will not develop others.

In Christian literature, these arguments were redeployed with less attention to the hand and more to the consequences of human reason: the capacity to dominate other animals. In his letter *On the Constitution of the Human Being,* for example, Gregory of Nyssa writes as follows: "But the human is marched into life naked of natural coverings, weaponless and poor, in need of everything useful, worthy, according to appearances, to be pitied, rather than considered blessed, being armed neither with projecting horns, sharp talons, hoofs, or teeth."[42] He details human weaknesses at some length before adding: "How, you might ask, has such a creature been allotted governance over everything? . . . The apparent neediness of our nature is the occasion for domination over all things that are under our control."[43] His reasoning is similar to that of Galen but goes one step further: if the human being had the swiftness of the horse, say, or the venom of the snake, then humans would not have developed other tools, strategies, and skills, there being no necessity to do so. It was precisely human weakness that provoked the human project of domination. Nemesius writes similarly: "So man has a need . . . of clothing because he has no natural covering, of a house because of the lack of proportion with regard to the environment and because of wild beasts, of medical care because of the change of qualities and the sensitivity with which the body has been endowed."[44] Where the human being lacks natural tools, he learns to take them from the animal. Weakness compels and encourages human beings to domination.[45]

Four aspects of human anatomy served the human purpose of this rational activity: upright stature; the hands; the vocal organs; and the brain. Each of these individual "proofs" was borrowed from Greco-Roman philosophical and medical writings. Early Christian authors discussed each in detail. With regard to the first three, their accounts were framed in comparative terms, juxtaposing human anatomy with that of other animals. When it came to the brain, however, other animals disappeared from view.

That upright stature distinguished animals from human beings was a conventional argument in Greco-Roman philosophy.[46] It was interpreted by philosophers and theologians alike as signifying the higher order of the human soul. In his *Exameron*, Ambrose writes that "animals and beasts have four legs, while birds possess two. Hence man has kinship with the winged flock, in that with his vision he aims at what is high. He flies as if 'on the oarage of wings' by reason of the sagacity of his sublime senses. . . . He is near what is celestial and is higher than the eagle, as one who can say: 'But our citizenship is in heaven.'"[47]

Ambrose is being poetic, but the point was a basic one in ancient thought. Although birds did *not* have citizenship in heaven, their occupation of the skies was a helpful symbol for the "true" home open to human beings. Basil of Caesarea, in the hexameral sermons that inspired Ambrose, writes that "being earthly, cattle are turned toward the soil. The human being, a creature of heaven, rises above them as much by bodily construction as by worthiness of soul."[48] Gregory of Nyssa uses the same idea to justify human kingship over the earth: "But the human being has an upright structure, reaching up to heaven, and looking upward also. These are signs of governance, indicating kingly value."[49] Nemesius similarly emphasizes stature as an index of one's position in earthly hierarchy, highlighting, like Basil, the "bent" posture of the quadruped: "But perhaps it is absurd that things which have no share in wisdom, and live only by natural impulse, that are bent towards the earth and display their servitude in their form, should be said to have been brought to be for their own sake."[50] That is to say, the "bent" stature of quadrupeds exhibited their servile function and indicated that their purpose lay in human need.

The upright stature of the human being was, as we have seen, a symbolic representation of cosmic hierarchy. In accordance with the twin doctrines of human exceptionalism and divine providence, the eminence of the human soul was mapped onto and measured through the literal eminence of the human body. Yet, the contribution of upright stature to human exceptionality was more than just symbolic: it was also deeply practical, insofar as standing on two legs gave humans the use of their hands. As Gregory writes: "For all other animals, the front limbs of the body are feet, because that which is bent over certainly requires structural support; but with regard to the constitution of the human body, the front limbs are hands."[51] The stature of the human body enabled the creation of hands, which are themselves practically and symbolically linked to human rationality: "the hands appear to be proper to the rational nature, and in this way the creator contrived an ease of movement for reason."[52] With the hands, one might carry out all manner of human activities: holding objects, working, writing, eating, and participating in religious rites.[53] Writing in particular, as a form of speech, demonstrated the adaption of the hands to "the requirements of reason," enabling the expression of mind in the sensible world.[54]

The appearance of irrationality in animals, some argued, was caused by their lack of hands for carrying out actions that would manifest their rational capacity. The hands were an organ especially suited for touch: "The whole body is the organ of touch," wrote Nemesius, "especially the interior parts of the hands, and even more than these the extremities of the fingers."[55] Furthermore, just as the palms and fingertips were the most sensitive parts of the body, so the human being was the most sensitive to touch among all animals: "Not merely for comeliness, but also on account of sensitivity of touch, in which man surpasses all other animals, [God] did not clothe us in a thick skin . . . nor in long, thick hair . . . nor in scales . . . nor in shells . . . nor in a pliable shell . . . nor in wings."[56] This sensitivity was considered the foundation of human knowledge, as well as the key to human weakness: "The sense of touch is not without its significance. It represents the keenest sort of pleasure and also gives an honest report of facts."[57] Sensitivity, as we saw in chapter 4, was a weakness both because of the physical softness it required and because of the psychological temptation it opened up. Once again, what distinguishes the human being is the careful balance required to achieve maximum intelligence within a (therefore) delicate frame.

The usefulness of the hands to the activities of the rational soul was not confined to the work of the hands themselves but enabled a further adaptation of human anatomy. "For if the human being had no share in hands," Gregory wrote, "then, exactly like quadrupeds, the parts of the face would be otherwise arranged in service of nutrition."[58] In a carefully orchestrated domino effect, the creation of hands allowed "articulate speech," through proper configuration of the "parts of the mouth." Thus, "since the hand has been bestowed upon the body, the mouth is at leisure to serve reason."[59]

The voice was a primary index of reason in ancient thought. As we saw above, Galen had argued that the bodily origin of squealing in a pig on the dissection table must be the same as the bodily origin of voice, and therefore also of the governing soul in the human being. As Nemesius wrote of the creator: "He linked articulate speech to thought and reasoning, making it a messenger of the movements of the intellect."[60] Ambrose made the same connection: "Men alone express with their lips what they feel in their hearts. Hence we make evident our tacit mental reflections with the speech that flows from our lips."[61] The construction of the mouth parts was essential for the manifestation of the rational soul. "What is the mouth of man," Ambrose continued, "but an avenue for discourse, a fount of disputation, a reception hall for words, a repository of the will?"[62] So also, Gregory of Nyssa:

> Since, then, the mind is a thing intelligible and incorporeal, its grace would have been incommunicable and untouchable, if its movement were not made manifest through some design. On this account, this instrumental constitution remained necessary, so that, touching the vocal organs in the manner of a plectrum, [the mind] might translate its internal movement through the kind of notes that have been struck.[63]

This instrument-like construction was shared in part with animals and birds, but was far superior in human beings, since the human mouth was not responsible for finding and gathering food.[64]

Yet, for all that the hands and the mouth and upright stature provided the conditions for the workings of reason, it was the brain that served as the primary instrument of the soul. "The brain," wrote Ambrose, "is the cause of all that we have discussed . . . the source of our nervous system and of all the sensations of voluntary movement."[65] In order to function properly as "the gathering point of all the senses," it was (like the human being among animals) the softest and most vulnerable of the bodily organs.[66] Nemesius, when describing how the soul worked through the body, distinguished three psychic faculties (imagination, thought, and memory), which he assigned to individual ventricles within the brain, identifying the *pneuma* within those ventricles and the nerves rooted therein as the instruments of the soul.[67] Gregory of Nyssa, although he denied that the soul was contained within the brain, nonetheless envisioned the brain as a charioteer, controlling the limbs through the nerves.[68]

Despite the centrality of the brain to the operations of the governing soul, there are no comparisons—as there are with other bodily parts—between human and animal brains. Ambrose does not suggest that the human brain, through material superiority, signifies "the sagacity of his sublime senses," nor Basil that the brain indicates "the dignity of [the human] soul." Nemesius, when he localizes rational thought in the middle cerebral ventricle, is apparently describing a *human* brain, but he does not make this explicit; nor does he explain what happens in the middle ventricle of the brain of a cow. While the bodily parts that support the manifestation of reason are described almost entirely through comparison, the animal brain—reason's very instrument—is passed over in silence.

ON THE ABSENCE OF ANIMAL BRAINS

Why do these authors never mention animal brains? If the brain was considered distinctively human, like hands, then we would expect theologians to boast of its design. If the brain was considered a shared feature, like mouth parts, then we might expect explanation of why the human brain performed activities that the animal brain could not. Its absence seems to signal some kind of consensus regarding how to negotiate two crucial boundaries: at a macrocosmic level, that between humans and nonrational animals, and at a microcosmic level, that between the brain and other parts of the body.

It is possible that the lack of reference to the comparative anatomy of the brain was an attempt to avoid positing human and animal cognitive capacities as the same kind of thing. By emphasizing the importance of brain anatomy for exclusively human qualities and by neglecting to mention that animals have brains too, early Christian authors perhaps sought to drive a wedge into the continuum between animal and human anatomy.

We might suggest, alternatively, that late antique Christian authors sought to locate the ultimate difference between human and animal intelligence in the soul alone, leaving the bodily instruments of reason roughly equal.[69] According to this argument, the comparisons between other bodily features (such as upright stature) were important clues to the construction of the human body for reason and governance, but were not themselves the organs that enabled or enacted intelligence. Perhaps the absence of the brain reflects the same concern that we saw in Isidore's response to Galen's *QAM* treatise: certain accounts of the brain threaten to undermine the need to theorize a rational soul.[70] Rather than compare specific organs of cognitive activity and risk reducing human intelligence to a kind of advanced animal quality, it is possible that Christian authors focused on the para-instruments and left the precise processes of reason unexplored.

Yet, in order to give anatomical structures credence as signifiers of function, it was necessary that no organism contain parts that did not serve it. What this means is that in order for the human body to be uniquely designed for reason, there needed to be something about its anatomy that served as a unique kind of instrument. We see this principle reflected in Nemesius' consideration of the possibility that animals have rational souls but lack the anatomical equipment to enact reason: he writes that it would have been absurd for God to have "fitted the body with a soul that was not suitable, but superfluous, useless and ineffective, since it is prevented throughout their whole life from carrying out its characteristic activities."[71] Anatomical structures were a reliable guide to intended function—here, rational ensoulment.[72] The reverse proposition also applied: just as God would not put a rational soul in a body incapable of manifesting reason, so God would not provide the instruments of reason for a nonrational soul. This would undermine the logic behind the teleological analysis of anatomy and its deployment toward proving the design of the human body as an instrument of the rational soul.

The design of the human body was certification of "citizenship in heaven." Just as the lack of hands and appropriate mouth parts signified lack of reason in other animals, the brain ought to have been a signifier of God's careful design: by the passage of spirit through the ventricles and the nerves, one could track the movements of the immaterial soul. The fact that animals lacked hands but, with some exceptions, possessed brains clashed with the basic principles of teleological anatomy—not when the brain was considered to be responsible for perception and voluntary motion, but specifically when the brain was understood as an organ of the kind of rational governance distinctive to the human being. It is possible, then, that the brain is absent from comparative accounts precisely because to include it would, among other things, have compromised its potential as a symbol and source of human reason and rule.

As Christina Shepardson has emphasized in relation to late antique Antioch, depictions of place tend to "reflect the interests and politics of their creators."[73] Given the basic analogies between the body and the city in late antique thought, we might understand the representation of places inside and on human and animal bodies as similarly shaped by the investments of theologians.[74] Early Christian authors were keen to put the brain on their map of the human body (qua rational, governing being) when considered in isolation, but they excluded it when mapping the relationship between human and animal forms.

The brain existed on the boundary between different modes of being—material and immaterial, instrument and agent (or, as in the metaphors we have examined, governor), body and soul. Exactly like the sponge, to which ancient medical authors had compared its texture and powers of absorption, the brain was a kind of hybrid object, both plantlike in its lack of sensitivity and voluntary motion, and distinctively human in its governing power and contribution to rational thought. As I have argued throughout this book, it was precisely insofar as it was a boundary object that the brain served as a useful microcosm of what it meant to be human, participating in both earthly and divine realms.

This ambiguity, useful for thinking "up" (i.e., in relation to the immaterial soul and to God), was perhaps less useful or desirable when setting the human alongside the animal. As a boundary object, the brain illustrated how the human could be a vulnerable, material body, while also manifesting divine reason (and, out of the combination of both, internal and external governance). In relation to animals, however, the brain highlighted the materiality and vulnerability of the human being, without any clear account of what, anatomically speaking, marked the human as superior. Given the increasing visibility of the metaphor THE BRAIN GOVERNS in late antiquity, and the role of that metaphor in legitimating human governance over one another and the earth, it is perhaps not surprising that animal brains vanished from the account. By neglecting to mention animal brains in comparative anatomical accounts that were organized around explaining the human being as a rational and governing being, Christian authors avoided the awkward insinuation that animal bodies might have the capacity for thought and governance also.

In the final two sections of this chapter, I turn to the political implications of the erasure of animal models from Christian accounts of the brain. First, we examine the brain as an agent and symbol of human hegemony in early

Christian thought. Finally, we turn to the traces and ghosts of these ideas in the modern phenomenon of "cerebral subject ideology," that is, the identification of the human subject with their brain.

THE BRAIN AS AGENT AND SYMBOL OF HUMAN HEGEMONY

Late antique Christian authors used anatomy to map animal, political, and cosmic hierarchies. While the brain had long been represented as a site of political leadership ("headship"), Christian authors used medical theory to develop the metaphor into a personification of the brain as agent of governance. This elaboration performed several functions: it justified axes of control as natural and divinely ordained; it mapped different kinds of hegemony onto one another, such that they became mutually reinforcing; and it established the importance of individual bodily and psychic discipline for the individual's role in social, political, and spiritual hierarchies.[75] Just as human rulers were supposed to serve as models of moral excellence for their subjects to imitate, so the brain too both governed and modeled governance.[76] The exclusion of the brain from arguments from comparative anatomy was effectively the exclusion of animals from accounts of the brain, lending scientific legitimacy to anthropomorphizing metaphors of the brain as a hegemonic organ.

Whereas the Platonist metaphor of the head as an acropolis typically assumed that the governing agent was the rational soul, early Christian authors sometimes compared the brain itself to human governors. We saw examples of this in chapter 4: John Chrysostom taught his congregants to think of the brain as a king who would be severely dishonored by the influx of fumes from drinking alcohol, or as a master assaulted by his overworked slave, whenever the stomach rebels against excess of food or drink.[77] The Platonist Christian theologian Gregory of Nyssa compared the brain to a charioteer in order to explain the mechanism by which the brain, via the nerves, enacted motor control—even though, in classic Platonist thought, the charioteer represents the rational soul.[78] Theodoret of Cyrrhus described the sick brain as struggling like a drowning man in the flood of "corrupt humors" (bodily fluids), projecting the lack of motor control experienced in mental illness onto the brain itself.[79] The personification of the brain in these texts plays upon THE BRAIN GOVERNS, suggesting that the brain actually performs the functions of the rational soul and does not merely, instrument-like, enable them. The brain in these texts is no "factory" or "storehouse." It is the steward and the foreman; it is the governing king; it stands in for the human being as a whole.

The elaboration of new anthropomorphizing metaphors of the brain was complemented by modes of engagement with medical theories of human brain function that associated the brain specifically with human cognition. Whereas Galen's experimental design involved the exhibition of animal brains performing nonrational functions such as consciousness, sensation, and voluntary motion, some Christian authors attributed human functions, such as reason and morality, to the brain. Toward the end of the fourth century, for example, the philosopher-turned-bishop Nemesius of Emesa wrote that rational thought operates from the middle ventricle of the brain.[80] John Chrysostom interpreted the scriptural "helmet of salvation" as the skull, designed like a helmet to protect the soft and vulnerable brain, which, he explained, is necessary for moral choice.[81] In the *Lausiac History,* Macarius of Alexandria committed himself to living without sleep in the open desert—until the extreme temperatures threatened to "dry out" his brain and send him mad, thus undermining the very self-control for which he was famed.[82] There are not many such references, but their range in terms of medical knowledge (ventricles, temperament) and presumed function (reason, morality, madness) and the lack of explication provided in each case suggest that they reflect a common knowledge and interpretation.

At the same time, Christian authors avoided reference to dissection, that is, to animal brains, as proof for brain function and specifically for the relationship between the brain and the *hēgemonikon,* the governing part of the soul. The central proof that they utilized in its place was the way that organic brain disorders caused disruptions to cognitive functions—reason above all. We have already seen this in numerous texts: Gregory of Nyssa's insistence that phrenitis can be caused by inflammation of membranes in the torso, proving that the mind is not contained within the brain; Nemesius' use of Galen's story about the phrenetic patient who throws glass vessels and then a slave out of a window in order to illustrate the theory of ventricular localization; Augustine's reference to mental illness as the key evidence for his own sketch of ventricular theory in his *Literal Commentary on Genesis.*[83] The rhetorical structures for explaining the relationship between the brain and the governing part of the soul assumed the primary association of the brain with human reason.

The brain, according to this representation, was necessary for distinctively human functions. If the brain was damaged, reason, morality, and self-control—that is, the faculties necessary for pursuing salvation—could be compromised. This claim was grounded in observation (head wounds affect cognition and behavior), but it was also motivated by theological concerns. As we saw in chapters 5 and 6, the brain provided a powerful example and symbol of the way that treatment of the body could affect the health of the soul and therefore the individual's access to salvation. The brain's vulnerability to physical harm both threatened the soul's ability to govern and also symbolized the vulnerability of the human soul as balanced between mortality and immortality and between morality and immorality—supremely capable of reason among animals, but subject to increased physical danger on that account and at risk of condemnation for immoral thoughts and deeds.

Theorizing and imagining the functions of the brain in anthropomorphic terms that prioritized THE BRAIN GOVERNS helped early Christians to explain how human beings could be self-governing animals, that is, how they could have free will within a world shaped by determination and design. It also provided an internal, bodily map—a microcosm—of the hierarchy of governance in the material world and in the cosmos as a whole. Early Christians, like their non-Christian predecessors and peers, devoted a great deal of attention to the parallels between bodily, political, and cosmic hierarchies. The governing power of the brain made it a lynchpin across all three.

Early Christian preachers adapted medical and philosophical arguments to support claims about human exceptionalism and divine providence: the consequence of this rhetorical strategy was the emergence of a new metonymic relationship between the brain and the human being, qua rational and governing body. As the part of the body responsible both for governing within the body and for the mode of rational thought that was assumed to enable human governance over other species, the brain became both the symbol and the agent of human hegemony.

Fundamental to this rhetorical strategy was the idea that what made the human being a suitable ruler over creation was physical vulnerability and a lack of brute strength. In this sense, the vulnerable brain served as a fitting analogy for the human being—or, perhaps more accurately, the concept of the brain was shaped by the notion that the human being was intrinsically vulnerable, and that this vulnerability was important to reason. Early Christian investment in the idea of the brain as representative of what it meant to be a human being was structured around a triangle comprised of governance, reason, and vulnerability.

The brain appears in early Christian texts as a rational, governing power that is also, in physical terms, the most vulnerable part of the body—its vulnerability explaining its intelligence and dominance. Examining the way that these representations of the brain framed what it meant to be human offers a new way in to understanding the role of the brain in the history of representations of human power and the management and regulation of who and what counts as a full human being. It is to some of these questions that we turn in the final section.

THE HEGEMONY OF THE BRAIN AND CEREBRAL SUBJECTIVITY

In the early Christian imagination, the brain could stand in for the idea of the human being, as we have seen both in anthropomorphizing metaphors and in the attribution to the brain of distinctively human activities. A similar association is pervasive within modern scientific and popular scientific thought, albeit not so much the identification of the brain with the idea of the human being as the identification of the brain with the individual human self, a phenomenon that has been called "cerebral subjectivity."[84] We see this both in understandings of what lends continuity to the human self (brain-in-a-vat experiments; the use of "brain death" to signify legal death; the popularity of colorful fMRI scans to represent personality and habits of thought) and in accounts of mental illness, where injury and impairment of the brain play a central role in understanding and narrating mental difficulties and transformations, despite our awareness that neither thinking itself nor the symptoms of mental illness more generally are confined to this organ.[85]

In this final section, I suggest that the origin of our association between the self and the brain has roots in the early Christian transformation of the brain into a distinctively human organ, a transformation that was motivated by the desire to develop arguments rooted in anatomy for the legitimacy and naturalness of exclusive human governance and salvation as a rational animal. This opens possibilities for further exploration into the relationship between the political investments of Christian humanization of the brain and cerebral subject ideology, which is similarly dependent upon bodily, moral, and spiritual hierarchies. To what extent did early Christian rhetorical strategies that humanized the brain shape ways of thinking about the brain and about human beings after late antiquity?

Historians have largely agreed that the phenomenon of cerebral subjectivity developed out of Enlightenment philosophy in seventeenth-century Europe.[86] This argument is rooted in the notion that the brain itself (that is, the structures and substance of the brain, rather than the soul that moved within its ventricles) was not important to concepts such as self, person, and mind prior to the experimentation on the brain that emerged during the Scientific Revolution. As I argued in chapter 4, this perspective prioritizes a modern conceptualization of the brain as a solid object and fails to observe the ways in which the premodern theory of ventricular localization imagined the brain as a musical instrument that operates precisely through the collaboration of physical structure, empty space, and the passage of air. More generally, as I have sought to show throughout this book, the brain was crucial to ways of thinking about what it meant to be a human being in the late antique period, and specifically within the framework of Christianity. As animal studies scholars have argued, the theory of human exceptionalism and superiority solidified in early Christian discourse, since Christian theologians needed animals to lack minds in order to lack morals and, by extension, the capacity for salvation.[87] This chapter has argued that early Christian preachers and theologians identified the brain with the human being (sometimes implicitly, sometimes explicitly, sometimes figuratively), and that this contributed to the formulation of an understanding of what it meant to be human (specifically a free, able-bodied Christian) as rational and (within limits) vulnerable, and on account of both of these characteristics qualified to govern and control the earth and to achieve salvation. This incorporation of the medical concept of the brain into Christian discussions about what it means to be human, formed during the emergence of Christianity as an imperial religion, laid the groundwork for cerebral subjectivity not only by establishing an association between the brain and the human being (albeit qua species rather than individual self) but also by implicating the brain in ideas about power, hierarchy, and control.

Within a modern context, cerebral subjectivity is inherently political. "Cerebral subject ideology," according to Vidal, identifies and values human beings through measurement of brain function, insofar as it reinforces both (1) "the alliance between the norms and ideals of individualistic autonomy and self-reliance" associated with classical liberalism and (2) "the prestige of the advanced technology supposed to demonstrate that we are our brains."[88] The implications of this are worth unpacking.

According to classical liberalism, each individual human being is free, not qua living creature, but specifically because of the human capacity for reason, which enables "autonomy and self-reliance" and so endows human beings with special value. As disability theorist Tobin Siebers has argued, the ideology of ability ("at its simplest the preference for able-bodiedness") became embedded in modern political thought with "the Enlightenment theory of rational autonomy, which represents the inability to reason as the sign of inbuilt inferiority."[89] A central problem with the liberal use of "reason" as a defining characteristic of the human being is that this requires categorizing, valuing, and according freedom in varying degrees, according to the degree of "reason" that can be measured.[90] The liberal idealization of "reason" as the defining characteristic of the free human therefore has implications within the study of disability, gender constructs, racism, and European settler colonialism. If, as Vidal argues, the widespread acceptance of the brain as a symbol for human selfhood reinforces the liberal equation of reason with human freedom, then we should expect to find links between cerebral subjectivity and these various power differentials that have been constructed around the hierarchy that liberalism legitimates. That is to say, we should expect the brain to factor into the logics of racism, misogyny, and colonialism.

Richard Devlin and Dianne Pothier explore the consequences of this in their account of critical disability theory and "dis-citizenship": "Liberalism tends to put great emphasis on the individual, assuming that the self is both sovereign and a foundational unit of analysis. However, critical disability theory forces us to reflect on a number of profound ontological questions. Who is a self?"[91] As they point out, the instability of the liberal concept of selfhood within the frame of disability means that "liberalism has the greatest difficulty in rejecting a hierarchy of difference" in this context: "In a utopian society, liberalism would not seek to abolish race or gender or sexual orientation. But it would seek to abolish disability, on the basis that human beings are not meant to 'suffer' disability. . . . Ridding society of disability, that is, ridding society of the defective and inferior other, is widely seen as understandable and perhaps socially acceptable behavior."[92]

The feminist philosopher Teresa Brennan describes the "self-contained" subject, whose origin she locates in Enlightenment Europe, as one of the greatest misconceptions of modern Western psychiatry.[93] The problem, she explains, lies in the idea that individuals are containers, sealed off from one another, and porous only in pathological conditions.[94] Her critique reveals two implications of privileging the "rational" and "autonomous" human subject. The first is psychiatric: the ideal of self-containment leads to the false pathologizing of affect, especially in women.[95] The second is political: "In science," she writes, "transmission between beings was neglected, while political philosophers denied that the fledgling individual was indebted to those that came before. It was born, this new individual, free and equal in the market place."[96] That is to say, classical liberal theories of citizenship minimize interdependence and promote individualism, rather than mutual support.

The idealization of rational autonomy as the defining characteristic of human identity risks dehumanizing people who are identified as having intellectual disabilities. If the human subject is by definition rational, and if rationality is thought to be measurable and differentiated among human beings, then human identity and value becomes a spectrum.[97] Further, if rationality is understood to be embodied in the brain, then the measure of humanity can be traced both in speech and behavior (the manifestations of reason) and through anatomical and physiological measures (the physical conditions for generating reason). Among the most famous examples of this in practice is the nineteenth-century white American physician Samuel G. Morton, who created a racial taxonomy based on skull capacity by measuring the quantity slightly space between the text obviously rooted in racism and supported by falsified results.[98]

As a contribution to and product of seventeenth-century philosophy and the invention of the scientific method, cerebral subjectivity is implicated in modern racism, misogyny, and ableism as axes of discrimination that rely on a projected lack of reason or cognitive capacity, as well as in the specific assumptions and prejudices of a neurotypical paradigm that privileges some modes of brain activity over others. In the crucible of the Enlightenment, the rational, able-bodied human being, as a male and as a white European, emerged as different—and superior—to other beings. This emergence provided the foundation for discrimination on various bodily grounds, especially race, gender, (dis)ability, and species.[99] Cerebral subject ideology supports the liberal privileging of the able-bodied, able-minded individual by identifying each person with their brain. It also legitimates embodied hierarchies, including those among human beings, as well as between humans and other animals, by establishing a physical and measurable site of personhood, and therefore also (within liberalism) of value.

Historically, reason and logic have served as a neurotypical norm. Yet, the neurodiversity movement that has emerged out of discussions and activism within the autistic community has to do fundamentally with the association of different emotional and relational styles with patterns of brain function (or "neurotypes").[100] As Victoria Pitts-Taylor has unpacked in her nuanced account of mirror neurons, the assumption that there are universal patterns of neuronal activity that underpin human empathy pathologizes neurotypes and emotional and relational styles that do not fit the norm.[101] Cerebral subjectivity is rooted in the identification of reason as *the* human quality, but it has extended to encompass emotionality also.[102] Within cerebral subject ideology, patterns of brain activity—rational, emotional, and relational—are understood to constitute the human subject, and some such patterns are valued over others as normative and healthy. The close bond between brain and subject and the idealization of specific kinds of brain activity as criteria for value qua (human) subject narrows the field of possibilities for inclusion within communities of mutual respect, value, and care.

Cerebral subject ideology arose within a different cultural space than that of what I have called the humanization of the brain in early Christianity. Yet, in both cases, the association between the brain and the human being involves the centering of rationality and self-regulation and reinforces existing power structures and hierarchies. We might think of this as the fulfillment of an intrinsic potential within the concept of a "chief" organ within the human body, but it is more likely, I think, that these resonances trace the underground influence of early Christian preachers on conceptualizations of the brain and the human being on the traditions of science and philosophy that developed in early modern Europe. The Latin translation movement of the late medieval period famously introduced ancient Greek medical and philosophical texts into medieval Europe (often via Arabic), but these texts arrived in a context shaped by familiarity with late antique Christian preachers—and, indeed, were often written by late antique Christian preachers, as in the case of Nemesius' treatise *On the Nature of the Human Being*, which was first translated into Latin in the eleventh century, and which became a touchstone in subsequent accounts of the brain. The correlation between the attachment to the brain as representative of the human and the normativization of certain modes of thinking, feeling, and regulating as sources of legitimacy for governance and claims to health (i.e., "salvation") is suggestive of the way that "natural" concepts such as the brain are molded by the pressures, agendas, and concerns that they travel through in their everyday usage within and beyond technical spheres. Behind modern neuromania lies a theology of human exceptionalism that, to the extent that it remains without critique, continues to shape the manner in which the modern (and especially the Western) subject relates to their brain.

CONCLUSION

In this final chapter, I have argued that the origins of our association between the human self and the brain have their roots in late antiquity. Specifically, I draw attention to the investment of early Christian preachers and theologians in the idea of the brain as representative of what it meant to be a human being—embodied but rational, vulnerable but (and therefore) suited to govern over the rest of creation. Thus, the brain was both a way of talking about human identity (a kind of microcosm or metonymy) and the part of the body that enabled uniquely human actions. At the core of my argument is the idea that this association between the brain and the human being laid the foundations for the identification of the brain with the human self, and that in so doing it established a particular understanding of what it means to be human. The brain shows up in early Christian texts as a rational, governing power that is also, in physical terms, the most vulnerable part of the body—its vulnerability explaining its intelligence and dominance. Examining the way that these representations of the brain framed what it means to be human offers a new way in to understanding the role of the brain in the history of representations of human power and the management and regulation of who and what counts as a full human being.

Conclusion

Early Christian authors used the concept of the brain in theoretical and pastoral texts in order to shape and sharpen ideas about ensoulment, salvation, and hierarchies of power. The ways in which they worked upon the idea of the brain both contributed to its conceptual development within medicine and philosophy and prepared audiences to understand the brain as an object relevant to problems of the self. The task of this book has been to explore how the introduction of Christian values and debates into the concept of the brain might newly inflect the stories we tell about how the brain became a central object of study in relation to human subjectivity.

At the core of early Christian engagement with the brain was the triad of vulnerability, governance, and reason. The vulnerability of the brain (and of the human being) was explained as enabling reason and demanding governance over both the self and others. This triad built on existing medical ideas about the brain to serve Christian pedagogical and rhetorical needs, including the promotion of moderate ascetic practice, the circumscription of the authority of "excessive" ascetic experts, and the justification of hierarchy and practices of exclusion within Christian ecclesial and political communities. It also offered a medical model for theological arguments about what it means to be human: powerful among animals and capable of self-rule and self-formation, but necessarily dependent upon God for protection and salvation.

We might ask ourselves how these adaptations of the brain as a conceptual object linger in contemporary neuroscience, including its popular manifestations: In what ways do we understand the brain to be an instrument of regulation, and over whom? How does the promise of salvation—which we might understand as release from mortality or from guilt—linger in our attachment to the brain? What role does vulnerability play not only within contemporary ideas about the brain (for example, in the need to preserve and strengthen its functionality) but also in how we think about power and responsibility? The discipline of neuroscience was created within Christianized intellectual communities, and among the assets that it inherited was a Christianized concept of the brain. My argument in this book has been that our treatment of the brain as a kind of Mini-Me or homunculus that we can work upon—that we must cultivate and tend to, that we might preserve in separation from the body in order to ensure personal immortality, that legitimates power differentials, hierarchies, and coercive rule—has roots in the Christianization of the brain as a conceptual object that served the theological and political needs of early Christian communities and their ruling men.

I began by arguing in Chapter 1 that an important motivation for early Christian attention to the brain was the cultural capital attached to knowledge of human anatomy more broadly in late antique society. The central actors in this study—preachers and bishops of the fourth and fifth centuries C.E.—were well-educated men who sought social prominence and mobility through public speech. The circulation of anatomical knowledge within elite circles during late antiquity suggests that when Christian intellectuals inserted the brain into their sermons, letters, and treatises, this was no surprise to their audiences. Steeped in a culture where medical ideas were developed and circulated by specialists and nonspecialists alike, Christian intellectuals were tapping into existing practices, and specifically into practices that were intended to accrue authority and cultural capital to the speaker.

Yet, early Christian authors did not simply reproduce medical ideas and transmit them in undoctored form. Rather, they elaborated the concept of the brain to support their own rhetorical program. It is important for us to have a sense, therefore, of what medical and philosophical texts and authorities were available to them in order to observe where and how they made revisions. Following common practice, however, early Christian authors rarely detailed their sources. In chapter 2, therefore, I laid out a kind of extended historical context, sketching the major theories of the brain in Greek medicine and philosophy prior to late antiquity. While the historical narrative I offered charts an increasing tendency to identify the brain as the organ of the *hēgemonikon*, a key insight that it brings to light is that the brain was simultaneously crucial as an organ responsible for bodily balance in relation to the four qualities (hot/cold, wet/dry) through its participation in cyclical processes of purgation. Contrary to common assumption in histories of the brain, this more physiologically centered role was closely entangled in the brain's responsibility for cognition and self-governance.

When late antique Christian intellectuals turned to medical and philosophical resources on the brain, they found images of the brain as a sponge, citadel, musical instrument, and plumbing system; they found the brain conceptualized as a gland, as a cooling system, as an interpreter, as the site of the *logistikon* and *hēgemonikon*, as the source of the nerves, and as the foundation for animal life. The story of the brain in early Christian thought must not be understood as a linear journey toward or away from modern understandings of the brain as the material organ of the mind. Instead, we can grasp it most clearly when we grasp that all of these conceptual resources were available to Christian authors as they constructed their own particular versions of the brain.

The period of late antiquity saw two major developments in how people thought about the brain: the introduction of ventricular localization as a model for the distribution of psychological functions and the anthropomorphization of the brain as a stand-in for aspects of the self. Both of these developments were grounded in medical ideas about brain function, especially the trend toward identifying the brain as the organ of the *hēgemonikon*, but each also offered distinctive figurative templates for early Christian authors. In chapters 3 and 4, I examined these two shifts in terms of two conceptual metaphors: THE BRAIN IS AN INSTRUMENT, and THE BRAIN GOVERNS. Neither metaphor was entirely new to Christianity, but the tension between them became more pronounced, revealing key questions and concerns about the extent of human self-determination, the possibility that the soul might be contained or replaced, and the consequences of failed self-governance both at the level of the individual and within political and ecclesial communities.

Chapters 5 and 6 explored different kinds and failures of self-management as understood in terms of the brain. I argued in chapter 5 that early Christian preachers developed a rhetoric of cerebral vulnerability in order to motivate ascetic practices among their congregations. The explicit aim of these practices was to preserve and improve the health of the soul; the implicit aim was to strengthen the bonds of Christian community through shared bodily practices. Key to this connection between the care of individual brains and the management of the communal body was the porosity of the brain, that is, its openness to the vapors that individuals breathed out, as well as the longstanding idea that its function included absorbing excess moisture from other parts of the body. It maintained the integrity of the whole not only through governance via the nervous system but also through participation in the exchange of bodily fluids that transformed its own matter, sometimes in risky ways. Unlike the governor within the citadel, the brain was never truly sealed off from the rest of the body. The vulnerability of the brain was not just the vulnerability of a soft mass or of an organ that required a delicate balance of temperature and humidity, but the vulnerability of an entity that functioned only through material connection to other body parts and animals.

Chapter 6 turned from the material vulnerability of the brain to the ways that its vulnerability was weaponized against religious opponents. This shift in perspective pivots around the attempt to manage ascetic practices: whereas chapter 5 showed how cerebral vulnerability was used to discourage gluttony and drunkenness, chapter 6 examined the ways that Christian authors emphasized the damaging effect of excessive ascetic practices on the brain and on mental health. This was, as I argued, a fundamentally political issue. By linking superlative ascetic practices to brain injury and disease, Christian authors sought to limit the extent to which any individual could pursue salvation or assert spiritual power outside the authorizing framework of the church. This rhetoric also proved useful in justifying punitive actions against "heretics" and "schismatics," since it was generally accepted in late antiquity (as today) that medical interventions did not require patient consent in the case of mental disorder. This co-option of medical ideas about mental disorder for religious polemic further laid the groundwork for the spiritualization and moralization of mental disorders as conditions that might require clerical attention.

Chapter 7 tied these threads together through a close reading of comparative anatomy in early Christian soundbites about the design of the human body for reason and governance. As I argued in this chapter, a key innovation of early Christian thought was the association of the brain particularly with the human being. We see this in the tendency toward anthropomorphization of the brain, in the attribution to the brain of cognitive activities considered definitive of human nature, and in the avoidance of any discussion of animal brains in early Christian accounts, despite the fundamental importance of animal models in medical literature. This "humanization" of the brain in early Christianity was, so I have argued, crucial to its usefulness for theorizing and legitimizing power over others through rational regulation of the embodied self.

NOTES

INTRODUCTION

1. All dates are C.E., unless otherwise stated.

2. Aug. *De orig. nat. an.* 4.5.6. All translations throughout this book are my own, except where indicated.

3. Mansfeld (1989) discusses the treatment of this question in ancient philosophical handbooks, specifically in relation to Aët. *Plac.* 4.5 (Diels 1879, 391–92). Van der Eijk (2005a) examines the medical background of the question. Gilbert (2014, 8–61) surveys the development of this question in medical, philosophical, and theological texts, focusing especially on the Hellenistic Jewish exegete Philo of Alexandria.

4. Thdt. *Cur.* 5.22.1–23.1.

5. Solmsen 1961, 180–81, with references; Long 1982, 47–49; Colish 1985, 27–28; Annas 1992, 60–69, esp. 61, with reference to DL 7.11 = SVF II, 828.

6. Kornmeier 2016; Long 1986, 171–72; Annas 1992, 62, with references to Aët. *Plac.* 4.21 = SVF II, 836 and Calc. *Comm. in Plat. Tim.* 220 = SVF II, 879.

7. Tertullian (c. 160–225) surveys the possibilities in *DA* 15.5. Annas (1992, 29n36) briefly discusses anachronistic attributions of the *hēgemonikon* in ancient texts.

8. See Aët. *Plac.* 4.2–7 (Diels 1879, 391), as presented in Mansfeld 1989, 314–20. There is useful discussion of the question in Tieleman 1996, xxxiv–xxxv; Runia 1999a, 232–33; Tieleman 2003, 259–60; A. Smith 2004, 206–08; van der Eijk 2005a, 123.

9. Manuli and Vegetti (1977) argue that the increasing dominance of brain and heart over blood represents political centralization.

10. Rocca 2003, 18–19; Knuuttila 2005.

11. Plato: Plato in general, see Manuli and Vegetti 1977, 77–99; Clarke and O'Malley 1996, 5–10. Medical writers: Frampton 2008, 117–26. Galen is never cited in these doxographic lists, perhaps because he worked after their formalization.

12. Aristotle: Tracy 1962, 46–47; Frampton 2008, 20–108, esp. 31; C. Smith 2010, 9–10. The Stoics: Long 1982, 48; Annas 1992, 69–70.

13. Gregory of Nyssa is an exception, although he nonetheless accepts the medical theory of the brain as the organ of sensory and motor function (see Wessel 2009, 32–39).

14. On the resurgence of Platonism in fourth-century philosophy, see Gersh and Kannengiesser 1992. On Platonism in late antique Christian thought specifically, see O'Meara 1981. On the influence of Galen, see Gilbert 2014. While Christian authors refer to Galen only very rarely, his arguments form the substructure of their accounts of the brain, especially in relation to the soul.

15. These examples are provided in Tert. *DA* 15.4 as evidence that the organ of the *hēgemonikon* is the heart.

16. On the organs of mental and emotional activity in the Hebrew scriptures, see North 1993 and M. Smith 1998.

17. Aug. *Trin.* 10.7.

18. In 1989, President George H. W. Bush announced that the 1990s would be the Decade of the Brain: *Project on the Decade of the Brain* (http://www.loc.gov/loc/brain, accessed November 11, 2021). See Goldstein 1994. In the early twenty-first century, we might be said to be living in the era of the nervous system and gut, both understood as extended networks that are easily imprinted by the assaults of the environment and the body's own systems of response and defense; perhaps unsurprisingly, the gut is frequently connected to both the nervous system and the brain in current thought. For a neurological account of the "enteric nervous system," see Gershon 1999; for a history of the psychoanalytic perspective and the development of a feminist account, see Wilson 2004a and 2004b, 31–48. My thanks to Katie Kleinhopf for this insight.

19. For critical response to the claim that brains are gendered, see especially Fine 2010; Jordan-Young 2011; Rippon 2019. On gut inflammation and the brain, see Mayer et al. 2014. Regarding the interpretation of brain imaging technology, see Dumit 2004; Vidal 2009, 22; Vidal and Ortega 2017.

20. Malabou 2008, 3, where Malabou defines "cerebrality" as "the causal value of the damage inflicted upon [cerebral] functions—that is, upon their capacity to determine the course of psychic life." The core text on the centrality of the brain and nervous system to trauma is van der Kolk 2014; Menakem (2017) develops van der Kolk's work to theorize racialized violence in the United States of America as a product of traumatized nervous systems.

21. Rose 2003, 46. See further at 54: "The sense of ourselves as 'psychological' individuals that developed across the twentieth century—beings inhabited by a deep internal space shaped by biography and experience, the source of our individuality and the locus of our discontents—is being supplemented or displaced by what I have termed 'somatic individuality.'"

22. Swaab 2015. See also the comments in Vidal 2009, 10. Consider also the following book titles: *The Private Life of the Brain: Emotions, Consciousness, and the Secret of the Self* (Susan Greenfield, published 2000); *Synaptic Self: How Our Brains Become Who We Are* (Joseph LeDoux, published 2003); *Tell-Tale Brain: A Neuroscientist's Quest*

for What Makes Us Human (V. S. Ramachandran, published 2011); *Connectome: How the Brain's Wiring Makes Us Who We Are* (Sebastian Seung, published 2012).

23. Bennett and Hacker 2003, 68–107 (the "mereological fallacy"); Mudrik and Maoz 2015.

24. Vidal 2009, 11–14; Vidal 2016, 90–91.

25. Vidal 2009, 6; Vidal and Ortega 2017.

26. Vidal 2009, 9–10; see also the arguments in Pitts-Taylor 2016. I discuss this in more detail in chapter 7.

27. Vidal 2009, 12.

28. See Borck 2012 on the rise and fall of new technological models for the functions of the brain.

29. James (2008) offers a good introduction to the formation of late antiquity as a period of study.

30. P. Brown ([1971] 1993) led this shift in perspective.

31. Inglebert 2012, 3 and *passim*.

32. P. Brown (1971) 1993 (the earlier edition specifies instead: "From Marcus Aurelius to Muhammad"). See, for example, the journal *Studies in Late Antiquity*, which is distinctive in its focus on "global late antiquity," rather than focusing on the regions surrounding the Mediterranean, as is the case of *Journal of Late Antiquity*, which uses the period c. 250–800.

33. For the period c. 200–600, see, for example, McGill and Watts 2018, 5. For the period c. 400–600, see, for example, Averil Cameron 1993 (c. 395–600); Cameron, Ward-Perkins, and Whitby 2000 (425–600).

34. Fowden 2014.

35. For discussion of this trope and its impact on modern scholarship, see Lizzi Testa 2017, ix–xx.

36. See the discussion in Lindberg 2010. Cf. Marx-Wolf 2015, 92–93; Marx-Wolf and Upson-Saia 2015, 257–60.

37. See the oft-cited historiographical critique in Nutton 1984, where late antique medical texts are described as being used by historians as "medical refrigerators" that preserve earlier ideas.

38. Studies of late antique medicine have flourished in recent years particularly through the collaborative projects undertaken at Humboldt University. One excellent example is Thumiger and Singer 2018, which focuses on mental illness from Celsus onward, effectively breaching the boundary between classical and late antique medicine, albeit with a strong focus upon the understudied authors of the late antique period. On Christian engagement with scientific and medical ideas, see Woloschak 2011 and the programmatic work of Marx-Wolf and Upson-Saia 2015, together with the dedicated journal issues they introduce.

39. P. Harrison 2006, 82. See Zucconi 2019 for an alternative approach to ancient medicine that decentralizes Greece and Rome.

40. Conrad (1995, 93) is representative: "The Arab-Islamic medical tradition was founded on Graeco-Roman medicine, the exponents of Arab-Islamic culture translated

into Arabic and so saved many classical texts which might otherwise have been lost, and the Islamic world ultimately passed this heritage back to Europe when its medical works were translated into Latin." Sabra (1987) offers a clear and critical discussion of this tendency. Pormann and Savage-Smith (2007) provide a counternarrative, constructing a detailed account of the emergence of Arab-Islamic medicine through engagement with Greek medical texts, but without centering Greece or positioning early modern Europe as its telos.

41. The most widely cited example from ancient Greek medicine is the Hippocratic text *On the Sacred Disease* (van der Eijk 2005b offers a useful discussion). See the discussions in Cunningham 1988; P. Harrison 2006. As P. Harrison (2015) argued, the opposition between science and religion that seems so obvious within the modern West is a product of Enlightenment debates, rather than an inherent contradiction between "scientific" and "religious" thought. See also the important discussion of this tension within the study of Islamic medical science in Fancy 2013, 2–11.

42. An early and important study of the appropriation of classical antiquity in British colonialist ideology was Goff 2005. There have since been several more detailed accounts of how classics underpinned British colonial systems, including the Caribbean (Greenwood 2010) and India (Vasunia 2013). For the reliance of white supremacism on classical allusions, see McCoskey 2018. On the implication of Eurocentric histories of science in colonialist and white supremacist projects, see Anderson 2003 (esp. 464) and Raj 2013.

43. On scientific pluralism as a philosophical paradigm, see Ludwig and Ruphy 2021.

44. The term "natural" is a minefield of its own, especially given the close relationship between science and technology. See, with regard to ancient Greek science, Lloyd 1991.

45. Marx-Wolf 2015.

46. See also Chiara Thumiger's observations of the increasing moralization of mental disorder and medicalization of desire and the will in late antique medicine, and the relationship between this shift and the rise of Christianity (Thumiger 2018a, 267; Thumiger 2018b, 270; see also Thumiger and Singer 2018, 22).

47. See, for example, Rocca 2003; von Staden 2005; Lo Presti 2008.

48. C. Gross (1995) frames Aristotle's denial of "the controlling role of the brain" as his "most egregious error."

49. Lo Presti 2008, 3–5. My translation.

50. Nutton 1984, 2.

51. Cf. King 1998, 2, and also more generally King 2013 and King 2019, for the cross-pollination of reception studies and history of ancient medicine.

52. Holmes 2010, 7–8.

53. An important example is Kuriyama 1999, which argues that Chinese and Greek medicine created different felt experiences of the body because theoretical preconceptions determine what physicians and patients feel and observe. See also the example explored in Lock 1993, which compares the Western medical concept "menopause"

with the Japanese concept *kōneki*, arguing that, while they are often equated, these are not the same thing, and that people have different embodied experiences of menstruation and aging, including different symptoms, depending on which framework dominates.

54. Fadiman (1997) offers a nuanced account of the impact of imposing Western medical concepts and norms onto a Hmong family that had recently arrived in California. At a more theoretical level, L. Smith (1999) establishes important groundwork for approaching anthropological research as a decolonizing project that does not center Western epistemological frameworks and interests; Kimmerer (2020) builds on this work to weave together Western plant biology with Indigenous expertise about plants and the natural world. Anderson (2008) explores biomedical science itself as a colonizing project, with a particular focus on the brain. Tallbear (2013) investigates the "co-production" or "con-constitution" of the concept of DNA as a criterion for belonging within Indigenous tribal groups.

55. Choudhury and Slaby (2012a and 2012b) lay the foundations for this field.

56. Choudhury and Slaby 2012b, 31; see also Pitts-Taylor 2016, which examines the political stakes of both neuroscience and critical neuroscience, and Vidal and Ortega 2017 for an exploration of what "cerebral subject ideology" looks like in practice.

57. Choudhury and Slaby 2012a, 2.

58. Choudhury and Slaby 2012b, 30.

59. Fitzgerald et al. 2014, 2.

60. Choudhury and Slaby 2012a, 9; Schmitz and Höppner 2014, 5–6; Pitts-Taylor 2016, esp. 5–8. Tuana (2008) charts a compelling path between realism and social constructivism (esp. 189–91) through the term "viscous porosity," through which she seeks to name both instability of ("natural") boundaries and the "sites of resistance and opposition" to easy fluidity and transformation (193–94). Choudhury and Slaby (2012b, 35) draw on the concepts of "biolooping" ("recursive loops between neurobiological and social/cultural processes") and "local biologies" (biological patterns and norms that exist at a local level, rather than being generalizable across a species) as principles for exploring how this interaction between "nature" and "culture" might be understood in relation to the brain.

61. P. Brown 1988 laid the groundwork; Bynum 1995b offers a more concise theoretical account of the significance of the body in early Christianity; Bynum 1995a explores the theme in much greater depth, with a focus especially upon resurrection.

62. Upson-Saia 2018; Mayer 2018.

63. Borck 2012; S. Gross 2015.

64. See E. Martin 2010, 379, for a discussion of theoretical pluralism in lay conceptions of the brain. Borck (2012, 118) examines how different technological metaphors reveal different aspects of the brain and issues a cautionary note regarding perceived complexity of the brain.

65. Choudhury and Slaby 2012a, 7. Cf. Emily Martin's famous analysis of "the egg and the sperm" in scientific texts, which is based on the premise that feminist science studies must "wake up sleeping metaphors in science . . . by becoming aware of when

we are projecting cultural imagery onto what we study," in order to neutralize "their power to naturalize our social conventions" (E. Martin 1991, 501).

66. Within conceptual metaphor theory, described below, a structural metaphor involves the projection of a complex conceptual structure (such as "health") from one domain (such as medicine) onto another (such as religion). See the useful discussion in Nyord 2017, 15–17.

67. On the figure of *Christus medicus*, see Arbesmann 1954.

68. Marx-Wolf 2015, 94.

69. Marx-Wolf 2015, 94–95.

70. Lakoff and Johnson 1980; see Mayer 2018 for a discussion of CMT as it applies to medicine and religion in late antiquity.

71. In CMT, metaphorical expressions are typically indicated through quotation marks (as here) or in italics; conceptual metaphors are usually marked through capitalization.

72. On CMT as controversial, see Gibbs 2017. For the quotation, and on the analysis of metaphorical expressions to uncover "preconscious thought," see Mayer 2018, 453. For a discussion of the widespread acceptance of this new understanding of metaphor as "belong[ing] . . . at the heart of thinking about language use in all its aspects" in relation to metaphor and allegory in the classical tradition, see Boys-Stones 2003 (1, for quotation).

73. See, for example, the articles collected in *Studies in Late Antiquity* 2.4 (2018).

74. Lakoff and Johnson 1980, esp. chap. 12. For discussion and development of this point, see El Refaie 2019, 18–46.

75. Upson-Saia 2018, 428. Cf. the important work of BeDuhn (1992) in relation to medical language within Manichaean texts. See also G. Smith 2008, 482–83, which articulates a methodological approach to demons that "begin[s] by taking what is said about their nature and activity as literally, as physically, as possible."

76. Quint. *Inst.* 8.6.4.

77. Averil Cameron 1991, 57.

78. Greg. Magn. *Cant. Cantic.* 2.1–3.15 (PL 79:473A6–8). On allegory as a form of metaphor in ancient rhetoric, see Boys-Stones 2003, 2, with reference to Cic. *Or.* 94 and Quint. *Inst.* 8.6.14. See also Quint. *Inst.* 8.6.44–47 for the explanation that one kind of allegory is composed of a series of metaphors, while another can be constructed without any metaphor whatsoever. See also Innes 2003, 19, on allegory as "sustained metaphor."

79. Froehlich 1984, 20–22. Sandwell (2011, 544) offers a clear and concise account of the differences between allegorical and literal exegesis, while taking into account the possibility that their polarization in modern scholarship has been overstated.

80. Amirav (2003, 33–44) explores the Alexandrian and Antiochene schools in detail, including their relationship to metaphor. See also F. Young 2003, and Martens 2008. Lim (1990) shows how exegetical practice might be tailored to context, arguing in particular that Basil of Caesarea rejected allegorical exegesis in his *Hexaemeron* because he did not consider it suitable for less experienced Christians. Stefaniw (2007)

argues that the practice of allegorical exegesis among Alexandrian intellectuals cut across different schools (Neoplatonist, catechetical, monastic) and was motivated by shared cultural assumptions and a shared orientation toward spiritual perfection, rather than by religious doctrine or specific cultic practices. Stefaniw (2016) examines the function of late ancient reading practices in ethical progression.

81. Mitchell 2009, 186.

82. V. Harrison 2007, 118: "One result of distinguishing between the spiritual meanings of a sacred text and the literal sense of the words that constitute it was that an enormous number of different, and sometimes rival, interpretations of the same texts became possible."

83. Stefaniw (2007) discusses the ways in which allegorical exegesis trained readers in constantly searching for the higher meaning behind the text.

84. Aug. *De orig. nat. an.* 4.5.6.

85. Greg. Nyss. *Op. hom.* 7 (PG 44:141.19–21).

CHAPTER 1. THE CIRCULATION AND PERFORMANCE OF MEDICAL KNOWLEDGE IN LATE ANTIQUITY

1. Evagr. *Or.* 72–73 (PG 79:1181.42–1184.4).

2. See Metzger 2018 for the role of demons in late antique medical texts.

3. Crislip 2013, 29: "While Galen or Oribasius would surely disapprove, for many ancient people disease could signify demonic invasion, the parasitic inhabitation of another being within one's own flesh." Cf. Grey 2005, 45; P. Brown 1972, 131–35 for the role of demons in troubling human health. See also G. Smith 2008, 508 (*pneuma* as the substance of demons) and 510 (demons as evil smelling).

4. On the medical background for the claim of late antique Christian clerics to be "physicians of the soul," see Marx-Wolf 2017. For the history of the concept of the brain as "instrument of the soul" in ancient medical and philosophical discourse, see chapter 2.

5. Ast. Am. *Hom.* 14.2.4.1–3. The overlapping effects of demonic invasion and drunkenness (palpation of blood vessels within the brain) reflect the vaporous nature of each.

6. See Holmes 2013 for the argument that the Hippocratic focus on nonhuman agency opened a gap for philosophers to develop a therapeutics of the soul. By late antiquity, the picture is even more complicated, and the three-part division I offer here is schematic only. For human agency and psychological causation in medical texts, see the contributions to the edited volume introduced by Thumiger and Singer (2018).

7. See in particular Wendt 2016. Gleason (2009) analyzes how this played out with regard to medical expertise.

8. Marx-Wolf 2018, 513: "It is also important to emphasize that the kinds of disciplinary boundaries we are accustomed to using today were far more permeable and fluid in Antiquity. This is especially the case when we look at the intersections between

what we would identify as medicine, natural science, philosophy, and theology or religion." See also Marx-Wolf and Upson-Saia 2015, 268–70, and Marx-Wolf 2015, 81.

9. De Wet 2019.

10. A. Jones 2009, 256.

11. Alan Cameron 1966 argued for 384, but Cameron 2011 (p. 243) for 382; Kaster 2011, I, xii–xxiv suggests c. 383.

12. Alan Cameron 1966, 27; Alan Cameron 2011, 327–28; Kaster 2011, 1:xv.

13. Kaster (2011, 1:xii) describes the *Saturnalia* as "an encyclopedic compilation quarried from mostly unnamed sources."

14. On the role of physicians in sympotic dialogues, see Kaster 2011, 1:xxxiv–xxxvii. For the historical Dysarius, see *PLRE* 1:275. Other examples of physicians in sympotic dialogues include the figure of Trypho in Plutarch's *Quaest. conv.* 3.1.3, similarly with reference to the brain.

15. Alan Cameron 2011, 231.

16. Kaster 2011, 1:xviii.

17. Chin 2008, 3: "Quintilian's account of rhetorical education places grammar at the outset of a process of subject formation that fits into a specific ideological framework, one based on predictable divisions between elites and non-elites, Romans and non-Romans, masculinity and its lack." The classic work on *paideia* in early Christianity is Jaeger 1961; central to current understandings of *paideia* as the driving force behind social relations in late antiquity is P. Brown 1992. More recently, see especially van Hoof and van Nuffelen 2014. On *paideia* as a shared cultural code, a practice of aesthetic appreciation, and a training in social mores exclusive to the upper class, wealthy, educated individuals, see Watts 2006, 1–23; Watts 2012, 468.

18. König 2012, 231, noting that the disruptive guest was a stock figure in sympotic literature.

19. Macr. *Sat.* 7.4.1.

20. Marx-Wolf and Upson-Saia 2015, 260.

21. On the explicit avoidance of classical literature in late antique Christian texts, see especially Chin 2008, 6: "These accounts are more than mere tropes of the dangers of classical literature; they also reveal the ways in which reading was understood as a cultural practice and an articulation of subjectivity." See Elm 2012 for the argument that contestations of literary knowledge and expertise formed the basis for the tensions between "Hellenism" and "Christianity" especially during and after the reign of Julian. Watts (2006, 16–20) similarly explores the influence of classical thought on fourth- and fifth-century Christian intellectuals; Watts 2012, 476. Stefaniw (2016, 238–40) explores continuities between the rejection of literary texts in Hellenic and Christian traditions of ascetic philosophy, revealing the centrality of mimetic ethics to ancient anxiety about texts and their impact on the soul.

22. Joh. Chrys. *Hom. in Stat.* 11.8 (PG 49:123.35–124.7). For discussion of this passage, see chapter 5.

23. Kaster 2011, 1:xxxiv–xxxvii.

24. See the final section of this chapter for further discussion of late antique handbooks.

25. Symm. *Ep.* 3.37, 9.44.

26. Symm. *Ep.* 9.44.1; *Ep.* 3.37.1. Macr. *Sat.* 1.7.1.

27. Macr. *Sat.* 7.9.4–5, 19–22.

28. Macr. *Sat.* 7.9.22.

29. Macr. *Sat.* 7.9.18.

30. Arist. *PA* 2.10, 656a23–24; see C. Gross 1995, 247–58.

31. Described in Aug. *Ep.* 137.1.1–2. For Volusianus, see PLRE 2:1184–85.

32. On the Christian connections of Volusianus, see P. Brown 1968, 113; P. Brown 2000, 298–99; O'Donnell 2005, 247–48; P. Brown 2012, 359–60. Brown consistently describes Volusianus as living in a "post-pagan" world, where "pagan" and "Christian" values and identities became increasingly enmeshed, rather than (as has often been projected) polarized.

33. Aug. *Ep.* 137.2.8.

34. PLRE 1:37–38. P. Brown 2000, 298–300; Reid 2008, 148fn464; Kaster 2011, 1:xxix; Alan Cameron 2011, 196–97. Cameron (2011, 260) suggests that the prominence of Volusianus in the early fifth century might explain the presence of his father in the *Saturnalia.*

35. See also the discussion of iatrosophists and Christian preachers in de Wet 2019.

36. Dio Chrys. *Or.* 33.6.1–5. On this speech, see Bowersock 2010, 83–85.

37. Dio Chrys. *Or.* 33.6.5–7.1.

38. Plato invoked the good physician as a model for the ideal rhetorician (Pl. *Phdr.* 270b–d, discussed in Pender 2005, 44–46). The earliest Greek medical texts emerged out of a cultural context defined by polemical and persuasive speech and not only responded explicitly to, but further shaped that context (Jouanna 2012b). See Thomas 2002 (building on the insights of Momigliano 1985) for a discussion of rhetorical and scientific writings in the fifth century B.C.E. as the context for the emergence of historiography. Agarwalla (2010) discusses the role of rhetoric in medical education during the fifth and fourth centuries B.C.E.

39. Jouanna 2012b, 50–52, including the observation that some ancient medical texts may in fact have been written by "sophists," rather than by "physicians." Laskaris (2002, 73–124) offers a detailed analysis of the Hippocratic text *On the Sacred Disease* as a "sophistic protreptic speech" (2). On Galen's use of rhetoric, see von Staden 1995; Mattern 2008, esp. 69–97; Gleason 2009.

40. For a clear statement of this division, see Temkin 1935, 425–26; Temkin 1962, 102; Plastira-Valkanou 2003, 191–92. On the iatrosophists as "pagan" intellectuals who followed Galenism, see Temkin 1973, 61–62. For a critical perspective on the apparent distinction between iatrosophists and practicing physicians, see Duffy 1984. Bowersock (2010) examines the evolution of rhetoric in medical practice and the emergence of the label "iatrosophist." Pormann (2010, 424–25) discusses iatrosophists in the context of late antique education. Marx-Wolf (2017, 86–87) describes iatrosophists as possessing

a kind of "hybrid identity" that encompassed various kinds of expertise. See also Marrou 1956, 190–94, for medically trained public intellectuals and teachers during the Second Sophistic period (i.e., the late first through early third centuries C.E.).

41. Watts 2009, 115: "Gessius [a iatrosophist] often came to be seen as the best representative of sixth-century Alexandrian pagan intellectuals because he was among the community's most publicly engaged members." The enduring prominence of Gessius reflects both his "personal characteristics" and the high cultural relevance of medical expertise.

42. Eun. *VS* 19–22.2.4. See especially the discussions in Temkin 1962 and Penella 1990, 109–17.

43. Eun. *VS* 19.1.1. See Bowersock 2010, 87, for this interpretation.

44. Eun. *VS* 19.1.1.2–3. On Alexandria as a center of medical education, see the comments in Amm. Marc. 22.16.18: "In place of all direct experience it is sufficient to commend mastery of [medical] skill if [a physician] has said that he was trained at Alexandria." Cf. Pormann 2010, 419–20; Watts 2015, 387.

45. Eun. *VS* 19.2–3: "Of his famous pupils, dividing up [their inheritance], some were bequeathed one or the other [of these skills], and others both; but whatever they had inherited of practice or speech, they excelled in."

46. Eun. *VS* 19.3.4–4.1 (a strategy not dissimilar, perhaps, to modern pharmaceutical advertising). For a survey of testimonies to Magnus, see Plastira-Valkanou 2003, which focuses especially on the satirical epitaph preserved as AP 11.281: "When Magnus descended to the Underworld, trembling Hades said, 'He has come to revive even the dead.'" Translation adapted from Plastira-Valkanou 2003, 189. Thphl. Protospath. *Ur. Pr.* 5.1–2 is more pessimistic about Magnus' medical skill: "Magnus, a doctor in words but inexperienced in action."

47. Eun. *VS* 19.5. See the discussion in Scarborough 2010, 236–37.

48. Eun. *VS* 21. On Oribasius, see Temkin 1962, 98–99; Baldwin 1975; Grant 1997; and now Musgrove 2017.

49. Marx-Wolf 2018, 517: "Few medical writers in this period were engaged in producing new and completely original work arising from their own research, experiments, and practice. . . . Only recently have historians begun to look at this literature on its own terms in order to discover the ways in which individual commentators and handbook writers innovatively engaged with earlier material." See also Nutton 1984, 2, for critique of traditional scholarly treatment of late antique compilers and encyclopedists. For illustration of these editorial practices in Oribasius, see Orib. *Coll. med.* 8.41 ("From the works of Diocese: Laxatives of the belly"), 8.42 ("From the works of Dieuches: Things that purge downward lightly"). Orib. *Coll. med.* 24.1 is titled "From the works of Galen: On the brain and cerebral membranes" and is constructed largely out of excerpts from Galen's *On Anatomical Demonstrations*, with gaps where Galen goes into detail or refers directly to the vivisection of animals.

50. On the formalization of the late antique medical curriculum, see Iskandar 1976; Pormann 2010, 424–25; Watts 2015, 387–88; Marx-Wolf 2017, 81–82.

51. Maxwell (2006, 11–40) explores the similarities between preachers and Hellenistic popular moral philosophers as public speakers attempting "to shape entire communities according to moral ideals" (11). See also Mayer 2015a, Mayer 2015b, and Mayer 2015c for a discussion of how early Christian therapeutics of the soul built upon philosophical concepts and strategies.

52. See especially Marx-Wolf 2017, which argues that the rising professional and social status of doctors contributed to the efficacy and attraction of the image of "the good physician" in late antiquity (esp. 80). See also A. Jones 2009, 252–60, for evidence in support of the argument that the social status of physicians rose in late antiquity, situated explicitly in contrast to earlier scholarship.

53. A. Jones (2009) discusses physicians in the imperial administration (256–57) and the clergy (258). Basil of Ancyra and Aëtius of Antioch are among the most famous late antique ecclesial leaders who trained in medicine.

54. On lay readership of medical texts, see Cañizares 2010, which focuses, however, on Hippocratic material and the classical period.

55. Greg. Naz. *Or.* 43.

56. On the educational paths of Gregory and Caesarius, see McGuckin 2001, 35–36, 44; Elm 2012, 21–27. On Basil's education in Athens, see Rousseau 1994, 27–60. Elm (2012, 168) suggests that "Gregory's knowledge [of learned medicine] exceeded the norm, possibly because of his brother Caesarius's profession." On Gregory's references to medicine and medical knowledge, see the detailed survey in Keenan 1941.

57. Greg. Naz. *Or.* 43.23.2.1–2.

58. Greg. Naz. *Or.* 43.23.5.1–3.

59. Greg. Naz. *Or.* 43.23.6.1–3.

60. Little has been written on Marcellus, despite his relevance to current interest in the social history of medicine in late antiquity. Key works include Stannard 1973; Meid 1996; Ewers 2009; Cilliers 2010.

61. Marc. Emp. *De med.* Pr. 3.

62. Orib. *Lib. ad Eun.* Pr. 1.1.1–4.

63. Orib. *Lib. ad Eun.* Pr. 1.4.1–2.

64. Although, as Marx-Wolf (2018, 519) notes, "in addition to the intense engagement among early Christian writers with medical knowledge, there is plenty of evidence that Christians became doctors. They also became teachers of medicine and compilers of medical knowledge."

65. Meanwhile, many of those we know to have had further education, including in medicine, such as Basil of Caesarea and Basil of Ancyra, barely give the brain passing mention: engagement with the medical concept of the brain did not, apparently, correlate with formal medical education.

66. Chin 2008, esp. 2: "The rise of formal grammatical study from the fourth century to the sixth coincides not only with the growth in numbers of identifiably Christian texts and people but also with a rich period of text-based magical practices, divination through books, and the like." Cf. Stefaniw 2016, 249: "This notion of the text as medium

of all that is valuable to human flourishing is not invented by Christians, but is also the driving force behind the practice of grammatical study and textual criticism throughout the ancient world."

67. Nutton 2012, 4–6.

68. Pormann 2010, 421–22.

69. Cilliers (2019, 219–30) makes a similar argument about the role of late antique North African medical authors in the preservation and transmission of Greek medical knowledge.

70. Quoted in Iskandar 1976, 241.

71. Cilliers (2019, 117–80) summarizes our knowledge of late antique North African medical authors and their texts.

72. For a survey of late antique Latin medical literature, see Sigerist 1958. For examples of late antique medical commentaries, see Davies and Westerink 1981; Duffy 1983; Duffy 1997; Dickson 1998.

73. Nutton 1984, 2–4; Marx-Wolf and Upson-Saia 2015, 259; Gäbel 2018, 318.

74. See the discussion in Sharples and van der Eijk 2008, 23–25.

75. For medical texts in particular, see Nutton 1984, 2–4; Pormann 2010, 421–25; Marx-Wolf 2017, 81–82. For interpretative strategies in relation to encyclopedic works, see Pormann 2004; van der Eijk 2010; Doody 2010.

76. Osborne 1987, 10.

77. For example, Galen's *On Theriac to Piso* and *Therapeutics to Glaukon*. See also the letters written by (or attributed to) various physicians that are collected in the opening to *On Medicaments* by Marcellus of Bordeaux (Cilliers 2010).

78. On Gregory's engagement with medical and scientific ideas, see Robin D. Young 1993; Bishop 2000; Ludlow 2009; Wessel 2009; Gilbert 2014.

79. Ladner (1958) discusses these questions in detail.

80. Greg. Nyss. *Op. hom.* 30 (PG 44:240.27–256.40), with "the constitution of our body" identified in the subtitle (PG 44:240.28–29): "A Brief, More Medical Account of the Constitution of Our Body" (Θεωρία τις ἰατρικωτέρα περὶ τῆς τοῦ σώματος ἡμῶν κατασκευῆς δι' ὀλίγων). On the representation of Galenic material in this section of Gregory's work, see Ladner 1958, 78 (including fn87, with references).

81. Greg. Nyss. *Op. hom.* 30 (PG 44:240.30–41).

82. Greg. Nyss. *Op. hom.* 30 (PG 44:240.41–46).

83. Amb. *Ex.* 6.9.61 describes "medical experts" (*medendi periti*) as the source for his knowledge about the brain. Aug. *Gn. Litt.* 7.13.30 refers to "physicians" (*medici*) in relation to the claim that *pneuma* flows through the whole body. Greg. Nyss. *Op. hom.* 12 (PG 44:157.44–46) cites "medical experts" (οἱ τῆς ἰατρικῆς ἐπιστήμονες) as his authority for an explanation of mental illness that does not necessarily involve the brain.

84. Greg. Nyss. *Op. hom.* 12 (PG 44:157.34–39).

85. Greg. Nyss. *Op. hom.* 30 (PG 44:240.50–241.1).

86. Greg. Nyss. *Op. hom.* 30 (PG 44:241.33–244.6).

87. Greg. Nyss. *Op. hom.* 30 (PG 44:244.45–53): "The consequences of the opposite condition [to normal] makes it crystal clear that the brain contributes most to life. For

if the membrane around it suffers any wound or lesion, death follows the injury immediately, and nature does not endure the wound for a millisecond. It is just like when a foundation is sunk and the whole building collapses with the part. That part which, when it suffers, clearly entails the destruction of the whole animal, must be properly agreed to hold the cause of life."

88. Greg. Nyss. *Op. hom.* 30 (PG 44:244.53–245.18).

89. Greg. Nyss. *Op. hom.* 30 (PG 44:249.47–252.1).

90. Greg. Nyss. *Op. hom.* 12 (PG 44: 157.34–39).

91. Ruf. *Anat.* 73.

92. Pl. *Phdr.* 246a–54e.

93. Greg. Nyss. *Op. hom.* 12 (PG 44:156.31–36, 160.47–49). I discuss this contradiction further in chapter 4.

94. Wessel (2009) offers a nuanced analysis of the tension between "Platonic dualism and . . . medical materialism" (27) in Gregory's text. See especially 32–39 for discussion of the *hēgemonikon*. See also Gill 2018 and Singer 2018 for the argument that Galen similarly maintained a distinction between medical texts (where he talked about brain health) and psychological or ethical texts (where he did not).

95. Wicher 1986, 33.

CHAPTER 2. THE HISTORY OF THE BRAIN IN ANCIENT GREEK MEDICINE AND PHILOSOPHY

1. Since my discussion in this chapter moves freely between centuries before and after the Common Era, I provide B.C.E. and C.E. designations for all dates.

2. For example: Finger 2000; Knuuttila 2005; Rocca 2003; van der Eijk 2005a; von Staden 2005.

3. Pl. *Phd.* 96a6–9. All translations of this text are from Grube, in Cooper and Hutchinson 1997. Translation adapted.

4. Pl. *Phd.* 96b3–8. Translation adapted. For discussion of the separation of sensation and knowledge in this passage, see Manuli and Vegetti 1977, 32–33; Laks 1999, 261.

5. This simplifies the complexity of Presocratic philosophical works. See Curd and Graham 2008, 5; Holmes (2010, 88) argues that the physicality of Presocratic philosophy can best be understood "in terms of a provocative shift of explanatory emphasis," rather than as a "philosophical discovery" or an "empirical grasp of the natural world." The term *Presocratic,* first attested in 1788, is problematic (Laks 2002, 17–25). See also Laks 2002, 18–19, for a discussion of the passage from the *Phaedo* cited here as a point of rupture between "Presocratic" and classical philosophy.

6. See Laks 1999 for a detailed study.

7. Runia 2008.

8. Empedocles/blood: Manuli and Vegetti 1977, 12; Laks 1999, 261. Diogenes/air: Manuli and Vegetti 1977, 44; Laks 1999, 252; Laks 2008b. See also the handbook answer

provided in Aët. *Plac.* 4.5: "What is the *hēgemonikon* of the soul, and in what part is it? . . . Diogenes [locates] it in the left ventricle of the heart, which is the one filled with *pneuma*. Empedocles [locates it] in the composition of the blood."

9. The priority of Alcmaeon is noted in Solmsen 1961, 151–52; Harris 1973, 4–10; von Staden 1989, 155; C. Gross 1995, 245; Rocca 2003, 22–23; Lo Presti 2008, 17–30. The neuroscientist Robert Doty (2007) makes much of Alcmaeon's innovation, claiming that "the locus of the mind is not betrayed [sc. in observing the brain itself] and, until the epochal discovery of Alkmaion (Alcmaeon, ca. 500 BC) in the city of Kroton in Magna Graecia, humanity was free to assign thought and mental experience to whatever entity they chose, anatomical or otherwise" (561). On Alcmaeon's contribution to medical theory more generally, see Nutton 2012, 47–49.

10. Manuli and Vegetti 1977, 29. On the fame of Croton as a medical center, see Hdt. 3.131. On Croton as a center for Pythagorean activity, see Kahn 2001, 6–7.

11. Wellmann (1929) identified Alcmaeon as the *pater medicinae Graecae*. On Alcmaeon's relation to Pythagoras, see Harris 1973, 9–10.

12. Manuli and Vegetti 1977, 9–10; Longrigg 1993, 60; Clarke and O'Malley 1996, 1–3; Ochs 2004, 10–11.

13. A 8 DK = Aët. *Plac.* 6.17.1. On "Aëtius" and the problematic history of reconstructing the text now attributed to him, see Mansfeld 1989; Mansfeld and Runia 1997; Runia 1999a; Runia 1999b.

14. Laks 1999. See Betegh 2007 for a discussion of Heraclitus of Ephesus (c. 535–475 B.C.E.) as the originator of the notion that the soul is the "centre of cognition" (4). Hippon of Rhegium (fifth century B.C.E.) was remembered as arguing that "the soul is sometimes brain, sometimes water," but the testimony is late, and no explanation is provided (Hippol. *Ref.* 1.16).

15. A 5 DK = Theophr. *Sens.* 26.4–6.

16. A 5 DK = Theophr. *Sens.* 25.7–8.

17. Lloyd 1975, 122.

18. On *pneuma* in Presocratic philosophy, see Lloyd 2007. On *pneuma* in early Christianity, see Troy W. Martin 2006, and also the comments in Wright 2019, 399–401.

19. Arist. *De an.* 1.2, 405a21–25: "Diogenes, and others similarly, [said that the soul is] air [ἀέρα], since he thought that this was of all things finest in composition and a first principle, and that because of this the soul possessed the faculty of knowing and moving. Insofar as it was the first [principle], from which everything else derives, it knows; and insofar as it is the finest in composition, it has motor power."

20. A 19 DK = Theophr. *Sens.* 39.1–2.

21. A 19 DK = Theophr. *Sens.* 39.3–5.

22. Harris (1973, fig. 2) and Laks (2008a, 96–97) provide diagrams of the network of *phlebes* as described by Diogenes. This is the basis for Diogenes' renown among modern physicians as the pioneer of vascular anatomy (for example: Crivellato et al. 2006; cf. Harris 1973, 20).

23. Rocca 2003, 23; Rocca 2012; Wee 2017, 157–58.

24. Von Staden (2005) further emphasizes the divergence of theories about the brain in antiquity, attributing it to "the competitive, agonal nature of Greek culture" (11); see p. 12 for a survey of Presocratic views on the brain.

25. On the Hippocratic corpus and the debates about the attribution of its texts, see W. Smith 1979; Craik 2015. On the legends of Hippocrates, see Pinault 1992.

26. Temkin (1991) discusses late antique reception of Hippocratic medicine and the figure of Hippocrates.

27. This is most clearly stated in Hipp. *Morb.* 4.40.9–11: "Each [part], unless it becomes diseased, naturally has the largest portion of its own [humor] from those already described—the head of phlegm, the heart of blood, and the spleen of water." See Lonie 1981, 59–60, 260. On phlegm itself, see Lonie 1981, 277–79.

28. In Hippocratic medical texts, there is no consistent account of the humors. See Lonie 1981, 54–62, with reference to the key Hippocratic articulation of the four canonical humors, as presented in Hipp. *Nat. hom.* 4.1–3: "The human body contains within itself blood and phlegm and both yellow and black bile, and these constitute the nature of the human body, and through these the human being feels pain and is healthy." Hipp. *Genit.* 3.3–4 presents a different set of four: "There are four kinds of humor: blood, bile, water, and phlegm." Cf. Hipp. *Morb.* 4.32.4–7: "Both women and men have four kinds of humor in their body . . . these are phlegm, blood, bile, and water." Bile and phlegm, as a pair, is the most regular component of Hippocratic humoral theory, and reflects the ambiguity regarding whether the humors are pathological substances (i.e., blood and water cannot be humors) or become pathological when out of balance (see Lonie 1981, 59–61). The canonization of black bile, yellow bile, phlegm, and blood was a consequence of Galen's attention to the Hippocratic text *On the Nature of the Human Being,* as discussed in Nutton 2012, 77–85. For a more general history of the humors, see Arikha 2007. For the continued importance of humoral theory in medieval and Renaissance medicine, see Siraisi 1990, 104–6. Humoral medicine is not confined to the ancient Mediterranean but can be traced globally in different systems of medical practice (Horden 2013).

29. For the association between phlegm and winter, see Hipp. *Salubr.* 5.2–3: "[It is necessary] to purge during the six winter months, for this season is more apt to produce phlegm than summer." See also Hipp. *Nat. hom.* 7.1–3: "During winter, phlegm increases in the human body; for of the components of the body it is most similar to winter in nature, being the coldest." On phlegm as cold and wet, see Hipp. *Morb. sacr.* 11.4–5, regarding the consequences of repeated seizures: "For the brain has become wetter than is natural and filled with phlegm." See also Hippocrates' *On Glands,* which describes the brain as a site of excess moisture and flux but does not explicitly identify that moisture as phlegm. For ambiguity regarding whether phlegm is cold or hot, see Lonie 1981, 278–79fn450.

30. Hipp. *Carn.* 4.1–3.

31. Described in *On the Sacred Disease, On Glands* (esp. *Gland.* 12), and *On Diseases* 2 (esp. *Morb.* 2.1 and 2.11).

32. Hipp. *Morb.* 2.11.1–4.

33. Craik 2012, 72. Craik (2001) describes a more general theory of flux as the principle behind many ancient diseases.

34. Hipp. *Morb.* 4.35.8–9: "The head, being hollow and positioned above just like a cupping instrument draws up the phlegm."

35. Hipp. *Gland.* 10: "As to the head, this too has (matter) like glands, the brain. For the brain is both white and loose-textured, just as glands (are) too, and accords the same benefits to the head as glands do (elsewhere). When, in accordance with my account, it is present, the brain giving relief removes the moisture and sends the excess from the fluxes away out to distant parts." All translations of this text are from Craik 2009, unless otherwise stated. See also the comments on glands in general at Craik 2009, 43. It is not clear from *On Glands* whether the brain itself *is* a gland or is only "like glands."

36. Finger 2000, 29; von Staden 2005, 13–19.

37. Vidal and Ortega 2017, 29, including the salient remark that *On the Sacred Disease* cannot be held as representative of the entire or even most significant Hippocratic perspective on the brain, as it often is (see, e.g., Gross 1995, 246; Frampton 2008, 31–34).

38. Hipp. *Morb. sacr.* 16.1–4: "On these grounds, I consider the brain to hold the greatest power in the human being. For, while it is in a condition of health, it is the interpreter of the things that come from the air: the air endows it with intelligence." Cf. *Morb. sacr.* 17.1: "Therefore I say that the brain is the interpreter of consciousness."

39. Hipp. *Morb. sacr.* 16.6–11: "The brain also disseminates consciousness: for whenever a human being draws *pneuma* in, it arrives first at the brain, and the air is thereby scattered to the rest of the body, leaving behind in the brain its zenith and whatever it has of intelligence and wisdom." For a nuanced discussion of the geological metaphors that shape this text, see Wee 2017, 152–64, with particular discussion of the movement of air in relation to the brain at 157–62.

40. Hipp. *Morb. Sacr.* 7.19–20: "Whenever the vessels [sc. between the brain and the other parts of the body] have been shut off from the air by phlegm and do not allow it through, this renders the human being without either voice or sense."

41. Hipp. *Morb. sacr.* 7.2–5.

42. Hipp. *Morb. sacr.* 14.15–20.

43. Craik 2009.

44. Hipp. *Gland.* 11.3–12.2: "There are natural fluxes to the point of secretion, by the ears, by the eyes and by the nose: these three. There are others by the palate to the trachea and to the esophagus. There are others by the vessels to the spine and to the hips: seven in all. These fluxes are impure matter going off from the brain. And if they did not go off, it would have been an ailment."

45. Hipp. *Gland.* 12.11–18.

46. See especially Thumiger 2017, esp. 22, for the observation that the distinction between "mental and physical" in the works of classical philosophers, such as Plato and Xenophon, "finds no match in the medical texts" of the period. See also Holmes 2013 for the argument that Hippocratic writers avoided offering therapies for the soul, thereby leaving a gap for philosophical experts to develop a new kind of therapy.

47. Hipp. *Morb. sacr.* 11.15–18.

48. Hipp. *Gland.* 10.2–5: "For the brain is both white and loose-textured, just as glands (are) too, and accords the same benefits to the head as glands do (elsewhere). When, in accordance with my account, it is present, the brain giving relief removes the moisture and sends the excess from the fluxes away out to distant parts."

49. Pl. *Phd.* 80b1–5: "The soul is most like the divine, deathless, intelligible, uniform, indissoluble, always the same as itself, whereas the body is most like that which is human, mortal, multiform, unintelligible, soluble and never consistently the same." Translation by Grube, in Cooper and Hutchinson 1997.

50. See Sheppard 2000 on cross-pollination among philosophical schools in late antiquity. On the inclusion of Aristotelian texts in the Neoplatonist curriculum, see Blumenthal 1996, 3 and 25–26. Blumenthal (1986) further discusses the absorption of Aristotelian concepts and theories into Neoplatonism. See T. Shaw 1998, 32–33, for the argument that Christian authors tended to blend a Platonist tripartite psychology with Stoic ethics.

51. Plato argues for the division of the soul into distinct parts or faculties in Pl. *Resp.* 4, 440–41, esp. 440e8–441a6, where the *logistikon*, the *thumoeides*, and the *epithumētikon* are clearly distinguished from one another as representing different roles and responsibilities within a civic community.

52. Pl. *Ti.* 70a2–7. All translations of this text are by Zeyl, in Cooper and Hutchinson 1997.

53. Pl. *Ti.* 70a7–d8.

54. Pl. *Ti.* 73c6–d1.

55. Pl. *Ti.* 69c5–6.

56. Pl. *Ti.* 69e1–2. Translation adapted.

57. Pl. *Ti.* 73c–d.

58. von Staden 2005, 16.

59. Pl. *Leg.* 12, 961d5.

60. Pl. *Leg.* 12, 964d5–6.

61. Pl. *Leg.* 12, 964e6–8.

62. Hier. *In Ezech.* 1.1.

63. For Aristotle's theory of brain function, see Clarke and Stannard 1963; C. Gross 1995; von Staden 2005, 17–18.

64. On the use of meteorological and geological metaphors in ancient accounts of disease, see J. Johnson 2017 (Babylonian medicine) and Wee 2017 (Greek medicine).

65. Arist. *Somn. uig.* 3, 457b31–458a5. Cf. Arist. *PA* 2.7, 653a2–8: "It is necessary to imagine—likening small things to large—that what happens is like the genesis of rain: for, as steam evaporates up from the earth and is carried by the heat toward the upper regions, whenever it enters into the region of air above the earth that is cold, it condenses back into water because of the cold and flows back down to the ground."

66. Although note that Aristotle describes the brain as "the driest of all the fluid parts of the body," being totally devoid of blood (Arist. *PA* 2.7, 652a34–b1).

67. Arist. *PA* 2.14, 658b2–5: "Among creatures, the hairiest with regard to the head is the human being; this is necessarily so on account of the wetness of the brain and because of the sutures (for wherever is wettest and hottest, there it is necessary that there be most growth)." The heat here seems to be the heat of vapors exiting via the sutures, rather than the temperature of the brain itself, which Aristotle considered to be cold.

68. Arist. *PA* 2.10, 656a13–29, where Aristotle indirectly references Plato's argument that the thin covering of the skull weakens the human being physically, but enhances the human being intellectually, by enabling acute sensations (Pl. *Ti.* 75a–b): here Aristotle argues that the brain "is not the cause [αἴτιος] of any of the sensations, being without sensation in itself, and also being just like an excretion" (656a23–24); instead, "the region around the heart is the source [ἀρχὴ] of sensations" (656a27–28). In *MA* 7, Aristotle also seems to make the claim that the heart is the source of motion, based on the expansion and contraction of *pneuma* in its vicinity (see especially the commentary in Nussbaum 1978, 351–52). As such, Nussbaum claims that for Aristotle, the heart is the "bodily *archē* of, or for, the soul" (1978, 153). See also Frampton's (2008, 20–108, esp. 31–39) extensive discussion of the functions of the heart and dismissal of the brain in Aristotle.

69. Frampton 2008, 80.

70. Arist. *MA* 7, 70 (on the heart) and 10 (on *pneuma*). Nussbaum 1978, 153; see also 351–52 for commentary on the relevant passages in Aristotle's *On the Movement of Animals*. For more extensive discussion, see Frampton 2008, 68–81. Hahm (1977, 155–56) discusses this theory with reference to specific passages.

71. Arist. *MA* 10, 703a4–6.

72. Arist. *MA* 10, 703a9–10, 14–16: "It is clear that all animals have connate *pneuma* and derive their strength from this. . . . And since the origin is for some animals situated in the heart, for some in an analogous part, it is clear that the connate *pneuma* is also there." All translations of this text are from Nussbaum 1978, unless otherwise stated.

73. On the impact of images, affections, and ideas on the expansion and contraction of the heart, see Arist. *MA* 7, 701b13–33. On the expansion and contraction of *pneuma* and its role in enabling movement, see *MA* 10, 703a19–22.

74. Arist. *MA* 7, 701b1–10: "The movement of animals is like that of automatic puppets that are set in motion by a small movement: the cables are released and the pegs strike against one another. . . . For they have functioning parts that are of the same kind: the sinews and bones. The latter are like the pegs and the iron in our example, the sinews like the cables. When these are released and slackened the creature moves." Translation adapted.

75. For Aristotle's theory of *pneuma*, see Solmsen 1957; G. Freudenthal 1995. On *pneuma* in the medical and philosophical tradition prior to Aristotle, see Lloyd 2007. Regarding later development of the concept, see Verbeke 1945 and, with a particular focus on the late classical physician Praxagoras of Cos, Lewis 2017.

76. Frampton 2008, 50: "The crux of the problem that plagued Aristotle's cardiosarcosinew model of sensorimotor function—and the problem that for centuries would

continue to plague most other counterproposals—was the difficulty of finding empirically well-delineated anatomical channels that could plausibly shuttle sensorimotor impulses between a centralized controlling source-organ and multiple peripheral sensory and motor end-organs." See also Gregoric and Kuhar 2014, 110–11.

77. Solmsen 1961, 177–78.

78. Praxagoras fr. 3 Lewis. See the discussion in Annas 1992, 21–22.

79. Solmsen 1961; von Staden 1989, 139–53 (on dissection), 155–61 (on the brain), 195–208 (for testimonies), and 237–39 (for discussion); von Staden 2005, 18–30, for a concise summary.

80. Annas 1992, 61–64.

81. The fragments of Praxagoras are collected in Steckerl 1958 and Lewis 2017.

82. Lewis 2017, 1–7.

83. Lewis 2017, 6–7.

84. Praxagoras fr. 16 Lewis. See the discussion in Lewis 2017, 166 and 292–93, for critical remarks.

85. Praxagoras fr. 3 Lewis. See the discussion in Lewis 2017, 219–22.

86. Frampton 2008, 69–81, esp. 79.

87. Rocca 2003, 32–33; Lewis 2017, 6–7.

88. Herophilus: von Staden 1989. Erasistratus: Garofalo 1988.

89. Longrigg 1988, 457–62; von Staden 1989, 139–53; von Staden 1992; Flemming 2005.

90. Longrigg 1988, 462–64; von Staden 1989, 158–61; see also Herophilus t. 75–79 von Staden (anatomy of the brain and skull) and t. 80–89 von Staden (nerves and eye); Rocca 2003, 36–38; von Staden 2000, 87–91.

91. Herophilus t. 77a, 77b, 78, 79 von Staden.

92. Herophilus t. 78 von Staden; Rocca 2003, 37.

93. Ruf. *Anat.* 71–75 = Herophilus t. 81 von Staden; Erasistratus fr. 288–89 Garofalo. On Erasistratus in general, see Longrigg 1988, 472–82. On Erasistratus' anatomy of the brain, see Garofalo 1988, 26–27 and (including the nerves also) von Staden 2000, 91–96.

94. We saw this in Gregory of Nyssa's *On the Constitution of the Human Being* (chapter 1, above).

95. See Tieleman 1996 on Chrysippus' psychology, including contextualization of the fragments of Chrysippus within the polemical arguments of Galen, which was a central site of their transmission. For the influence of Praxagoras on Chrysippus, see Tieleman 1996, 83–86, 189; Rocca 2003, 32–33.

96. Hahm 1977, 163–66.

97. Hahm 1977, 163–65.

98. Hahm 1977, 159; von Staden 2000, 102. Chrysippus' predecessors in the Stoic school held slightly different views. See Hahm 1977, 157–61 for discussion.

99. Hahm 1977, 163.

100. Gal. *PHP* 3.10–11. All translations of this text are from De Lacy 2005, unless otherwise stated. The translation here is adapted. For discussion, see Hahm 1977, 159.

101. On the differentiation of *pneuma* during this period and the challenge of identifying who first articulated which distinction, see von Staden 1989, 253–54, esp. fn52–53; Rocca 2003, 61–64; Rocca 2012, 635–36. Rocca (2012) discusses the historiographical "reconstruction" of a tripartite *pneuma* (psychic, vital, natural) in Galen, arguing that in fact Galen did not consistently uphold a concept of natural *pneuma*. See also Sharples and van der Eijk 2008, 101fn505, for a brief discussion of psychic *pneuma*, with references to Hellenistic medical and philosophical texts.

102. Estimates run to 10 percent of extant Greek literature prior to the fourth century C.E. (Holmes 2009, 554).

103. Temkin 1973; Nutton 1984; García-Ballester 2002.

104. Hankinson 1991.

105. Discussed at length in Tieleman 1996. On the text *On the Opinions of Hippocrates and Plato*, see Hankinson 2006, esp. 232–33.

106. Gal. *PHP* 7.1.5.4–5.

107. For discussion of this argument and Galen's counterargument, see Hankinson 1991, 215–18, 232; Tieleman 1996, 42–44.

108. Hankinson 1991, 215–16, esp. 215.

109. Gleason 2009, 98–100.

110. See the description in Gal. *Praen.* 5.9–21 and Gal. *AA* 8.3, and cf. Gal. *AA* 11.4, with discussion in C. Gross 1998; Frampton 2008, 198–200; Gleason 2009, 97–100, Mattern 2013, 157–60. See French 2006, 26–27 for Vesalius' imitation and critique of this experiment.

111. Dissection of ox brain removed from body: Gal. *AA* 9.1–9, esp. 9.1. Dissection of the brain of an ape: Gal. *AA* 9.10. Dissection of the brain within a living animal: Gal. *AA* 9.11–13, esp. 9.11.

112. Gal. *AA* 9.1 (2:707.4–708.2 K.).

113. Gal. *AA* 9.11. Cf. Gal. *PHP* 7.3.15–16.

114. Gal. *PHP* 7.3.32–33: "This was not the least reason why Erasistratus mistakenly believed that the animal immediately becomes motionless when the meninx is cut; for he saw that oxen wounded at the first vertebra become motionless as soon as the meninx is severed. But this results not from the injury to the meninx but from the exposure of the posterior ventricle. This is evident from the fact that when any other part of the meninx is wounded no such effect is produced."

115. Gal. *AA* 9.12.22–23. Translation from Duckworth 1962. This portion of the text is no longer extant in Greek. Cf. Gal. *PHP* 7.3.17–18, where the same progression from slight to serious injury is described in relation to cutting the cerebral ventricles. Notably, Galen here makes a comparison to the effects of pressure on the brain ventricles, as observed in cases of trepanation.

116. Gal. *PHP* 7.3.19–22. See the discussion in Hankinson 2006, 235–36; Debru 2008, 272; Rocca 2008, 252–53; Gleason 2009, 101–2.

117. On Galen's concept of *pneuma*, including his engagement with its Stoic theorization, see Rocca 2003, 59–66.

118. Rocca 2003, 65.

119. Rocca 2003, 245–48.

120. Hankinson 2006, 235.

121. Debru 2008, 272.

122. Rocca 2003, 59: "Pneuma is a theoretical construct that may be used in a physiological system without undue difficulty. . . . Pneuma is a broad church."

123. Gal. *PHP* 7.3.21–22. Translation adapted.

124. Nutton 2013, 299.

CHAPTER 3. THE INVENTION OF VENTRICULAR LOCALIZATION

1. All other dates in this chapter are C.E., unless otherwise noted.

2. In general, historians working on late antiquity use the phrase "ventricular localization," while medievalists and early modern historians prefer "cell doctrine" or "cell theory." I use these terms interchangeably. "Ventricular" comes from the Latin word *uentriculum*, "little stomach," from *uentres* ("stomach"), and was in use in antiquity. "Cell" comes from the Latin word *cella* ("room") or *cellula*, "little room." Late medieval authors sometimes used *uentriculum, uentres, cella,* and *cellula* without distinction (Stratton 1931, 128).

3. Clarke and O'Malley 1996, 463; C. Gross 1999, 30–36; Manzoni 1998; Grunert 2002; Green 2003; Knuuttila 2005; Finger 2000, 53–55.

4. Manzoni 1998, 119. Cf. Finger 2000, 53: "The most significant conceptual change about brain function to take place during the Dark Ages seems to have occurred in the fourth or fifth century. At this time, some scholarly Christians began to present the hollow ventricles of the brain as the abode of the rational soul. The brain substance forthwith assumed a secondary role to that of its cavities."

5. Manzoni 1998, 117. See the summary in Clarke and O'Malley 1996, 463, introducing Nemesius' account of ventricular localization: "[Nemesius' work] was an interesting attempt to interpret Greek scientific knowledge of the human body from the standpoint of Christian philosophy."

6. Marx-Wolf 2015, 91.

7. Vidal 2009, 12.

8. Rocca 2003, 247.

9. Hippolytus' authorship of this work is contested, but there is a consensus that it must have been written during the early part of the third century by a Christian theologian living in Rome. I continue to use the name "Hippolytus" for the sake of concision. See Secord 2013, 217fn1.

10. Secord (2013) discusses Hippolytus' familiarity with contemporary anatomical demonstrations.

11. The six references: in a fragment assigned to the Presocratic philosopher Hippon of Rhegium, as identical with the soul (1.16.1–2); as an analogue for Adam (as the source of all humans) (5.7.35.2–4, 5.8.13) and for Eden (as the source of all rivers) (5.9.15.1–4); as a model for the cosmos (4.51.10–14, 5.17.11–12).

12. Hippol. *Haer.* 4.51.8, terms from Litwa 2016, 187.

13. Hippol. *Haer.* 4.51.9, terms from Litwa 2016, 187.

14. Hippol. *Haer.* 4.51.10.1–11.1.

15. Hippol. *Haer.* 4.51.11.1–3. Note that the Greek terms in Hippolytus' account recall language from the Hippocratic texts *On the Sacred Disease* and *On Glands,* highlighted above in chapter 2. The observation that the functional brain should be unmoved was as old as Alcmaeon of Croton, who warned that "the senses . . . are incapacitated if [the brain] is moved [κινουμένου] or changes position" (A 5 DK = Theophr. *Sens.* 26.5).

16. Hippol. *Haer.* 4.51.11.3–4.

17. Hippol. *Haer.* 4.51.11.4–12.6.

18. On Galen's vivisections as performances, see von Staden 1997a; Gleason 2009.

19. Arist. *Rhet.* 3.11, 1411b24–30: "By 'making them see things' I mean using expressions that represent things as in a state of activity . . . 'Thereupon up sprang [ᾄξαντες] the Hellenes to their feet,' where 'up sprang' gives us activity as well as metaphor, for it at once suggests swiftness." Translation adapted from Barnes 1984. See Webb 2009, 85–86. On present participles as a tool for "zooming in" on action, see Panagiotidou 2016, 140.

20. [Longin.] 15.2.2–3.

21. [Longin.] 15.11.2–3. See Goldhill 2007, 4–7.

22. Goldhill 2007, 4, on Plutarch's evaluation of ekphrasis in Thucydides.

23. See the discussion of this in Secord 2013.

24. Hippol. *Haer.* 5.17.11.1–12.5.

25. Hippol. *Haer.* 4.51.13.1–2.

26. Hippol. *Haer.* 4.51.12.6–13.1: "The end of which [vessel] terminates in the reproductive organs, and from this seed is excreted, going from the brain through the loins."

27. E.g., Is. 40:22: "He stretches out the heavens like a canopy [καμάραν], and spreads them out like a tent to live in." NIV translation. See also Litwa 2016, 311fn328.

28. Gal. *UP* 8.14 (3:675.8–12 K.). All translations of this text are from May 1968, unless otherwise stated.

29. Gal. *UP* 8.14 (3:675.29–676.5 K.).

30. Gal. *UP* 8.14 (676.17–677.2 K.). Translation adapted.

31. Gal. *UP* 8.14 (3:677.2–7 K.).

32. Miller 2018, 155–90.

33. Robert M. Young 1970 (describing cerebral localization in the nineteenth century); Manzoni 1998, esp. 116–19; Martensen 2004 (focusing on seventeenth-century developments in cerebral localization); Finger 2000 (esp. chaps. 4 and 5).

34. An important exception is Grunert 2002.

35. See Rocca 2003, 245–47, for the argument that Galen does not describe a theory of ventricular localization.

36. Nem. *Nat. hom.* 8 (Morani 63.2–5, 7–11).

37. Aët. Amid. *Med. coll.* 6.2.1–17.

38. Herophilus t. 138 von Staden = Gal. *UP* 8.11 (3:667.12–16 K.). Translation adapted from May 1968.

39. My account here is dependent upon the analysis of von Staden 1999, 177–87, with reference to the middle ventricle at 183–84. See also the brief discussion in von Staden 1989, 389.

40. von Staden 1999, 181.

41. Phot. *Bibl.* 211 (Bekker 169b13–16).

42. von Staden 1989, 389; von Staden 1999, 182–84.

43. von Staden 1999, 194.

44. Phot. *Bibl.* 185 (Bekker 130b15–18).

45. Phot. *Bibl.* cod. 211 (Bekker 168b31–32).

46. Phot. *Bibl.* cod. 185 (Bekker 130b20–22).

47. Wicher 1986, 32–33.

48. Telfer 1955, 208–9; Sharples and van der Eijk 2008, 2–3.

49. The letters complimented Nemesius on his philosophical and rhetorical acumen, and the poem attempted to convince Nemesius (perhaps with some success) to convert to Christianity. See van Dam 2002, 86–87. Van Dam 1996, 61–62, argues against identifying these two Nemesii.

50. Jaeger 1914; Skard 1937; Skard 1938; Skard 1939; Skard 1942; Halton 1989; Streck 2001; Debru 2005; Sharples and van der Eijk 2008; Wessel 2010.

51. Nem. *Nat. hom.* 6 (Morani 56.2–4). All translations of this text are from Sharples and van der Eijk 2008, unless otherwise stated.

52. Nem. *Nat. hom.* 12 (Morani 68.11–13).

53. Nem. *Nat. hom.* 13 (Morani 69.18–20).

54. Nem. *Nat. hom.* 13 (Morani 69.16–18).

55. Nem. *Nat. hom.* 13 (Morani, 69.20–25).

56. Nem. *Nat. hom.* 13 (Morani 69.25–70.3).

57. Nem. *Nat. hom.* 13 (Morani 70.21).

58. Nem. *Nat. hom.* 13 (Morani 70.24–71.3).

59. Nem. *Nat. hom.* 8 (Morani 64.1–2).

60. Nem. *Nat. hom.* 8 (Morani 64.4–7).

61. Nem. *Nat. hom.* 8 (Morani 64.8–13).

62. Nem. *Nat. hom.* 8 (Morani 64.9). See the comments in Sharples and van der Eijk 2008, 112fn552, with reference to Gal. *PHP* 7.5.13.

63. Nem. *Nat. hom.* 8 (Morani 64.9–11).

64. For a discussion of ancient debates about whether the nerves are solid or hollow, see Wright 2016, 73–76. According to Rufus of Ephesus, Erasistratus considered sensory nerves to be hollow, with the implication that motor nerves were not (Herophilus t. 81 von Staden = Ruf. *Anat.* 71–75; Erasistratus fr. 288–89 Garofalo).

65. Nem. *Nat. hom.* 8 (Morani 64.11–13).

66. 1 Cor. 12:21. NIV translation.

67. Joh. Chrys. *In 1 Cor. hom.* 31 (PG 61:261.27–35).

68. For more detailed discussion of this interpolation, see Wright 2017 and 2018.

69. P. Brown 2000.

70. Gourevitch and Gourevitch (1998) argue that Augustine was familiar with the work of Caelius Aurelianus, a late antique medical author from North Africa. See also Keenan 1936; Keenan 1939; Retief 2010; Cilliers 2019.

71. Aug. *Gn. litt* 7.17–9.

72. This exegetical habit was inspired by the work of the Jewish theologian Philo of Alexandria (see Runia 2001).

73. Aug. *Gn. litt.* 7.3. Translation from Hill 2002. Elsewhere in quotations from *Literal Commentary on Genesis,* I use my own translations.

74. After running through various accounts of the nature of soul, Augustine concludes that it must be understood as incorporeal, and therefore not composed of any bodily element(s), but that it moves the earthly body through the medium of the lighter elements, air and fire. In order to articulate this medium, he draws upon medical doctrine of a "fiery air" that pours from the brain into narrow channels to the sensory organs, thereby animating the whole. Whilst he does not name *spiritus* here, it is clearly to this substance that he refers.

75. Aug. *Gn. litt.* 7.17.

76. Aug. *Gn. litt.* 7.18.

77. Aug. *Gn. litt.* 7.18. Augustine's use of the metaphor *uigere* (to flourish, bloom) is perhaps an allusion to Cicero's phrase *memoria uigere,* "to flourish in memory," which refers to the training of one's memory to retain the main points of a speech.

78. Aug. *Gn. litt.* 7.18.

79. Aug. *Gn. litt.* 7.18.

80. Pl. *Ti.* 45a7–b1.

81. Aug. *Gn. litt.* 7.19.

82. Aug. *Gn. litt.* 7.20.

83. Frampton 2008, 257; C. Smith 2014, 6.

84. Green 2003, 140.

85. Wicher 1986.

86. Gal. *UP* 8.6. See my discussion in chapter 2.

87. Temkin 1962, 104.

88. Thphl. Protospath. *Opif. hom.* 4.5.11–15, 4.8.8–11.

89. Thphl. Protospath. *Opif. hom.* 4.31.1–9.

90. Thphl. Protospath. *Opif. hom.* 4.31.9–13.

91. Thphl. Protospath. *Opif. hom.* 4.31.13–18.

92. Thphl. Protospath. *Opif. hom.* 4.31.19–24.

93. Thphl. Protospath. *Opif. hom.* 4.31.24–32.

94. Frampton 2008, 253, 258.

95. Greg. Nyss. *Op. hom.* 12 (PG 44:161.7–19).

96. Greg. Nyss. *Op. hom.* 12 (PG 44:161.9–24).

97. Gal. *UP* 7.11 (3:553.12–17 K.) and 7.13 (3:561.2–4, 7–11 K.), and see also the musical metaphors for the brain in Gregory's description of the cerebral membrane that descended down the spine as "flute-like" (αὐλοειδῶς), adding that it granted impulse

and power to the bones and "joints" (ἁρμονιῶν, also "harmonies"), at *Op. hom.* 30 (PG 44:249.51–252.1).

98. See, e.g., Nem. *Nat. hom.* 1 (Morani 4.20–24).

99. Greg. Nyss. *Op. hom.* 12 (PG 44:156.33–34.

100. Greg. Nyss. *Op. hom.* 12 (PG 44:156.50–157.1).

101. Greg. Nyss. *Op. hom.* 12 (PG 44:157.41–47).

102. See van der Eijk 2005a, 119–21; McDonald 2009a, 12–13, 82–85; Thumiger 2017, 46; Wright 2020.

103. Arist. *NE* 1.7, 1098a7–12; Plot. *En.* 1.4.16.23–27.

104. Pl. *Phd.* 85e–86, 91e–95a; Arist. *De an.* 1.4, 407b27–408a28; for Plotinus, see Rich 1963.

105. Taylor 1983; E. Wagner 2001.

106. Isid. Pel. *Ep.* 4.125 (PG 78:1197C–1204A). The full address is "To Proeschius, learned physician" (Προεσχιῳ σχολαστικῳ ἰατρῳ) or, as Temkin (1991) renders it, "To Proeschius Scholasticus, physician" (205fn43). It is possible that σχολαστικῳ ἰατρῳ carried a similar meaning to "iatrosophist," i.e., "medical sophist."

107. Gal. *QAM* (4:767.1–2 K.).

108. The title given to the letter, "About the same thing," clearly refers to the title of the previous letter, "About the soul."

109. Gal. *QAM* 3 (4:772.17–773.4 K.).

110. Gal. *QAM* 3 (4:774.19–775.2 K.). Translation from Singer 2013.

111. Isid. Pel. *Ep.* 4.125 (PG 78:1197C).

112. Isid. Pel. *Ep.* 4.125 (PG 78:1197C).

113. Isid. Pel. *Ep.* 4.125 (PG 78:1197C, 1200A): τῇ κράσει τοῦ σώματος ἕπονται αἱ τῆς ψυχῆς δυνάμεις.

114. The model of soul as "harmony" is not what Galen is arguing for in *QAM*, but rather reflects a traditional mode of the soul/body relationship that Isidore conflates with Galen's argument.

115. Isid. Pel. *Ep.* 4.125 (PG 78:1200B).

116. Isid. Pel. *Ep.* 4.125 (PG 78:1201A). Galen frames *QAM* similarly as a discussion of the relationship between bodily *krasis* and the virtue (although not the mortality) of the soul. See García-Ballester 1988, esp. 127–30.

117. Isid. Pel. *Ep.* 4.125 (PG 78:1201B): "If the soul were immortal, he says, as Plato wishes, why does it separate whenever the brain becomes violently cold, excessively dry, or excessively wet?" Cf. Gal. *QAM* (4:775.4–8 K.): "If it is immortal, as Plato wishes, why does it separate whenever the brain becomes violently cold, excessively hot, excessively dry, or excessively wet?"

118. Most Platonist interpretations of Galen's localization model ignored his theory of temperament. See Hankinson 1991 and 2006. Donini (2008) examines the contradiction between the theory of temperament in *QAM* and Galen's tripartition of the soul in other texts, such as *On the Opinions of Hippocrates and Plato.*

119. Isid. Pel. *Ep.* 4.125 (PG 78:1200A): "But he ought not to put his mind to this [question]. For, following medical dogma and wishing to exhibit his own proper skill,

he did not give heed to the truth. Let this man chatter on about the treatment of bodies, since he is a craftsman in this (for I will not diminish his worthiness in this regard) but let him not contend with wiser men regarding the soul; let him not enter a contest in which he is untrained and unpractised."

120. Yet, medical, philosophical, and theological authors continued to note the plurality of the tradition: Lact. *Op. dei* 16.1–5; Aug. *Trin.* 10.7; Cael. Aur. *Acut.* 1.8.53–54; Nem. *Nat. hom.* 2 (Morani 16.11–17.15); Thdt. *Graec. aff. cur.* 5.22–25.

121. Gilbert (2014) suggests a tendency toward "cardiocentrism," especially in Origen's wake (3–4). Gilbert's own work shows, however, that theologians could not be divided simply into cardiocentric and encephalocentric camps. More often they supported both positions, depending upon rhetorical context and goals.

122. Isid. Pel. *Ep.* 4.125 (PG 78:1201D–1204A).

123. Isid. Pel. *Ep.* 4.125 (PG 78:1204A): "This does not demonstrate that the soul is not immortal, but rather that its faculties are impeded [ἐμποδίζεσθαι], just as a musician is not excellent if he has a discordant lyre [ἄμουσον λύραν], nor does he produce harmonious song [ἐναρμόνιον . . . μέλος] if he falls into the sea."

124. Isid. Pel. *Ep.* 4.125 (PG 78:1200A): "Neither let an athlete judge music."

125. Gal. *UP* 8.2 (3:614.9–615.9 K.), discussed above.

126. I discuss this argument further in chapter 2.

127. Gal. *UP* 8.4 (3:629.8–18 K.).

128. LSJ s.v. I.1. On *skindapsos* as a nonsense word: May 1968, I, 395fn35, with reference to similar usage in Gal. *Diff. febr.* 2.6 (7:348 K.) and *Diff. puls.* (8:662 K.); Rocca 2003, 83; Morison 2008, 133–35, although see also 134fn25.

129. LSJ s.v. II.3; L&S s.v. I.B. Other meanings included the sinews and bow strings.

130. Amb. *Ex.* 6.9.61. Translation adapted from Savage 1961.

CHAPTER 4. THE GOVERNING BRAIN

1. See my discussion in chapter 2.

2. Pl. *Ti.* 69c–70e.

3. Pl. *Ti.* 70a4–7. All translations of this text are by Zeyl, in Cooper and Hutchinson 1997. This translation is adapted.

4. Pl. *Leg.* 12 (964e1–965a2).

5. Pl. *Ti.* 73c6–d2.

6. Hom. *Il.* 1.194–200.

7. Heraclit. *All.* 17.8. Translation adapted from Russell and Konstan 2005.

8. A Middle Platonist philosopher by the name of Alcinous is not otherwise known. The origin for the identification of "Alcinous" as Albinus is Freudenthal 1879. Dillon (1993, ix–xiii) argues against this identification.

9. Alc. *Did.* 17.4.1–6.

10. Alc. *Did.* 17.4.6–10.

11. Runia 1995.

12. For this list, see Runia 2001, 336. The passages in question are *Leg.* 2.91, *Leg.* 3.115, *Agr.* 46, *Somn.* 1.27, *Somn.* 1.32, *Spec.* 3.111, *Spec.* 3.184, *Spec.* 4.92, *Spec.* 4.123, *Opif.* 139.1–9, *Det.* 33, *Det.* 85, *Conf.* 19.

13. Ph. *Leg.* 3.115.4–8.

14. Ph. *Somn.* 1.32.

15. On Gregory's familiarity with Philo's *On the Creation of the World,* see Gilbert 2014, 29 and, on the localization of the *hēgemonikon* in Philo more generally, 28–61.

16. Greg. Nyss. *Op. hom.* 12 (PG 44:156–57).

17. Gal. *PHP* 2.4.17. All translations of this text are from De Lacy 2005, unless otherwise stated.

18. I discuss this text in greater detail in the next chapter.

19. Joh. Chrys. *Ep. 1 ad Tim.* 13 (PG 62:570.35–39).

20. Joh. Chrys. *Ep. 1 ad Tim.* 13 (PG 62:570.39–41).

21. Pl. *Ti.* 69d6–e3.

22. For further discussion, see chapter 5.

23. On the hexameral genre, see Robbins 1912 (58–59 on Ambrose in particular). On Philo's exegesis of the creation narrative in Genesis, see Runia 2001. On Basil's *Hexameron,* see Lim 1990 and Sandwell 2011.

24. Teleology (the notion that everything is constructed for the sake of a certain end, or *telos*) is particularly associated with Aristotle. On the incorporation of Aristotelian teleological into ancient medical theories, see von Staden 1997b.

25. On teleological explanations of human anatomy, especially in Galen, see Schiefsky 2007b. See Sandwell 2011, 546, for teleological explanations in hexameral literature.

26. For Christian reception of Galenic teleology, Siraisi 1997, 4 (giving the example of Lactantius); Lloyd 2003, 234; M. Johnson 2005 (esp. chap. 1); Sharples and van der Eijk 2008, 13. D. Martin (2004, 123–24) contrasts the "conservative" teleology of Galen (that is, the demiurge must work within the constraints imposed by nature) with the Christian understanding of God as transcending natural constraints. As Stefaniw (2016) has compellingly argued, late antique Christian arguments about the order of created things provided the foundation for an ethical imperative regarding how to live within that created order. That is to say, teleological accounts of human anatomy did not simply support explanations of human nature but supported pastoral care also.

27. Compare, for example, Amb. *Ex.* 6.9.55 with Cic. *DND* 2.142–43, on the eyes as sentries posted in the citadel of the skull.

28. Robbins (1912, 58–59) notes that the final book of the *Exameron,* devoted to the construction of the human being, is unlike the remainder of the text in that it has no obvious source. Basil of Caesarea similarly borrowed from Greek natural philosophy and medical science in his *Hexameron.* See Sandwell 2011, 548.

29. Amb. *Ex.* 6.9.61. All translations of this text are from Savage 1961, unless otherwise indicated.

30. Amb. *Ex.* 6.9.57. Translation adapted. The term *consultator* refers to a person who consults a jurist for an opinion in a legal matter (Berger 1953, 412; Chroust 1955, 527fn2). It is possible that it is here a scribal error for *consul* or *consulares.*

31. Amb. *Ex.* 6.9.57 (translation adapted).

32. Amb. *Ex.* 6.9.55.

33. Holmes 2013, 168–72; de Wet 2019, 427–28. See also Galen's *On the Affected Parts* 3, regarding the influence of the stomach upon the brain.

34. For further discussion, see chapter 5.

35. Joh. Chrys. *In Matt.* 44.7 (PG 57:472.13–17).

36. De Wet 2015; de Wet 2019, 433.

37. Greg. Nyss. *Op. hom.* 30 (PG 44:249.45–47).

38. Greg. Nyss. *Op. hom.* 30 (PG 44:251.57–252.1). J. Warren Smith (2000) explores this image elsewhere in Gregory's corpus. Schiefsky (2007a, 87–89) and Berryman (2009, 213–15) discuss a similar analogy in Greg. Nyss. *Anim. et res.* (PG 46:35.45–36.15).

39. Arist. *MA* 10, 701b1–10. Berryman (2009, 211) discusses a variation on image in the writings of the Stoic emperor Marcus Aurelius: "Marcus Aurelius makes frequent use of the comparison to puppets worked by strings. The term he uses is etymologically connected to *neura,* the term used first for the sinews that move an animal's limbs and, later, the nerves. Marcus Aurelius uses the puppet image to claim that our impulses pull us around." For further discussion of Aristotle's theory of voluntary motion and its influence on later theories of the nerves, see chapter 2.

40. Pl. *Phdr.* 246a–b, 247b–248b, 253c–254e, 255e–256a. For analysis of a more conventional adaptation of the charioteer metaphor in Gregory's *On the Soul,* see Wessel 2010, 373–75. On the popularity of the charioteer metaphor in Christian ascetic writings, see T. Shaw 1998, 86fn19, citing Basil of Ancyra, Evagrius, Gregory of Nyssa, Basil of Caesarea, John Chrysostom, and Jerome. As Shaw explains, the metaphor as used in these ascetic texts represents abstinence and self-control.

41. Gal. *Caus. resp.* (4:469.10–14 K.), translation from Furley and Wilkie 1984.

42. Greg. Nyss. *Op. hom.* 12 (PG 44:156.31–36).

43. Greg. Nyss. *Op. hom.* 12 (PG 44:160.47–49).

44. Gregory's negotiation here echoes that of Plotinus, who argued that the brain was not the seat of the discursive phase of the soul (for the soul is omnipresent, although its functions may be dispersed), but at the same time recognized the brain as the center of the nervous system. See Rich 1963, 10; Tieleman 1998.

45. Amb. *Ex.* 6.9.55.

46. For detailed discussion of this metaphor in Theodoret, see Wright 2018.

47. 1 Cor. 12:28 (NIV translation).

48. Joh. Chrys. *Princ. Act. hom.* 3.3 (PG 51:92.22–31).

49. This is the same elision of head and brain that we saw in Ambrose's *Exameron.*

50. Eph. 4:15–16 (NIV translation).

51. Joh. Chrys. *In Eph. hom.* 11 (PG 62:84.4–24).

52. Joh. Chrys. *In Eph. hom.* 11 (PG 62:84.26–32).

53. See my discussion in chapter 2.

54. See, for example, Galen's cure of Pausanias, who had injured his back, but whose fingers were impaired, in Gal. *Loc. aff.* 3.14 (8:213.10–214.6 K.).

55. Joh. Chrys. *In Eph. hom.* 11 (PG 62:84.38–42).

56. On the role of the body/community analogy in "boundary maintenance," see Fournier 2016. Contemporary analysis of how the body/society metaphor enables discussion and negotiation of social boundaries is grounded in Douglas 1966, which explores in particular how bodily fluids, such as saliva or semen, represent "boundary pollution" within the social order (125–27).

57. Joh. Chrys. *In Eph. hom.* 11 (PG 62:84.42–49).

58. Mitchell (1991) points out that Paul's verb καταρτίζειν, used in reference to conflict and resolution within early Christian communities, means not only "to put in order, restore" in a political sense, but also "the knitting together of broken bones or dislocated joints" (74–75). Laird (2013, 133) notes a similar image in Chrysostom's sermon *On the Incomprehensibility of the Nature of God*, where he interprets a reference to a dislocated bone as indicating "erring Christians in his congregation," who "are seen to be part of the body, but crippled and not functioning as they ought. This corresponds with his view of them as sick rather than dead, as semi-Christian, on the edge within, or close outside the Christian fold, but defective in their understanding." In his exegesis of Ephesians, Chrysostom appears to take a harder line.

CHAPTER 5. THE RHETORIC OF CEREBRAL VULNERABILITY

1. *Il.* 3.298–301.

2. Archibald G. Brown, "A Sermon Delivered on Lord's-Day Evening, June 20th 1869," in Brown 1873, 73.

3. Joh. Chrys. *In 1 Tim. hom.* 13 (PG 62:567.60–570.64); [Joh. Chrys.] *De prec.* (PG 64:461.37–44).

4. Greg. Nyss. *Op. hom.* 30 (PG 44:244.44–51).

5. Brain injuries invariably lead to death in the *Iliad* (8.85–86, 11.95–98, 12.184–86, 16.345–47, 17.295–98, 20.398–400), which would likely have been among the first literary or performance contexts in which ancient Greek and Roman individuals encountered wounds to the head. Head wounds are also identified as being often fatal in Hippocratic medical texts (*Prorrh.* 2.12.1–3, 2.14.1–7; *Aph.* 6.18; *Coac.* 400, 499; *Morb.* 1.3.1–7; *VC* 2.1–10, 2.14–18). See also [Alex.] *Pr. Suppl. prob.* 1.10 (Kapetanaki and Sharples): "Why do those who have been struck hard on the temples die? Because this muscle grows out from the brain itself, and therefore is close to it. So the brain, being affected together with it and feeling pain with it and being influenced by the blow together with it, contracts, and along with it the psychic *pneuma* is compressed and thickened, and so the soul, not being provided with its proper instrument, departs from the body; for the destruction of a bond effects the release of what was intertwined." Translation from Kapetanaki and Sharples 2006.

6. As Gregory indicates, this wounding could affect the brain substance itself or the cerebral membrane that surrounded it.

7. Arist. *PA* 4.10, 687a23–b; Gal. *UP* 1.2 (3:3.3–5.8 K.); Bas. *Hex.* 6.1.37–42; Greg. Nyss. *Op. hom.* 7 (PG 44:140.49–144.9); Amb. *Ex.* 6.6.36; Nem. *Nat. hom.* 1 (Morani 8–14). See the discussion in Robbins 1912, 56.

8. Galen discusses this principle at length in *On the Usefulness of the Parts* 1.2–8 (3:1.6–21.18 K.). On teleology in ancient medicine and philosophy, see my discussion in chapter 4.

9. For further discussion, see chapter 7.

10. Joh. Chrys. *De stat.* 11.11 (PG 49:125.23–30).

11. See Gal. *Thras.* 19 (5:840.2–5 K.) for the notion that the health of the human body requires continual correction of balance to maintain health.

12. The earliest reference to this notion is B 4 DK: "Alcmaeon [says] that the essence of health is the balance [ἰσονομία] of the powers: wet, dry, cold, hot, bitter, sweet, and the rest, and that monarchy among them is the author of disease." See also the Hippocratic text *On the Nature of the Human Being.* Galen formalized existing concern with a balance of qualities in, among other works, his treatises *On the Art of Medicine, On Mixtures,* and *That the Faculties of the Soul Follow the Mixtures of the Body.* For discussion, see García-Ballester 1988, esp. 130–33; Mattern 2008, 102–5. Van der Eijk (2015) 77–79 surveys theories of mixtures prior to Galen.

13. Isid. Pel. *Ep.* 4.125 (PG 78:1200B).

14. Isid. Pel. *Ep.* 4.125 (PG 78:1201B), quoting Gal. *QAM* 3 (4:775.3–7 K.).

15. Joh. Chrys. *De stat.* 11.8 (PG 49:123.35–40).

16. Pl. *Ti.* 75a7–b7. All translations of this text are from Zeyl, in Cooper and Hutchinson 1997. Translation adapted.

17. Pl. *Ti.* 75b7–c5.

18. Thdt. *Interpret. ep. i ad Cor.* (PG 82:328.51–54).

19. 2 Cor. 12:9–10 (NIV translation).

20. Joh. Chrys. *De stat.* 11.8 (PG 49:123.40–51).

21. Gal. *UP* 8.9 (3:656.6–660.17 K.), excerpted by Oribasius, *Med. coll.* 24.1.12.1–14.1.

22. Gal. *UP* 8.9 (3:659.1–4 K). All translations of this text are from May 1968. Translation adapted.

23. Gal. *UP* 9.1 (3:688.17–18 K.): "But first, before the skin was put on, she covered [the brain] with bone like a helmet (κράνος)." Translation adapted.

24. Thdt. *De prov.* 3.27 (PG 83:601.4–9). See my discussion in Wright 2018.

25. Thdt. *De prov.* 3.27 (PG 83:601.9–11). Cf. Orib. *Coll. med.* 24.14.3–4: "Again, in this density, the external surrounding bone, which is called the cranium [κρανίον], is positioned just like a helmet [κράνος]."

26. Joh. Chrys. *In Heb. hom.* 5.8 (PG 63:54.6–14).

27. Gal. *UP* 8.6 (3:636.16–637.2 K.). On the softness of the brain and sensory nerves, see Siegel 1970, 177–78; von Staden 2000, 115–16; Rocca 2003, 83–86. Chrysostom may have accessed this text through its inclusion in Oribasius' fourth-century encyclopedia: Orib. *Coll. med.* 24.1.

28. Gal. *UP* 8.6 (3:636.14–16 K.): "In substance the brain is very like the nerves, of which it was meant to be the source, except that it is softer."

29. Arist. *De an.* 2.12 (424a17–25), which is indebted to Pl. *Tht.* 190e5–196c5 (see Everson 1997, 56). Cf. SVF II, 56; DL 7.50.2–3. There is ongoing debate regarding the

question of what kind of physical "alteration" Aristotle thought must take place within the sensory organ: for discussion, see Sorabji 1974, especially the survey of positions at 63–64; Burnyeat 1992; Nussbaum and Putnam 1995; Everson 1997, 56–102; Magee 2000. Regarding the Stoics, see Sambursky 1959, 25–26; Annas 1992, 72–74; Lesses 1998, 5; SVF II, 53, 55, 56, 59. For Galen, see von Staden 2000, 115; Rocca 2003, 84fn15. Siegel (1970, 20) notes that for Galen, "the concept of 'changes' . . . evidently seemed not to contradict the basic idea of Epicurus who spoke of the 'stamping' [*typosis*] of the visual picture onto the air," with reference to DL 10.49.

30. As, for example, in Descartes' pineal gland, on which see Krell 1987 and Hatfield 2000.

31. Amb. *Ex.* 6.9.61. Translation from Savage 1961.

32. Greg. Nyss. *Sanct. Pasch.* 9.258.20–27.

33. Greg. Nyss. *Sanct. Pasch.* 9.258.27–28.

34. Dean-Jones 1994, 55–58; King 1998, 47–50; Flemming 2000, 158. King (2013, esp. 31–48) argues that women's bodies are characterized not primarily by "female" genitalia, but by the softer, warmer, and wetter texture of their flesh. Ascetic practices were thought to "dry out" and to "harden" female flesh, such that they might be perceived as transformed into men. See Elm 1994, 113–20 (with regard to Basil of Ancyra); T. Shaw 1998, 220–51. On the masculinizing effects of asceticism in general, see Castelli 1991; G. Clark 1998b; Hunt 2012, 63–77; Vogt 1993. Cf. Rousselle 1988 on the ways that ascetic practices were thought to reduce desire.

35. This word first appears in Philo and a handful of contemporary philosophical texts, after which it is the preserve of Christian ascetic writings.

36. Ph. *Op. mund.* 165–66, esp. 165.3–5: "For in us the intellect has the role of man, while sense-perception has that of woman. Pleasure encounters and consorts with the senses first, and through them she deceives the ruling intellect as well." Translation from Runia 2001.

37. Toner 2015, 164: "Senses such as smell were thought to pose a moral risk to Christians, in that they could enter and corrupt the body via temptation and entice the soul away from the path of life." Toner balances the corrupting potential of sensory input against the medicinal and restorative power of smell.

38. G. Smith 2008, 496: Through their constitutional affinity with the human soul (that is to say, their pneumatic quality), demons have the power to instigate "psychological (which is to say quite physical) 'movements' in a person's soul."

39. On "pollution" as an illness model in early Christianity, see D. Martin 1995, esp. 139–61. Douglas (1966) established a framework for talking about "pollution" in conceptualizing health and disease, although she described the process not as the use of ideas about pollution to structure disease categories, but rather as the appropriation of "the laws of nature . . . to sanction the moral code," focusing upon illnesses thought to be caused by moral transgression (3). Parker 1983 is fundamental for the history of pollution in antiquity and examines the relationship between pollution and disease at 235–56. See also Jouanna 2012a for a clarifying account of the differentiation of religious and medical concepts of pollution (*miasma*) in ancient Greece.

40. On vainglory in Chrysostom, see Leduc 1969; Leyerle 2001, 48–49; Roskam 2014.

41. For the relationship between sensory input and susceptibility to affections, see Harvey 2006.

42. Joh. Chrys. *Inan.* 715–21.

43. Chrysostom identifies "four gates" in the walls of the body: "eyes, tongue, hearing, smell, and, if you like, touch" (*Inan.* 361–62). The "tongue" is described as a gate through which pass not the sensory impressions of taste but the "drones" of speech (366–455). The "ears" are a gate through which might pass dangerous and alluring tales, but by means of which the child might also be fruitfully instructed (456–713). Much less space is devoted to the topic of smell (714–27), but Chrysostom attends most closely in this paragraph to the intertwined physiological and psychological effects of sensory experience. Following his discussion of smell, Chrysostom deals briefly (728–75) with the gate of the "eyes," focusing in particular upon the problem of female beauty. He then concludes his discussion with a fifth gate, "not of such a kind as the others, insofar as it pervades the whole body"—that is, touch (776–83). Chrysostom remarks only that touch deceives, since it appears closed, but is in fact open to all comers; in order to protect the child, "we must allow this [gate] to be familiar with neither soft clothing nor bodies," in order that "we might render it firm" (779–81).

44. Gal. *UP* 8.6 (3:647.11–13 K.). Translation adapted.

45. Siegel (1970, 140–57) discusses Galen's teachings on smell. In contrast to the passage discussed here, Chrysostom states in his homily *In 1 Cor. hom.* 10.7 (PG 61:86.28–62) that the nostrils are the organs of smell but that they quickly transmit their perceptions to the brain.

46. Gal. *UP* 8.6 (3:647.8–11 K.); Gal. *Inst. od.* 4.7–9; cf. also Gal. *SMT* 4. (11:698.8–11 K.).

47. Orib. *Coll. med.* 24.6; Nem. *Nat. hom.* 11 (Morani 67.13–20): "Smell comes about through the nostrils and penetrates as far as the limits of the frontal cavities of the brain. For these are very vaporous in their nature and readily receive vapors. . . . But the brain has not sent a nerve of sensation to smell as it has done to the other senses, but it satisfies its need and receives the exhalation of vapors with the ends of its own nerves." Translation from Sharples and van der Eijk 2008.

48. Harvey 2006, 103–4.

49. Harvey 2006, 129, for divine fragrance, and 161 for ambiguity regarding the effect of smells; see also 162: "An ascetic rhetoric of sensory control thus permeated late antique homiletics and writing, even as Christian practices became more sensorily demanding. . . . Ascetic rhetoric provided means by which to grasp the volatile situation and reconfigure its structure." Woolgar (2006, 117–46) examines the transformation of late antique thinking about smell in late medieval England, highlighting the association between good odors and sanctity, bad odors and sin; in late antiquity, as Harvey has made clear, the picture was more complex.

50. Totelin 2015, 29.

51. Laks (1999) explores the relationship between perception and thought in early Greek philosophy. A. Smith (2004, 8) discusses the relationship between external perception and internal perception in the writings of Plotinus.

52. Cf. G. Smith 2008, 508: "The substance of thought [sc. *pneuma*] is what makes it possible to talk, all in the same breath, about material constitution, fine-material physics, and the relationship of demons to the self."

53. For a detailed examination of "psychophysical causality" in Stoic philosophy, see Sedley 1993. For the material alteration of the soul by vaporous and airy substances, with reference to a thinker of a different period, see Sutton 2000, 704.

54. G. Smith 2008, 510. Cf. 501 for a fourth-century love spell that invokes myrrh as a demon formed of *pneuma* and therefore can act directly upon the *pneuma* within the brain.

55. Evagr. *Prakt.* 39.

56. See also Caciola 2003, 148–49, for medieval accounts of how internal vapors rising into the brain could cause women to experience visions of demons.

57. Joh. Chrys. *Inan.* 715–21.

58. Simp. *In Cat.* (CAG 8:402. 22–26). Translation adapted from Gaskin 2014. See the comments on this passage in Ahonen 2018, 361.

59. Berryman 2009, 193–95. See also 196, where Berryman emphasizes that *tonos* was "a technical term for a property of matter in general, important in explaining its ability to transmit impulses and convey complex forms by physical contact."

60. In his treatise *On the Movement of Muscles,* Galen writes that "nerve [νεῦρον] or sinew [τόνος] stems from the brain or spinal marrow." He explains the existence of two words for the same organ as descriptive of the "pushing [νεύειν] and pulling [τείνειν] motion" necessary for movement. See Gal. *Mot. musc.* 1 (4:369.6–8 K.). My translation uses the English terms suggested in Goss 1968, 2.

61. Annas 1992: 53: "Soul, then, is not just *pneuma,* but a specific level of *pneuma,* with the degree of tensions required for it to function as *pneuma psuchikon,* the *pneuma* of a soul, unifying a body and enabling it to perceive and act in certain ways." See Hahm 1977, 170–73, for discussion of the origins of *tonos* as a Stoic term.

62. Graver 2007, 70–71.

63. Nussbaum 1994, 317–18.

64. Nussbaum 1994, 318fn3. Cf. Graver 2007, 116: "Given Stoic notions of the relation between systematicity of judgment and an optimal level of tension in the mind's material substrate, it would be natural enough for him [sc. Chrysippus] to describe all the specified conditions as various ways in which pneumatic tension might be relaxed to the point of impairment."

65. Trompeter 2016, 98: "If, assuming the existence of psychic *pneuma,* psychic properties are in Stoic doctrine material conditions, which come to be through the *tonos* of the *pneuma,* this means that all movements of the will of the unified soul, all its rational deeds and not-deeds, come about, finally, through the strength or weakness of its *pneuma.*" My translation. See also Sedley 1993, 326 (the Stoic soul is neither more

nor less than "a specially attuned portion of *pneuma*"); Tieleman 2003, 112 (emphasis upon psychic *tonos* as "physical"); Graver 2007, 114 (insanity, like dreams, might be caused "nonmysteriously, through the relaxing of pneumatic tension").

66. Gal. *Loc. aff.* 4.3 (8:233.2–3 K.). Discussed briefly in Rocca 2003, 191; Trompeter 2016, 104–5.

67. Trompeter 2016, 92–99, 106 (*tonos* as a function of *thumos*), 88–92 (on the importance of *tonos* and *thumos* in maintaining a healthy relationship between the parts of the soul). See also Schiefsky 2012, 337.

68. See Gill 2006 for *pneuma* as the bridge between psychological and physiological causality.

69. Greg. Nyss. *Op. hom.* 30 (PG 44:249.45–47, 249.58–252.1): "The [force] that is considered to come down from the cerebral membranes and the brain . . . renders our earthen statue active and mobile, as if by some mechanism . . . just like a charioteer himself, endowing the impulse and force of each movement and stasis upon all the junctures of the bones and joints and the branches of the muscles."

70. See my discussion of this text in chapter 4, above.

71. Schiefsky 2007a, 88.

72. Bassiri (2012, 245) identifies a similar ambiguity in Descartes' theorization of the pineal gland: "The pineal would need to facilitate, as no other object could, the operational commensurability between Descartes' two ontologically incommensurate domains and to constitute the site of an absolutely metaphysical encounter too expansive to be satisfied or delimited by mind or matter alone."

73. For example, ointments could be "warming" (ἀναθερμαινόντων) or "cooling" (ἐμψυχόντων), as Clement mentions in passing at *Paed.* 2.8.68.3.1–2.

74. Clem. *Paed.* 2.8.67.2.1–3.

75. On changing perspectives on professional massage and the use of oil in early Christianity, see Bond 2015.

76. Clem. *Paed.* 2.8.68.1.3–6.

77. On *hexis* in Stoic cosmology, see Hahm 1977, 163–68.

78. Clem. *Paed.* 2.8.68.7–9.

79. Clem. *Paed.* 2.8.70.3.1–4.

80. Theophr. *Od.* 46, 49–50.

81. See, for example, Gal. *Loc. aff.* 5.6 (8:342.10–16 K.): "But, following indigestion, these [people] appear to be taken seized violently by the aforementioned symptoms. Most of them are affected in their spleen, such that one might deduce that a toxic serum streams from this organ into the stomach. Whatever symptoms that affect the brain or the eyes follow upon the vaporization of evil humors."

82. Bas. *In eb.* (PG 31:453.6–9). I am grateful to Susan Holman for pointing out this reference.

83. Bas. *Ep.* 210.3.9–11.

84. Aug. *Mor.* 2.44.16–19.

85. Ast. Am. *Hom.* 14.2.4.2–3.

86. [Joh. Chrys.] *De prec.* (PG 64:461.37–41). Cf. Petr. *Sat.* 47.6, where Trimalchio claims that preventing oneself from releasing wind will send up "vapors" (the Latin borrowing *anathymiasis*) into the brain, creating a disturbance throughout the body.

87. [Gal.] *Rem.* (14:317.12–318.6 K.); Orib. *Coll. med. lib. incert.* 35.10; Orib. *Lib. ad Eun.* 4.1.15–16; Aët. Amid. *Med. lib.* 4.29.5–8, 43.1–10; Steph. *Comm. Gal. Glauc. Ther.* 1.263.25–264.8. Like perfume, wine could also be construed as beneficial (see, for example, Penniman 2015, 197).

88. [Alex.] *Pr.* 1.96.4–7.

89. NIV translation.

90. Joh. Chrys. *In 1 Tim. hom.* 13 (PG 62:568.28–34).

91. For example: Gal. *Loc. aff.* I.7 (8:66–67 K.); Phil. *In eb.* 155; Bas. *Ep.* 210.6, *In eb.* (PG 31:448.15–17); Amphiloch. *Or.* 7.74–76; Joh. Chrys. *In Eph. hom.* 13 (PG 62:93.53–94.16), which similarly compares the "darkness of understanding" (ἡ σκοτομήνη τῆς διανοίας) to corrupt humors that enter the eye and obscure vision; Thdt. *De prov.* 6 (PG 83:645.42–46).

92. For further discussion, see chapter 7.

93. LSJ, s.v. ὁ σκοπέλος: (1) lookout place: hence peak, headland, promontory; (2) watchtower. Cf. s.v. σκοπέω: (1) behold, contemplate, examine, inspect, look out, watch.

94. Cic. *N.D.* 2.56; Amb. *Ex.* 6.9; Bas. *Hom. attend.* 36.19–37.1, where the eyes take the "highest look-out spot" (τὴν ὑψηλοτάτην σκοπιὰν); Aug. *En. Ps.* 41.7 where the mind looks out through the "window" of the eyes.

95. Arist. *Top.* 108a11 and *De an.* 412b17–22; Phil. *Op. mund.* 30.5–6; Gal. *Opt. doct.* (1:52.1–3 K). See Leyerle 1993, 162 for the privileged connection between eye and soul.

96. Hom. *Od.* 12.73–75. For later commentary on this passage, see the following: Aristonic. *Sign. Od.* 73–75; Eustath. *Comm. Hom. Od.* 2.8.16–31. For its literary reception, see esp. Apoll. *Arg.* 4.924–29.

97. On the continued importance of Homer in late antique education, as well as in literary and intellectual culture, see, for example, Lamberton 1989; P. Brown 1992, 39; MacDonald 1994; Frank 2000; Cribiore 2001, 34–35, 140–43, 194–97; Sandnes 2011; Maciver 2012; Niehoff 2012; Rylaarsdam 2014, 96–99.

98. For Libanius as the teacher of Chrysostom, see Hunter 1989; Malosse 2008; Tonias 2014, 20–24.

99. Lib. *Ep.* 650.5.

100. Joh. Chrys. *In Joh. hom.* 2 (PG 59:35.11–18).

101. Siegel 1970, 59–65.

102. Gal. *Loc. aff.* 1.2 (8:20.13–16 K.): "For when certain vapors are carried up from [the mouth of the stomach] into the eyes, the visual power [Siegel 1976, ad loc.: 'pneuma'] encounters them and produces the kind of sensory effects as happens in the case of suffusion." Concern regarding the rising of vapors from the stomach into the eyes recurs throughout this text. Cf. the longer discussion of eye diseases at Gal. *Caus. symp.* 1.2.1–10 (7:86–101 K.). Eye diseases were common in antiquity (Birley 1992, 111–13; Trentin 2013, 89). For a summary of treatments, see Cels. *Med.* 6.6.1.

103. For the relationship between eye and soul, see Arist. *De an.* 2.1, 412b17–22, with Polansky 2007, 165–67.

104. Cf. Arist. *De an.* 2.1, 413a8–9. On this passage, see Bos 2003, 123–30; Polansky 2007, 168–70. See also Tert. *DA* 8.17–18. See also the passage already discussed in Isid. Pel. *Ep.* 4.125 (PG 78:1204) in chapter 4.

105. Joh. Chrys. *In 1 Tim. hom.* 13 (PG 62:568.36–45).

106. The collocution of λογισμοί (thoughts) and θορυβεῖν (to raise a tumult; to throw into disorder) is common in late antique writings, but typically the phrasing is such that one is "thrown into disorder" *in* one's thoughts, or that one's thoughts "throw [others] into disorder"; it is unusual for the thoughts themselves to be personified. For example: Orig. *In Joh.* 10.25.148.5: Jesus "dispels the tumultuous plots [thoughts]" (λογισμοὺς θορυβοῦντας διασκεδάσαι); Eus. *Comm. in Ps.* 11 (PG 23:841.10–11): "I have become disturbed in my thoughts" (ἐθορυβούμην τοῖς λογισμοῖς); Athan. *Ep. ad Amun* 70.7: "thoughts disturb me" (λογισμοί με θορυβήσωσιν); *Exp. in Ps.* 72/73 (PG 27:329.38): "I have become disturbed in my thoughts" (ἐθορυβούμην τοῖς λογισμοῖς). Exceptions, although not exact, are to be found mostly in Chrysostom's homilies *On Lazarus,* where the phrase indicates mental distress, typically caused by what one hears: Joh. Chrys. *Laz. conc.* 3.1 (PG 48:993.3–4), where shameful words, entering through the ears, "have sent our thoughts into tumult" (ἐθορύβησεν ἡμῶν τὸν λογισμόν), and 5.5 (PG 48:1025.41–42): God's command to Abraham to sacrifice Isaac was sufficient "to send his thoughts into tumult" (θορυβῆσαι αὐτοῦ τὸν λογισμὸν). One other exception with which Chrysostom was perhaps familiar is Bas. *In Ps. 1* (PG 29:212.39–40): "[The psalm] relieves the panic and surge of thoughts" (τὸ θορυβοῦν καὶ κυμαῖνον τῶν λογισμῶν καταστέλλων).

107. Hier. *Ep.* 61.3. This letter was followed up by a notoriously vituperative (even for Jerome) treatise *Against Vigilantius,* as well as Letter 109, written to a mutual acquaintance, in which Jerome once again questioned the health of Vigilantius' brain.

108. LSJ, s.v. ὁ ἄντλος: (1) "hold of a ship, bilge-water, flood"; (2) "bucket"; (3) "heap of corn."

109. Chrysostom also emphasizes, as we have already seen, the psychological effect of bilge-water, sending one's soul and one's thoughts into panic. Cf. Joh. Chrys. *In Act. apost. hom.* 16 (PG 60:133.26–30) for the "flood" of luxury that sends the sailors and captain into tumult.

110. Water in the brain was a commonly recognized medical problem, although it was typically cured by surgery (see, for example, Aët. Amid. *Lib. med.* 6.1), rather than by ascetic practice.

111. Joh. Chrys. *In 1 Tim. hom.* 13 (PG 62:570.18–39).

112. Ancient physicians did not teach a doctrine of blood circulation (Fancy 2013); instead, blood was generated by the liver out of the food that had been consumed and was dispatched throughout the body to nourish the various parts (Boylan 2007).

113. Strikingly, Galen describes diarrhea through comparison to excretions from the brain: Gal. *Caus. symp.* 3.11.2 (7:262.18–263.5 K.): "For example, the brain is the cause of both *catarrh* [excess of mucus flowing to the mouth] and *coryza* [excess of

mucus flowing to the nose], as a homeomerous part being brought to an imbalance by cooling and similarly by sun-stroke and being heated as an organ. Diarrhea is the sort of affection that occurs in the stomach in disordered digestion, like each kind of thing spoken of in the brain." Translation adapted from Johnston 2006.

114. See my discussion of this metaphor in chapter 4.

115. Gal. *PHP* 6.5.30.1–3. Translation from De Lacy 2005.

116. Rocca 2003, 100. For use of terminology from civil engineering in medical contexts, see van Tilburg 2015, 3–22. See also Wright 2018 for analysis of a metaphor comparing the brain to an urban aqueduct in Theodoret of Cyrrhus.

117. Gal. *San. tu.* 5.5 (6:338.3–4 K.).

118. Gal. *Alim. fac.* (6:608.4–5 K., 6:616.4–7 K.); Paul. *Epit. med.* 1.73.11–13.

119. Leyerle 2009.

CHAPTER 6. INSANITY, VAINGLORY, AND PHRENITIS

1. See Elm 1994, 115, for a similar point in Basil of Ancyra's *On the True Purity of Virginity.*

2. McDonald 2009b, 113; see also further discussion in McDonald 2009a.

3. Prud. *Ham.* 123–24.

4. On madness as the medicalization of deviance, see Conrad and Schneider 1980.

5. This practice was adopted at the highest levels of Christian politics, and not with phrenitis alone. See, for example, Constantine's use of the word "madness" (μανία) to describe Donatist Christians in his letter to Caecilian of Carthage (Eus. *HE* 10.6.5).

6. On the assumption that perpetrators of mass shootings suffer from mental illnesses, see Metzl and MacLeish 2015. Betus, Kearns, and Lemieux (2021) discuss the influence of racial and religious identities on the likelihood that media reports will discuss mental illness in relation to terrorist acts; see in particular their suggestion that the greater the number of fatalities, the more likely media coverage is to reference mental illness (1148).

7. Merideth 1999, 153: "Disease retained its traditional negative connotations as something that needed to be healed and Christianity was the 'medicine' that cures." See also Crislip 2013, 3–4, quoting Adolf Harnack: "Christianity never lost hold of its innate principle; it was, and it remained, a religion for the sick. Accordingly it assumed that no one, or at least hardly any one, was in normal health, but that men were always in a state of disability" (*Die Mission und Ausbreitung,* 78, trans. Moffatt, *Mission and Expansion,* 109). The cure, as Crislip clarifies, was salvation. For the reinvigoration of this metaphor in contemporary theology, see Charry 2010, 50: "Augustine's therapeutic soteriology is the primary handhold for the current effort to reclaim a Christian doctrine of happiness."

8. For contemporary reflection upon this question, see the essays collected in Freeman and Goodenough 2009.

9. Rafter (2008) discusses the history of scientific investigation into whether certain features of the brain produce "criminal" activity. Henne and Ventresca (2020) show

the prominence of this question in accounts of the American football player Aaron Hernandez's murder of Odin Lloyd, which can be divided into those that emphasized psychological causation and those that privileged degenerative brain injury sustained by Hernandez in the course of his sporting career.

10. On this question in modern, Western culture, see Choudhury and Slaby 2012b, 39: "Intensified media representation coupled with audiences increasingly trained, through continuous exposure, to be receptive to easy-to-digest narratives of self-objectification ('your brain made you do it') contribute to the distorted images of the person—as lacking in free will, possessing skewed decision-making powers, being driven instead by automatized emotions, and thus as not genuinely responsible for their acts (while simultaneously making them responsible for 'managing' their brains)." Our capacity (and perhaps responsibility) for brain-management is suggested by the concept of "neuroplasticity," that is, the notion that brains are continually reshaped through activity and experience, and that animals can therefore intentionally transform their brains (Schwartz and Begley 2003; and see the critique in Pitts-Taylor 2016, 17–42; cf. the discussion of the "brain fitness" movement (neurobics) in Vidal and Ortega 2017, 42–57. Also relevant here are the theories and therapies that address posttraumatic stress disorder via changes in the nervous system (see, especially, van der Kolk 2014).

11. Praxag. fr. 22 Lewis and Diocl. fr. 72 van der Eijk.

12. Gal. *Caus. symp.* 2.7.2 (7:202.11–13 K.). Translation adapted from Johnston 2006.

13. Gal. *Trem. palp.* (7:641.9–10 K.).

14. Alex. Trall. *Ther.* 13.509.11–13.

15. Aët. Amid. *Med. lib.* 6.2.1–3.

16. See the discussion in McDonald 2009a, 1, and Thumiger 2017, 47.

17. Studies of the word *phrēn* tend to focus upon its appearance in Homeric texts, where it does have both anatomical presence (although this is difficult to locate with consistency or precision) and mental function. Sullivan (1988) discusses the psychological function of the *phrēn* in Homeric texts. See also Ireland and Steel 1975, 183–95.

18. Gal. *Loc. aff.* 5.4 (8:327.13–16 K.).

19. Greg. Nyss. *Op. hom.* 12 (PG 44:157.42–47).

20. Cael. Aur. *Acut.* 1.1.8.53–54. Translation adapted from Drabkin 1951. Caelius' Latin phrase *animae regimen* translates the Greek term ἡγεμονικόν.

21. Van der Eijk 2005a, 119–23; Urso 2018, 293.

22. Mansfeld 1989, 321–22.

23. Pigeaud 1987, 126–27.

24. See E. Clark 1997, 215, for the observation that ascetic writers often report that renunciation, especially of food, sleep, and human company, can lead to madness. Gal. *Loc. aff.* 3.7 (8:165.17–166.1 K.) reports a case of a young man who nearly lost his memory and who damaged his rational faculty "through love of toil and sleeplessness during his studies." Another example of both sleeplessness and excessive study leading to fear that the cerebral membranes might be damaged can be found in Joh. Chrys. *Ad Stag.* 2 (PG 47:450.15–18).

25. See Krueger 1996, 61, on the circulation and popularity of the *Lausiac History*.

26. There are useful introductions to the *Lausiac History* in Brakke 2006, 134–44; Meyer 1965, 3–16. Harmless (2004, 275–308) provides broader contextualization.

27. On Kellia, see Harmless 2004, 275–76. For an introduction to Macarius of Alexandria, see Vivian 2004.

28. Pall. *Hist. laus.* 18.3.1–4. All translations of this text are from W. Clarke 1918. Translation adapted. On late antique sleep asceticism and its medical roots, see Dossey 2013.

29. See especially Perkins 1995 on the role of suffering in early Christian identity formation, and G. Clark 2005 on the question of whether bodily injury and illness was an ascetic aim. Crislip (2013, especially 15–35) contrasts suffering caused by ascetic behaviors (for example, injury) to unprovoked bodily illness, and argues that the latter could be utilized as a form of ascetic practice.

30. Pall. *Hist. laus.* 18.3.4–8.

31. Crislip 2013, 35.

32. Nonetheless, "playing mad" was a recognized strategy amongst, in particular, desert ascetics. In some contexts, (the appearance of) insanity might represent the most authentic renunciation of the things of this world. Krueger (1996) provides an extended discussion, exemplified by Symeon the Holy Fool, whose seventh-century biography was to become the origin for a literary tradition. Palladius (*Hist. laus.* 34.1–2) provides an earlier example of a nun who feigns madness, and so is rejected by her companions.

33. Krueger 1996, 57–71.

34. C. Johnson 2014, 606 (for quotation) and 593, for a definition of "holy foolishness" as "the attribution of hidden sanctity behind behavior that appears outwardly hostile or disturbed."

35. Paul. Nic. *Med. lib.* 10.2–10.

36. Joh. Chrys. *Hom. in Stat.* 11.11 (PG 49:125.26–30).

37. Gal. *QAM* 3 (4:774.19–775.2 K.): "Now, if the reasoning form of the soul is mortal, it too will be a particular mixture, [namely] of the brain [κρᾶσίς τις ἐγκεφάλου]." Translation from Singer 2013.

38. Gal. *Ars med.* 8 (1:326.10–11 K.). Translation from Singer 1997. *The Art of Medicine* was one of four Galenic texts used to teach medicine in late antique Alexandria (Temkin 1962, 102–3).

39. See Dossey 2013, 214fn18, with further references.

40. Thumiger 2017, 177.

41. See, however, Thumiger 2017, 184–88, for a discussion of insomnia as a symptom of mental illness in general.

42. Gal. *Hipp. prorrh.* (16:494.5–6 K.).

43. Gal. *Loc. aff.* 5.4 (8:329.17–330.2 K.).

44. Alex. Trall. *Ther.* 13.509.25–27.

45. Cf. McDonald 2009a, 40–41: "Any deviation from one's normal sleeping pattern is thought to be indicative, *or even causative* of some sort of mental or physical disturbance" (emphasis added). See also Lo Presti 2015 for a detailed account of the

relationship between sleep and epilepsy. The material causes of sleep are, as Lo Presti shows, rooted in the brain.

46. Valantasis 1995; E. Clark 1999. See also Bynum 1995a, 90–91, for a discussion of scholarship (especially P. Brown 1988 and E. Clark 1990) on the question of whether ascetic practices might produce social distinctions in the eschaton. Caner (2002) discusses at length the social tensions exacerbated by voluntary poverty.

47. This is illustrated by the *Life of Saint Syncletica* 53, which is quoted and discussed in Castelli 1992, 140–41. See also Crislip 2013, 105, on chapters 49–52 of the same text: "Syncletica reads the illness of the ascetic as a possible sign of demonically inspired asceticism. In fact this type of ascetic self-hurt is a 'disease' (*nosos*), the 'ultimate and chief of all evils,' brought on 'through an excess of asceticism.'"

48. Brakke 2006, 68–69; Crislip 2013, 81–108.

49. See, for example, the description of Tilby 2005, 149, in relation to Evagrius of Pontus, whose theorization of the passions as *logismoi* ("[intrusive] thoughts") was to become influential: "For Evagrius vainglory is the most subtle of the thoughts to afflict the monk because it flourishes particularly in those who try to live good lives. Vainglory resonates with the nagging sense that virtue ought to be rewarded. It seeks publicity and praise. The demon of vainglory even brings to the monk's imagination the sound of admiring crowds as the sick and hysterical receive healing through his ministry."

50. See Wright 2015 for discussion of how the threat of vainglory might discipline a monk's ascetic practice.

51. Crislip 2013, 84.

52. For this distinction, which was first systematically theorized by Galen, but which has its roots in Hellenistic medicine and philosophy, see chapter 2. A different set of resonances is suggested in Hunt 2012, 11: "Within the Christian tradition a natural/contra-natural dichotomy is inferred in analyzing how the desert Fathers, for example, seek to integrate the materiality of the human body within the totality of Christian experience."

53. Pall. *Hist. laus.* 18.17.1–4.

54. Pall. *Hist. laus.* 18.17.4–9.

55. Pall. *Hist. laus.* 18.18.1–8.

56. Hipp. *Int.* 39.3–13: "When the patient is on the verge of death, he sees keenly, talks confidently, and demands something to drink and eat; if anyone gives it to him, and he eats it, he soon gives up the ghost, unless he vomits." Translation from Potter 1988.

57. W. Clarke 1918, 83.

58. Hsch. *Lex.* 1705.

59. Luc. *Dial. mort.* 6.4.12–3.

60. The Greek word used here (λογισθῇ) evokes the Evagrian term *logismos* ("thought"), which describes the category of psychological conditions of which vainglory is one example (Corrigan 2009, 73–101).

61. On the flight of Roman aristocratic women to the shores of North Africa, see P. Brown 2000, 286–87. I use Hombert's (2000, 121) date for this treatise.

62. Aug. *B. uid.* 15.19. Cf. Sen. *Ep.* 15.1: "Without [philosophy], the soul is sick. The body too, even if it has great strength, is strong no differently from the body of a madman or a person suffering from phrenitis [*furiosi aut phrenetici*]." Augustine did not invent the connection between phrenitis and the illness of the soul, but he did exploit it more than any other ancient author.

63. This is a schematic and partial description of Pelagius' views. For an in-depth account, see the discussion and texts collected in Rees 1998. See also P. Brown 2000, 340–53, for an account of the conflict between Pelagius and Augustine over the lives of aristocratic women in the years following the sack of Rome. Allen and Neil (2013, 115–18) discuss Pelagius and Pelagianism in relationship to religious and ethnic conflict in the early fifth century.

64. On Demetrias and the letters she received from famous theologians in these years, see Jacobs 2000; Kurdock 2007; Cain 2009, 160–66. For the date of Jerome's letter, see Cain 2009, 160. On "holy women" in late antique texts, see E. Clark 1998.

65. See Cain 2009, 165, which describes Jerome as "grooming" Demetrias as an exemplar of "Hieronymian-style" female asceticism. On Jerome's relationship with other ascetic women, see Miller 1993; Cain 2009, 102–5; Crislip 2013, 81–84.

66. Hier. *Ep.* 130.17.

67. Hier. *Ep.* 130.17.

68. Cobb (2008, 92–123) argues that female martyrs were both masculinized (in order to establish the power of Christianity over its enemies) and feminized (in order to reinforce gender norms within Christian communities).

69. Hipp. *Mul.* 1.25–28: "I say that a woman's flesh is more spongelike and softer than a man's: since this is so, the woman's body draws moisture both with more speed and in greater quantity from the belly than does the body of a man." Translation from Hanson 1975.

70. King 2013, 73–96. See also Hipp. *Vict.* 1.34: "The males of all species are warmer and drier, and the females moister and cooler, for the following reasons: . . . males use a more rigorous regimen, so that they are well warmed and dried, but females use a regimen that is moister and less strenuous, and in addition purge the heat out of the bodies every month." Translation from W. Jones 1931.

71. As discussed in Galen's *On Mixtures* and *QAM.*

72. Hipp. *Gland.* 10 describes the brain as the largest of the glands within the body, responsible for absorbing and redistributing excess moisture.

73. Hipp. *Aër* 10.31–33.

74. Cobb 2008, 102; Dean-Jones 1994, 83–85.

75. Gal. *Hipp. epid. 6* (17b:4.5–12 K.).

76. [Aris.] *Pr.* 897b23–26.

77. Arist. *GA* 5.3, 783b26–30. All translations of this text are from Reeve 2019, unless otherwise stated.

78. Arist. *GA* 5.3, 784a2–4.

79. Arist. *GA* 5.3, 784a4–7.

80. Vind. *Gyn.* 18. Translation from Cilliers 2005.

81. A 13 DK = Aët. *Plac.* 5.3.3.

82. [Gal.] *Def. med.* 439 (19:449.14–16 K.).

83. Thumiger 2018b.

84. Nem. *Nat. hom.* 25 (Morani 87.10–15): "But other animals avoid intercourse when they are pregnant, while a woman always receives it. . . . For women have free will about intercourse after conception as in other matters." Translation from Sharples and van der Eijk 2008. Cf. also Holmes 2012, 79: "Being a woman was viewed . . . as a condition dictated by nature. Masculinity, by contrast, is something you have to work at."

85. Evagr. *Or.* 72–73 (PG 79:1181.42–1184.4).

86. On the corporeal nature of demons, see G. Smith 2008. Smith demonstrates that late ancient demons are made of *pneuma,* that is, the same substance as the human soul. "Their constitutional affinity with the soul may have offered special access to a person's thoughts or inclinations, allowing the instigation of psychological (which is to say quite physical) 'movements' in a person's soul" (G. Smith 2008, 496).

87. Aug. *B. uid.* 15.19.

88. For further development of the ideas in this section, see Wright 2020. Anti-Manichaean polemic: *Util. cred.* 18.36. Anti-Jewish polemic: *S. dom. m.* 1.19.57; *En. Ps.* 35.17.20–28; *En. Ps.* 58, *s.* 1.7.17–20 and *s.* 2.5.67–71; *En. Ps.* 63.3.17–24; *En. Ps.* 65.4.66–68; *En. Ps.* 68, *s.* 2.5.41–45; *En. Ps.* 70, *s.* 1.14.72–73 and 20.20–55; *En. Ps.* 96.2.27–29; *En. Ps.* 134.22.25–28; *Ep. Io. tr.* 8.10–11; *Io. eu. tr.* 7.19.1–6 and 17.15.27–29; *S.* 16A; *S.* 77.4; *S.* 80.4; *S.* 111.2; *S.* 175.3; *S.* 284 (PL 38:1292.17–30 and 1293.16–18); *S.* 386 (PL 39:1697.12–15); *S.* 229E (Morin 1:468.15–18); *S.* 313B (Morin 1:74.9–10); *S.* 4D.6; *S.* 25D.18. Anti-Donatist polemic: *C. Cresc.* 4.50.61; *Ep.* 89.6; *Ep.* 93.1–2; *Ep.* 185.2; *S.* 47.17.436–38; *S.* 99 (PL 38:599.16–20); *S.* 359 (PL 39:1595.49–1596.16); *En. Ps.* 34, *s.* 2.13.23–34. Anti-Pelagian polemic: *Nat. et gr.* 7.7; *Ep.* 157.2; *B. uid.* 15.19; *Gr. et pecc. or.* 2.7.8; *C. Iul.* 4.27. Against badly behaved Christians: *En. Ps.* 39.8.1–25; *En. Ps.* 98.5.22–25. Against pagans: *S.* 87 (PL 38:538.21–43); *Io. eu. tr.* 7.2.1–8; *S.* 25D.18 (also listed above, under "Anti-Jewish polemic"). Other occurrences of phrenitis: *Ep.* 7.2; *Quant. an.* 22.38 and 22.40; *Gn. litt.* 12.12–21; *Cura mort.* 12.14; *Ciu.* 19.4.44–58. I have checked this list against that compiled in Gourevitch and Gourevitch 1998, 516–17. I do not include, as they do, instances where Augustine refers to symptoms of phrenitis (for example, fever) without naming the condition itself. This is because various mental illnesses involved fever of some kind.

89. A recent exception is the work of Chiara Thumiger, who similarly pointed out the significance of Augustine in the development of phrenitis as a "heavily moralised" disorder in her lecture "*Quasi Phreneticus:* Metaphorical and Technical Interactions in the History of the Ancient Disease Concept *Phrenitis*" (King's College London, November 8, 2017). I am very grateful to Thumiger for sharing the handout from this lecture, which I was unable to attend in person. Kolbet (2010) and Couenhoven (2013) each deal with Augustine's role as healer of souls, but do not discuss phrenitis in any depth. The single exception is Gourevitch and Gourevitch 1998, a brief but precise study providing an account of phrenitis as it appears in Augustine's corpus. The authors

emphasize that Augustine is most interested in the *phreneticus* ("phrenetic patient") and the "sacred drama" between doctor and disease, using the noun form "phrenitis" on only a couple of occasions (Gourevitch and Gourevitch 1998, 505). They also emphasize Augustine's knowledge of medical, especially Methodist, accounts of the disease, and suggest that Augustine was familiar with the works of Caelius Aurelianus (510). Despite drawing attention to the Christian symbolism that permeates Augustine's account of phrenitis (511), however, Gourevitch and Gourevitch do not examine the question of how phrenitis fits into Augustine's theological and pastoral framework.

90. See Gourevitch and Gourevitch 1998, 510–11, for the suggestion that Augustine's use in this text of *iter* ("passageway") and *uia* ("path") to describe physical connection between brain and sensory organs points to a Methodist understanding of the disease (that is, the blockage of *poroi*), rather than a Galenic concern with the nerves. Yet, Augustine's discussion of the role of the brain in controlling sensory and motor action (*Gn. Litt.* 7.13), and his description of ventricular localization (*Gn. Litt.* 7.17) earlier in the treatise, suggest that he is working with a Galenic model. O'Daly (1987, 80–81) also understands Augustine's references to *uiae* and *iter* in *Gn. Litt.* 12 to refer to the nerves.

91. Aug. *Gn. Litt.* 12.20.

92. Aug. *Quant. an.* 22.38.

93. [Alex.] *Suppl. prob.* 1.5 (Kapetanaki and Sharples 2006, using their translation). We might also translate *neura* as "sinews," since, like the Latin word *nerui*, it could carry both meanings.

94. Solignac 1962, 662; P. Brown 2000, 24.

95. Aug. *B. uid.* 15.19.

96. Aug. *En. Ps.* 58, *s.* 1.7.7–11.

97. On the overlap in Augustine's polemic against Pelagians and Jews, see Cary 2008, 23.

98. The definition of "grace" that I use in this chapter derives from Karfíková 2012, 64: "Augustine calls this help [from God] 'grace' (*gratia*), rendering by the word deliverance from the fear of punishment, forgiveness of sins on account of penitence, and *righteousness bestowed on the grounds of the faith in mercy, not one's acts*" (emphasis mine).

99. Aug. *En. Ps.* 70, *s.* 1.1.54–56.

100. Aug. *En. Ps.* 70, *s.* 1.1.17–20. Cf. Aug. *Ep.* 157.7, where the verb recurs in a similar context.

101. Aug. *En. Ps.* 70, *s.* 1. 20.20–23.

102. On the violence of phrenetic patients, see Urso 2018, 307. See also Elm 2012, 168, describing how physicians of the soul face "extraordinary resistance" in their patients.

103. Amundsen 1982, 331: Fourth-century Christian authors "inherited and exploited to the fullest the positive metaphorical value of the idea of the physician as one who unselfishly succors the ill, enduring unpleasant tasks in caring for the unhealthy, often administering necessarily painful means for effecting a cure."

104. Cf. Cels. *Med.* 3.18, 98.33. This was a common theme in ancient medical texts.

105. Aug. *En. Ps.* 70, *s.* 1.14.72–73.

106. Cf. Aug. *Beata u.* 2.16, in an exchange between Augustine and his mother: "She remarked: 'Tell us who these Academics are and what they want.' When I had provided an explanation, briefly but clearly enough that none of them might depart in ignorance, she said: 'They're epileptics' (*caducarii sunt*)." Translation adapted from Schopp 1948. Like the "Jews," and the excessive ascetic practitioners, the Academics, who practice skepticism, are branded as proud, chiefly for their "restraint and detachment" and their "avoidance of error." I am grateful to Catherine Conybeare for pointing out the relevance of this passage.

107. On Augustine's anti-Jewish polemic, see Fredriksen 2010, 311: "A glance at the subject index under Jew or Judaism in any volume of Augustine's sermons reveals the familiar themes of *adversus Iudaeos* invective: Jews are blind, hard-hearted, fleshly, stubborn, and prideful; they murdered Christ; they are exiles; they carry the church's books; they are saved only by conversions."

108. Rotelle 2000, 23–24.

109. Cary 2008, 21–23.

110. Meconi 2014, 695: "While the Bishop of Hippo was not the first Catholic preacher to transform pagan Aesculapian imagery into Christ the healer, Rudolph Arbesmann's classic opens by maintaining that, 'Augustine easily holds the first place among those patristic writers of the West who made use of the *Christus medicus* figure.'" As Meconi suggests, the classic account of the medical metaphor in Augustine's writings and more generally is Arbesmann 1954. Cf. Thomas Martin 2001, 222fn9, for references to works dealing with Augustine's use of a "healing paradigm." Augustine's development of the *Christus medicus* trope remained influential into the medieval and renaissance periods (Henderson 2006, 113).

111. For the importance of late antique Christian preaching in shaping the imaginations and moral ideals of their communities, see Maxwell 2006, esp. 11–41 and 88–117, where the Christian preacher is compared to the pagan philosopher in their responsibility for educating nonliterate and nonelite groups through public speech. On Augustine's approach to preaching, and his cultural context, see Sanlon 2014.

112. Aug. *S.* 175.3.

113. As Ruddy (2004, 92) puts it, "Christ, as the antidote to human pride, serves the dual role of physician and medicine." The notion that persuasive speech is a kind of medicament thrives throughout the Greco-Roman philosophical tradition. For its role in fourth-century preaching, see especially Kolbet 2010, Rylaarsdam 2014, Mayer 2015a, and Mayer 2015c.

114. Aug. *S.* 77.4.

115. In this, Augustine echoes and tweaks the Stoic teaching that everybody but the sage is insane. See Ahonen 2018, 346 and passim.

116. I am grateful to Mel Webb for this suggestion. On the role of the Eucharist in constructing ecclesial membership and identity, see especially Harmless 1995. Augustine's reference to the medicinal blood of Christ as consumed by members of the church stands in contrast to the "symbolic" conception of the Eucharist that was assigned to Augustine in the Middle Ages (Crockett 1989, 88–98). Penniman (2015) discusses the Eucharistic wine as a medicament.

117. Aug. S. 25D.18.

118. Matt. 5:39: "If anyone slaps you on the right cheek, turn to them the other cheek also." NIV translation.

119. Lancel (2002, 275–304) provides an account strongly sympathetic to Augustine of the conflict between Donatists and Catholics in the late fourth and early fifth centuries. The discussion by Peter Brown (2000, 209) is brief but illuminating, and far more balanced in its consideration of both Catholic and Donatist parties: "Briefly, the Donatists thought of themselves as a group which existed to preserve and protect an alternative to the society around them. They felt their identity to be constantly threatened: first by persecution, later, by compromise. Innocence, ritual purity, meritorious suffering, predominate in their image of themselves. They were unique, 'pure': 'the Church of the righteous who are persecuted and do not persecute.'" O'Donnell (2005) offers a similarly impartial overview of the development of Donatism (210–15) and the Donatist/Catholic conflict (215–43). Allen and Neil (2013, 118–21) present the evidence for Donatism based on Augustine's epistolary evidence, contextualized within a broader frame of religious crisis and conflict in late antiquity. For discussion of the violent confrontations between "Donatists" and "Catholics" in fourth- and fifth-century North Africa, see also Gaddis 2005, 103–30 and 131–50, and B. Shaw 2011.

120. On the use of "Caecilianist" to describe the position that became known as "Catholic," see O'Donnell 2005, 210.

121. This distinction was presented influentially but also controversially in Frend 1952, which argued that Donatism represented local (read "less Romanised") North African resistance to imperial (Romanized, i.e., Catholic) authority. (For critique, see O'Donnell 2005, 211: "[Frend] still thought of catholicism as the norm and Donatism as the divergence.") P. Brown (1968) challenged Frend's notion that the strength of Donatism in the mid-fourth century reflected the rise of local North African identity. B. Shaw (1992) offered a nuanced revision, suggesting that Donatists were not so much a resistance group as the local orthodoxy, prior to the introduction of state intervention and the imposition of state-sanctioned Christianity in the late fourth and early fifth centuries. Maureen Tilley stood at the forefront of revisionist Donatist history, arguing in particular that the Donatist movement must be investigated not only through the writings of its opponent Augustine, but also through the meager but extant remains of its own texts: Tilley 1996; Tilley 1997; Tilley 2006; Tilley 2007. See also O'Donnell 2005, 209, for the difficulty that late antique scholars have in evading the powerful rhetoric of Catholic orthodoxy that emanates from Augustine's texts: "As we recognise the polyphony of early Christian voices, even the best late-antique scholarship remarkably often accepts the notion of a single unitary 'catholicism' in late antiquity, surrounded by heresies. But that catholicism is something that was invented and propagated, and Augustine's own history is a part of that process."

122. P. Brown 2000, 207–39, esp. 210 ("Until the time of Augustine, the tide of feeling in this debate had flowed consistently towards the Donatist attitude") and 222 ("From 393 onwards, Augustine and his colleagues took the offensive against the Donatist church"); see also B. Shaw 1992, 13. See P. Brown 1964, 108–9, with references,

for the traditional (and, according to Brown, inaccurate) view that Augustine was "converted" to the utilization of repressive legal measures against the Donatists only after the "Edict of Unity" in February 405.

123. See, for example, *S.* 47.6–8, in which Augustine suggests that Donatist bishops seek to distinguish the "sheep" from the "goats," rather than leave this judgement to God. Cf. P. Brown 2000, 215: "The basic Donatist idea was of a Chosen People, that had preserved its identity without compromise with the 'impure' world." Gaddis 2005, 105: "The Donatists sought to separate themselves, a pure and zealous minority, from a corrupt world and especially from the corruption of imperial power."

124. Cf. Lancel 2002, 288: "In any case, added Augustine, 'it was not the penalty that made the martyr, it was the cause.'" Lancel refers to *C. Cresc.* 3, 51, noting parallel sentiments in *Ep.* 89.2 and *Ep.* 108.5.

125. Aug. *En. Ps.* 34, *s.* 2.13.10–13. See Gaddis 2005, 131–50, for Augustine's rhetoric of "disciplinary violence" against Donatist Christians. Punishment for an *actor* or *procurator* who allowed for a meeting of "heretics" on an estate without the owner's knowledge was to be "bound with lead" and "sentenced to work in the mines." See the edict of Honorius and Theodosius on February 22, 407, at *Cod. Theod.* 16.5.40.

126. Aug. *En. Ps.* 34, *s.* 2.13.

127. Pl. *Protag.* 354a3–7: "You who say that some painful things are good, do you not say that such things as athletics and military training and treatments by doctors such as cautery, surgery, medicines, and starvation diet are good things even though painful?" Translation by Lombardo and Bell, from Cooper and Hutchinson 1997. Compare Pl. *Gorg.* 479a6–b1, where Socrates discusses those who avoid seeing a physician when they are sick from fear of pain.

128. Gomory, Cohen, and Kirk 2013, 120fn1: "Only pediatricians and psychiatrists treat persons who do not seek their services." Cf. Aug. *En. Ps.* 35.17.20–25: "For he was a doctor, and he had come to cure a phrenetic patient. Just as a doctor does not care about whatever he hears from the phrenetic patient, but rather about how the phrenetic patient might grow healthy and become well—indeed, does not care even if he receives blows from that man—the one giving the other fresh wounds; the other heals the old fever, so also the Lord came to the sick man, came to the phrenetic."

129. Maxwell 2006, 12: "In Late Antiquity, Christian preachers attempted to shape entire communities according to moral ideals traditionally associated with philosophers and their circles." See 12–41 for a detailed discussion of the relationship between preacher and philosopher.

130. Maxwell 2006, 41.

131. P. Brown 2000, 365: "To him [sc. Augustine], a bishop's duties were not only 'pastoral'; they had also become 'medicinal.'" See also Elm 2012, 166–71, with reference to Gregory of Nazianzen, who understood the philosopher to be a "physician of the soul."

132. Mayer 2015a; Mayer 2015b; Mayer 2015c.

133. Sorabji (2000) explores the Christian reception and transformation of Stoic psychology, in particular the role of the "passions." For "passions" and "affections" more

generally in Greco-Roman philosophy, see also Brunschwig and Nussbaum 1993; Braund and Gill 1997.

134. See, for example, John Chrysostom's letter *To Stageirios, being harassed by a demon,* in which Chrysostom urges Stageirios to unlearn his despondency, through reorientation of the *doxae* (opinions, judgments) that motivate him (discussed in Wright 2015). On anger, see especially Gal. *Aff.* 1.4 (5:16.4–21.4 K.), where learned restraint from anger is described as a form of *askēsis* (5:21.5 K.). For the psychophysiological aspect of affects, see Arist. *De an.* 1.1, 403a25–b3.

135. Although note Elm 2012, 168, where it is observed that, according to Gregory of Nazianzen, "only a trained physician ought to attempt to cure himself."

136. Thus, Augustine famously writes in *Conf.* 8.7.21–22: "Grant me chastity and continence, but not yet!" He theorizes this vacillation in greater detail some paragraphs later (Aug. *Conf.* 8.9.9–11) as the division of the will, such that "[The mind] orders, I said, what it should will: it would not command if it did not will; and it does not do what it commands. It does not, in fact, wholly will: it does not, therefore, wholly command." Strikingly, Augustine describes his behavior in this moment of vacillation as akin to that of a person suffering from an illness that impedes voluntary movement of the limbs, such as paralysis (*Conf.* 8.8.15–7, 30–33). I am grateful to Catherine Conybeare and Kristi Upson-Saia for bringing these passages to my attention.

137. Nussbaum 1994, 317: "The patient [in philosophical therapeutics] must not simply remain a patient, dependent and receptive; she must become her own doctor." Although note Plutarch's analysis of psychic illnesses as entailing subjects' ignorance of their own condition, and his explicit reference to phrenitis, in Plut. *Mor.* 500–1 (discussed in Wright 2020).

138. Lancel 2002, 303.

139. On the identity of Boniface, see Lancel 2002, 303, and B. Shaw 2015, 50–55. Hombert (2000, 133) lists 417 as the date of this letter. According to Allen and Neil (2013, 130), Augustine "regarded [this letter] as a book," titled "*The Correction of the Donatists.*"

140. Of this letter, Lancel (2002, 302–3) writes as follows: "Augustine felt no need to elaborate a theory of coercion in religious matters, but he wanted at least to clarify his ideas on its legitimacy." On Augustine's ambivalent justification of religious coercion, and the history of its reception, see P. Brown 1963 and 1964. Cf. Gaddis 2005, 133: "an overtly coercive paradigm came to define the Catholic and imperial approach to the Donatist problem."

141. Aug. *Ep.* 185.2.

142. Lancel 2002, 303: "It was, as we would say nowadays to signify the intolerable, wanting to make someone happy in spite of himself; and that is what the Donatists said, too, declaring that one should not be forced into good." Gaddis (2005, 137) highlights the "therapeutic" aspect of the punishments that Augustine requested from imperial authorities: "Donatist violence was to be answered not with violent persecution but with a steady coercive pressure that used fines, legal disabilities, and confiscations to bring recusants into the Catholic church. It was not retributive punishment but

rather disciplinary correction, a paradigm that justified coercive force out of the necessity to 'save' the Donatists from the consequences of their own error."

143. Lancel 2002, 290. See B. Shaw 2011, 822–24, for a presentation and discussion of the surviving sources on the "Edict of Unity." Gaddis 2005, 106–11 discusses the context and consequences of this event.

144. *Cod. Theod.* 16.5.38.

145. Ebbeler (2012, 154) notes that, following this edict, "Augustine largely abandoned his efforts to initiate corrective correspondences with Donatist Christians and resorted to other tactics to force unification." P. Brown (2000, 231) situates Augustine's treatise against Cresconius amid a host of other works defending the Edict of Unity: "Augustine, in replying to his persistent critics, wrote the only full justification, in the history of the Early Church, of the right of the state to suppress non-Catholics."

146. On the date of Cresconius' letter, see Willis 2005, 54. Hombert (2000, 353) dates Augustine's treatise to 405–6 or 406–7.

147. He mentions the "Edict of Unity" directly at C. *Cresc.* 3, 43.47, 44.48, 47.51.

148. Aug. C. *Cresc.* 4.51.61.

149. Gourevitch and Gourevitch 1998, 511.

150. Aug. *S. dom. m.* 1.57.

151. Joh. Chrys. *Ad Stag.* 2 (PG 47:451.17–19).

152. Hier. *Ep.* 130.17.

153. See B. Shaw 2011, 195–259, for discussion of Augustine's response to the "Circumcellions," 630–74 for the identification of the Circumcellions in the historical record, 633–38 for the name "Circumcellions," and 828–39 for a review of the historiographic construction of Circumcellion identity.

154. Gaddis 2005, 125–30, on the violence of the Circumcellions as a response to imperial repression.

155. Lancel (2002, 301–2) refers to the Circumcellion and the Donatists as "fanatics" and "outlaws," engaged in "terrorism." In contrast, O'Donnell (2005, 221) emphasizes mutual participation in violence and the difficulty of getting a clear view on the Circumcellions, as presented solely through the eyes of their enemies: "It is tempting to try to equate them to modern terrorists, but in fact their behavior is not unlike that of the stereotypically British football fan of our own day, and they may well have been as socially diverse (despite some common tendencies) as contemporary hooligans. No one in antiquity speaks up for them, and we see them only through the eyes of their enemies, chiefly Augustine, who credits them with organizational loyalty that may overstate the case. . . . But there was plenty of violence to go around, and not all of it from Donatists against Caecilianists." Cf. P. Brown 2000, 225: "Both churches, by that time, had a record of violence. . . . Compared with the mounting pressure of the Catholic persecutions, the violence of the Circumcellions would always seem erratic and aimless; and in Hippo at any rate, such violence reached a climax only as an answer to the use of force by the Catholics."

156. Aug. C. *Cresc.* 3.51.61.

157. Hippo Diarrhytus was the site of particular conflict. See O'Donnell 2005, 221: "Florentius, the fire-breathing bishop of Hippo Diarrhytus (modern Bizerte, east of

Augustine's Hippo), kept his opponent, the Donatist bishop, imprisoned for many years and tried to have him executed." For the date and location of this sermon, see Hill 1995, 207fn1; see also Hombert 2000, 167fn337.

158. Aug. *S.* 359.7.

159. Vincentius had been appointed as heir to Rogatus, leader of the "Rogatists." The Rogatists had split off from the Donatists, apparently in dispute over resistance to imperial authority, but remained distinct from Augustine's Catholic party. See P. Brown 2000, 239; Lancel 2002, 169; O'Donnell 2005, 46. For the date of this letter, see Hombert 2000, 286–87.

160. Aug. *Ep.* 93.2.446.26–447.5.

161. Aug. *Ep.* 93.2.447.5–11.

162. Aug. *Ep.* 93.2.447.11–13.

163. Tying down the patient was common in ancient treatment for phrenitis, according to Augustine's contemporary, the North African medical writer Caelius Aurelianus, *Acut.* 1.1.9.65: "Now if the patient is seen trying to jump out of bed in a fit of insanity, it will be better to use the aid of a large number of attendants who can hold him back gently. . . . If, however, there is no one to hold the patient back in this way, or if the patient is fired up by the sight of attendants, use bonds. But use wool or cloth to protect the places where the ropes are tied, lest the harm done to the sick person be greater than the advantage gained in quietening them down." Translation adapted from Drabkin 1951. Gourevitch and Gourevitch (1998, 508) take Augustine's emphasis upon tying up the patient to indicate his familiarity with the challenges of contemporary psychiatric practice. Cf. P. Brown 2000, 234: "Augustine's view of the Fall of mankind determined his attitude to society. Fallen men had come to need restraint. Even man's greatest achievements had been made possible only by a 'strait-jacket' of unremitting harshness."

164. See, in particular, Gorgias' *Helen* and Plato's *Phaedrus*. Laín Entralgo (1970) focuses on the continuity between verbal charms and the verbal "medicine" of philosophy. Elm 2012, 172–76, esp. 174: "A philosopher's principal work as physician of the soul was to use the therapeutic power of words to aid the *logos*, word or reason, in maintaining a harmonious balance of the soul." See also the useful survey in Thumiger 2020. Gill (2013) offers a glimpse of what this might have looked like in practice.

165. P. Brown 2000, 344–46 and 360–63; O'Donnell 2005, 253–55, 264, 282.

166. Aug. *Gr. et pecc. or.* 2.6.7.

167. Aug. *Gr. et pecc. or.* 2.7.8.

168. Castelli 1992, 137.

169. Hunt 2012, 53. Castelli (1992, 140) frames this from the opposite perspective, emphasizing that *even though* asceticism is a bodily practice, it is oriented toward the health of the soul.

170. Bynum 1995a.

171. Hunt (2012, 17) considers the "transformation" of pagan philosopher into Christian holy man to be one of privatization, a turning inward from public office to the cultivation of the self.

172. Singer (2018) discusses the differentiation (and ambiguity) of cerebral and ethical illness in the works of Galen.

173. See Wetzel 2012 for an overview of Augustine's teachings on original sin.

174. P. Brown 2000, 369.

175. O'Donnell 2005, 261, summarizes with customary crispness: "a stereotype of Pelagianism: generous support for human free will against an Augustinian/Pauline acceptance of divine predestination." See also P. Brown 2000, 367–69. On Augustine's development of theories of grace and the will through disputes with the Donatists, meanwhile, see Karfíková 2012, 133–55.

176. On the importance of spiritual discipline for theories of salvation in the late fourth century, see P. Brown 1988; O'Donnell 2005, 264–71.

177. Charry 2010, 35. For a brief account of Augustine's response to the question of why some are not saved, see Karfíková 2012, 186. See Couenhoven 2013 for an argument that Augustine came, in the end, to reject free will as a defense of theodicy.

178. Charry 2010, 61.

179. See, for example, Stump 1996.

180. See Ahonen 2018, 361–62, for a discussion of this problem in Stoicism.

CHAPTER 7. HUMANIZING THE BRAIN IN EARLY CHRISTIANITY

1. On this text and the question it examines, see chapter 1, above.

2. Tert. *DA* 15.2.

3. It also relies, of course, on the assumption that the organ of the *hēgemonikon* can be only the heart or the brain, which is a useful window into the standardization of these options by the second century C.E. but is less relevant to the argument here.

4. Gal. *UP* 8.2 (3:614.12615.9 K.). All translations of this text are from May 1968.

5. Gal. *UP* 8.2 (3:615.9–620.3 K.).

6. Gal. *UP* 8.4 (3:630.6–8 K.).

7. Tert. *De res. mort.* 15.16.

8. Tert. *DA* 15.6.

9. Hier. *In Matt.* 1.537. Translation from Scheck 2008.

10. Hippol. *Haer.* 4.51.10.1–11.1.

11. A similar tension marked early modern attempts to reconcile comparative anatomy with theories of the human soul. See the chapters collected in Buchenau and Lo Presti 2017, especially Crignon 2017.

12. See Arist. *PA* 4.10 (686a24–687b25), with reference to upright stature and hands. On the comparison of mouths, see *PA* 3.1 (661b6–26).

13. See *PA* 2.7 (653a27–b8, the human brain is largest in order to counteract the great heat of the heart) and 2.14 (658b2–10, the human brain is wettest and therefore the human head is hairiest); *HA* 1.16 (494b24–29, the human brain is biggest and wettest); GA 2.6 (744a26–31, the human brain is biggest and wettest because of the purity of heat around the heart; the human temperament enables the human being to

be most intelligent among all animals); *Sens.* 5 (444a28–33, the human brain is biggest and wettest, and this is why humans alone enjoy fragrant smells).

14. Erasistratus fr. 289 Garofalo = Gal. *PHP* 7.3.10. All translations of this text are from De Lacy 2005. Translation adapted.

15. Gal. *UP* 8.12 (3:673.10–674.1 K.).

16. For a more detailed introduction to Galen's animal dissections, see chapter 2.

17. On the public demonstrations, see Hankinson 1991; Gleason 2009.

18. Gal. *AA* 9.11.

19. Gal. *PHP* 7.3.15–16.

20. Gal. *AA* 9.12.22–23. Translation from Duckworth 1962.

21. This demonstration has been reconstructed from sparse references. The evidence is Gal. *Praen.* 5.9–21, *AA* 8.3, and *AA* 11.4. For the reconstruction, see Gross 1998; Frampton 2008, 198–200; Gleason 2009, 97–100; Mattern 2013, 157–60.

22. Tieleman 1996, 38–40. The source for this summary of the Stoic argument is Galen's *On the Opinions of Hippocrates and Plato.*

23. Hankinson 1991, 215–23; Frampton 2008, 146–89.

24. On the authority of Galen's writings in late antiquity, see Temkin 1973, especially 61–70. Galen's works were still canonical in the sixteenth century, when Vesalius finally refuted Galen's arguments about anatomy and physiology by carrying out animal dissections described by Galen himself (Siraisi 1997; French 2006, 26–27).

25. We might compare this to the principles of contemporary behavioral neuroscience and its use of animal experimentation, and the philosophical and methodological questions that this practice raises. See Insel 2007; Rose and Abi-Rached 2013, 82–109.

26. Patterson 2002, 16–23.

27. Sorabji 1993. Miller (2018) nuances this assessment.

28. Nem. *Nat. hom.* 1 (Morani 5.9). All translations of this text are from Sharples and van der Eijk 2008. Ladner (1958, 71–72) situates Nemesius' work within late antique philosophical theories of the relationship between humans and other animals.

29. Nem. *Nat. hom.* 1 (Morani 11.3–5).

30. Nem. *Nat. hom.* 1 (Morani 6.18–20).

31. See especially G. Clark 1998a, and the critical discussion in Miller 2018, 3–4. Ladner (1958, 67) discusses these arguments in Gregory of Nyssa's *On the Constitution of the Human Being.* See, for illustration, Greg. Nyss. *Op. hom.* 4 (PG 44:136.18–22): "The master craftsman created our body just like a tool for activity suitable for rulership, preparing it both by advantages of the soul and by the very structure of the body, so as to be in a suitable condition for rulership."

32. Nem. *Nat. hom.* 1 (Morani 13.23–26): "If the rational part in us rules the non-rational part in us, how is it not reasonable that it should also have mastery over the non-rational things external [to us] and that they should have been given to serve its needs? For it is the natural role of the non-rational to serve the rational, as was shown with regard to ourselves."

33. Nem. *Nat. hom.* 1 (Morani 4.22–24): "Thus he joined everything to everything harmoniously and bound them together and collected into one thing intelligible and things visible, by medium of the generation of man." The classic account of this "chain-of-being," a theory closely associated with Aristotle, is Lovejoy 1936. Cf. Amb. *Ex.* 6.9.54, where the size of the human being represents its intermediary position: "the very appearance of the body is gentle and pleasing without those extremes of size and of insignificance which might lead either to dread or to indifference."

34. Amb. *Ex.* 6.9.55. I discuss this text in chapter 4.

35. Joh. Chrys. *In Eph. hom.* 11.11 (PG 62:84.4–49). I discuss this text in chapter 4.

36. Greg. Nyss. *Op. hom.* 8 (PG 44:148.27–36): "Since, indeed, the human being is a rational animal, it was necessary that the instrument of the body be prepared appropriately for the use of reason. Just as we can observe musicians performing music in accordance with the form of their instruments, and not piping through lyres, nor strumming flutes, in the same way, it was necessary that the preparation of the instruments correspond to reason, so that, when struck by the parts associated with voice, it might naturally resound for the use of words."

37. Amb. *Ex.* 6.9.54. Translation from Savage 1961.

38. Arist. *PA* 4.10, 687a23–26.

39. Arist. *PA* 4.10, 687a11–13.

40. Gal. *UP* 1.2 (3:3.3–7 K.). All translations of this text are from May 1968. Translation adapted.

41. Gal. *UP* 1.4 (3:8.1–9 K.). Translation adapted.

42. Greg. Nyss. *Op. hom.* 7 (PG 44:140.49–55).

43. Greg. Nyss. *Op. hom.* 7 (PG 44:141.19–21).

44. Nem. *Nat. hom.* 1 (Morani 9.8–13).

45. Ladner 1958, 67–68, with reference to Greg. Nyss. *Op. hom.* 7 (PG 44:140–44). Cf. Gal. *UP* 1.4 (3:8.6–9 K.): "For if he had been born with a natural weapon, he would have that one alone for all time, and just so, if he had one natural skill, he would lack all others." We might trace echoes of this logic in the rhetoric used to legitimate violence within modern imperialism, where the violence of the aggressor has often been explained as a response to the extraordinary or brutish violence of the "savage," in contrast to the reasoning and "softness" of the occupying force. K. Wagner (2018) offers a useful analysis of the construction of British military practice as "soft" and "humane," especially in contrast to the violence of "savage warfare." Hokowhitu (2004) dissects the colonialist construction of Māori and Polynesian men as "physical" (i.e., suitable primarily for warfare and sports) and its afterlife in contemporary New Zealand rugby. The legacy of these narratives also lives on, for example, in disproportionate police violence against Black men, especially in the United States.

46. See the discussion in Sharples and van der Eijk 2008, 48fn238. Van der Eijk (1997, 245–46) discusses this in detail in relation to Aristotle. Ladner (1958, 68) identifies the upright posture of the human being as the essential feature of "the [human] body's share in divine image-likeness."

47. Amb. *Ex.* 6.9.74.

48. Bas. *Hex.* 9.2.31–34.

49. Greg. Nyss. *Op. hom.* 8 (PG 44:144.14–16).

50. Nem. *Nat. hom.* 1 (Morani 13.11–13).

51. Greg. Nyss. *Op. hom.* 8 (PG 44:144.21–24).

52. Greg. Nyss. *Op. hom.* 8 (PG 44:149.12–14).

53. Amb. *Ex.* 6.9.69.

54. Greg. Nyss. *Op. hom.* 8 (PG 44:144.27–28).

55. Nem. *Nat. hom.* 8 (Morani 65.13–15).

56. Nem. *Nat. hom.* 1 (Morani 8.15–21). All elided material in this quotation provides comparison to different animal species. Cf. Nem. *Nat. hom.* 8 (Morani 65.9–11): "In this [i.e., touch] and also in taste he is superior to other living beings, even though he is inferior in the three other [senses]." For the medical background to this claim, see Gal. *Temp.* 1.9 (1:563.14–564.2 K.): "Of such a kind also is the human skin, being at the precise midpoint between all the extremes, hot, cold, hard, and soft, and, within this category, the skin on the hand in particular. For this part was meant to be the yardstick of all perceptible [objects], crafted as it was by Nature as the organ of touch proper to the most intelligent of animals." Translation from Singer, van der Eijk, and Tassinari 2018. See also the comments in Sharples and van der Eijk 2008, 113fn561.

57. Amb. *Ex.* 6.9.64.

58. Greg. Nyss. *Op. hom.* 8 (PG 44:148.44–47).

59. Greg. Nyss. *Op. hom.* 8 (PG 44:149.10–12). See Ladner 1958, 68–69 (with references), for an account of these anatomical features and their interrelationship in Gregory of Nyssa's *On the Constitution of the Human Being*, and the suggestion that the philosopher Posidonius of Apamea (c. 135–51 B.C.E.) was the origin of this theory of a cause-and-effect relation between the different anatomical features that support human reason.

60. Nem. *Nat. hom.* 1 (Morani 4.20–22).

61. Amb. *Ex.* 6.9.68.

62. Amb. *Ex.* 6.9.68.

63. Greg. Nyss. *Op. hom.* 9 (PG 44:149.24–31).

64. On ancient philosophical treatments of the problem of birdsong, see Justin E. H. Smith 2017.

65. Amb. *Ex.* 6.9.61.

66. Amb. *Ex.* 6.9.61.

67. Nem. *Nat. hom.* 6–13 (Morani 55–71).

68. Greg. Nyss. *Op. hom.* 30 (PG 44:249.47–252.1).

69. This is explicitly the case for early modern thinkers: see Cellamare 2017 and Crignon 2017.

70. See my discussion in chapter 3.

71. Nem. *Nat. hom.* 2 (Morani 36.6–9).

72. This argument operated at the level of the species, not the individual; that is to say, disability did not preclude the presence of the rational soul. Cf. Nem. *Nat. hom.* 14 (Morani 71.13–15) on "immanent" reason: "For both those who are dumb from birth

and those who have lost their voice through accident or disease are none the less gifted with reason."

73. Shepardson 2014, 171.

74. On the analogy between the human body and the city in late antique thought, see, for example, Amb. *Ex.* 6.9.

75. Stefaniw 2016, 236–37.

76. Stefaniw 2016, 251: "In the late antique imagination, the civil order was a continuation of the cosmic order, and both the governance of the cosmos and of the empire depended on a copy-model structure according to which those in authority could and should provide for the moral guidance and betterment of their subjects."

77. Joh. Chrys. *In Ep. 1 ad Tim.* 13 (PG 62:570.18–37) and *In Matt.* 44.7 (PG 57:472.11–20).

78. Greg. Nyss. *Op. hom.* 30 (PG 44:249.47–252.1).

79. Thdt. *Haer.* 5.9 (PG 83:481.14–19).

80. Nem. *Nat. hom.* 12 (Morani 68.3–13). See my discussion in chapter 3.

81. Joh. Chrys. *In Ep. ad Heb.* 5.8 (PG 63:54.6–14). See my discussion in chapter 5.

82. Pall. *Laus. Hist.* 18.3. See my discussion in chapter 6.

83. Greg. Nyss. *Op. hom.* 12 (PG 44:157.41–47); Nem. *Nat. hom.* 13 (Morani 70.21); Aug. *Gn. litt.* 7.18.

84. For the term "cerebral subjectivity," see Vidal 2009; Vidal and Ortega 2017. See also Rose and Abi-Rached 2013; Pitts-Taylor 2016, 3–4.

85. E. Martin 2010.

86. See my discussion of cerebral subjectivity in the introduction.

87. See, for example, Patterson 2002, 20. Berkowitz (2015, 38–40) offers a more nuanced account. As Miller (2018) argues, the overall claim is too simplistic a rendering of late ancient Christian engagement with animals.

88. Vidal 2009, 9–10.

89. Siebers 2008, 12.

90. Devlin and Pothier (2006) argue that this is the case for disability in general. Sherry (2013) argues that acquired brain injury is marginalized even within disability studies.

91. Devlin and Pothier 2006, 16.

92. Devlin and Pothier 2006, 11.

93. Brennan 2004, 2, 16–19.

94. Brennan 2004, 24: "In theories of psychiatry and psychoanalysis, the healthy person is a self-contained person."

95. Brennan 2004, 12–15.

96. Brennan 2004, 17.

97. Siebers 2008, 89–90.

98. Morton is discussed most influentially and controversially in Gould 1996, 83–88; see for brief review Mitchell and Michael 2019.

99. See DeLeon 2010, 5–8, for the argument that understanding "speciesism" can scaffold understanding of human-to-human oppression also. Among the most prom-

inent early animal studies scholars was Carol Adams, who asserted the parallelism between the oppression of women and the oppression of animals as "meat" (Adams 1990). See also the remarks in Gruen and Weil 2012. Note that animal studies and disability studies scholars do not always agree, because some animal studies scholars (most famously Peter Singer) have argued that "able-bodied" animal life should be preserved over "disabled" human life. See, for a measured but clear response, Siebers 2008, 92.

100. See the essays collected in Kapp 2020.

101. Pitts-Taylor 2016, 82.

102. As discussed most influentially in Damasio 1994.

WORKS CITED

Adams, Carol J. 1990. *The Sexual Politics of Meat: A Feminist-Vegetarian Critical Theory.* Bloomsbury Revelations Series. New York: Bloomsbury.

Agarwalla, Pankaj K. 2010. "Training Showmanship: Rhetoric in Greek Medical Education of the Fifth and Fourth Centuries BC." In *Hippocrates and Medical Education,* edited by Manfred Horstmanshoff, 73–85. Leiden: Brill.

Ahonen, Marke. 2018. "Making the Distinction: The Stoic View of Mental Illness." In *Mental Illness in Ancient Medicine,* edited by Chiara Thumiger and P. N. Singer, 343–64. Leiden: Brill.

Allen, Pauline, and Bronwen Neil. 2013. *Crisis Management in Late Antiquity (410–590 CE): A Survey of the Evidence from Episcopal Letters.* Supplements to *Vigiliae Christianae* 121. Leiden: Brill.

Amirav, Hagit. 2003. *Rhetoric and Tradition: John Chrysostom on Noah and the Flood.* Traditio Exegetica Graeca 12. Louvain: Peeters Publishers.

Amundsen, Darrel W. 1982. "Medicine and Faith in Early Christianity." *Bulletin of the History of Medicine* 56, no. 3: 326–50.

Anderson, Warwick. 2003. "How's the Empire? An Essay Review." *Journal of the History of Medicine and Allied Sciences* 58, no. 4: 459–65.

———. 2008. *The Collectors of Lost Souls: Turning Kuru Scientists into Whitemen.* Baltimore: Johns Hopkins University Press.

Annas, Julia. 1992. *Hellenistic Philosophy of Mind.* Berkeley: University of California Press.

Arbesmann, Rudolph. 1954. "Christ, the *Medicus Humilis* in St. Augustine." In *Augustinus Magister* 2: 623–29. Paris: Études augustiniennes.

Arikha, Noga. 2007. *Passions and Tempers: A History of the Humours.* New York: Ecco.

Baldwin, Barry. 1975. "The Career of Oribasius." *Acta Classica* 18: 85–97.

Barnes, Jonathan, ed. 1984. *The Complete Works of Aristotle: The Revised Oxford Translation.* Bollingen Series, 71.2. Princeton, NJ: Princeton University Press.

Bassiri, Nima. 2012. "Material Translations in the Cartesian Brain." *Studies in History and Philosophy of Biological and Biomedical Sciences* 43, no. 1: 244–55.

BeDuhn, Jason David. 1992. "A Regimen for Salvation: Medical Models in Manichaean Asceticism." *Semeia* 58: 109–34.

Bell, T. A., ed. 1997. *John of Alexandria. Commentary on Hippocrates' "On the Nature of the Child."* Berlin: Akademie Verlag.

Bennett, M. R., and P. M. S. Hacker. 2003. *Philosophical Foundations of Neuroscience.* Oxford: Blackwell.

Berger, Adolf. 1953. "Encyclopedic Dictionary of Roman Law." *Transactions of the American Philosophical Society* 43, no. 2: 333–808.

Berkowitz, Beth. 2015. "Animal." In *Late Ancient Knowing: Explorations in Intellectual History*, edited by Catherine M. Chin and Moulie Vidas, 36–57. Oakland: University of California Press.

Berryman, Sylvia. 2009. *The Mechanical Hypothesis in Ancient Greek Natural Philosophy.* Cambridge: Cambridge University Press.

Betegh, Gábor. 2007. "On the Physical Aspect of Heraclitus' Psychology." *Phronesis* 52, no. 1: 3–32.

Betus, Allison E., Erin M. Kearns, and Anthony F. Lemieux. 2021. "How Perpetrator Identity (Sometimes) Influences Media Framing Attacks as 'Terrorism' or 'Mental Illness.'" *Communication Research* 48, no. 8: 1133–56.

Birley, Anthony R. 1992. "A Case of Eye Disease (*Lippitudo*) on the Roman Frontier in Britain." *History of Ophthalmology* 5: 111–19.

Bishop, Jeffrey P. 2000. "Mind-Body Unity: Gregory of Nyssa and a Surprising Fourth-Century CE Perspective." *Perspectives in Biology and Medicine* 43, no. 4: 519–29.

Blumenthal, H. J. 1986. "Body and Soul in Philoponus." *The Monist* 69, no. 3: 370–82.

———. 1996. *Aristotle and Neoplatonism in Late Antiquity: Interpretations of the De Anima.* Ithaca, NY: Cornell University Press.

Bond, Sarah E. 2015. "'As Trainers for the Healthy': Massage Therapists, Anointers, and Healing in the Late Latin West." *Journal of Late Antiquity* 8, no. 2: 386–404.

Borck, Cornelius. 2012. "Toys Are Us: Models and Metaphors in Brain Science." In *Critical Neuroscience: A Handbook of the Social and Cultural Contexts of Neuroscience*, edited by Jan Slaby and Suparna Choudhury, 113–33. Chichester: Wiley-Blackwell.

Bos, A. P. 2003. *The Soul and Its Instrumental Body: A Reinterpretation of Aristotle's Philosophy of Living Nature.* Leiden: Brill.

Bowersock, G. W. 2010. "Iatrosophists." In *Historiae Augustae colloquium Genevense in honorem F. Paschoud septuagenarii: Les traditions historiographiques de l'antiquité tardive; Idéologie*, 83–91. Bari: Edipuglia.

Boylan, Michael. 2007. "Galen: On Blood, the Pulse, and the Arteries." *Journal of the History of Biology* 40: 207–30.

Boys-Stones, George, ed. 2003. *Metaphor, Allegory, and the Classical Tradition: Ancient Thought and Modern Revisions.* Oxford: Oxford University Press.

Brakke, David. 2006. *Demons and the Making of the Monk: Spiritual Combat in Early Christianity.* Cambridge, MA: Harvard University Press.

Braund, Susanna Morton, and Christopher Gill, eds. 1997. *The Passions in Roman Thought and Literature*. Cambridge: Cambridge University Press.

Brennan, Teresa. 2004. *The Transmission of Affect*. Ithaca, NY: Cornell University Press.

Brown, Archibald G. 1873. *East London Tabernacle Pulpit*. London.

Brown, Peter R. L. 1963. "Religious Coercion in the Later Roman Empire: The Case of North Africa." *History* 48, no. 164: 283–305.

———. 1964. "St. Augustine's Attitude to Religious Coercion." *Journal of Roman Studies* 54, no. 1–2: 107–16.

———. 1968. "Christianity and Local Culture in Late Roman Africa." *Journal of Roman Studies* 58, no. 1–2: 85–95.

———. (1971) 1993. *The World of Late Antiquity, AD 150–750*. Revised ed. London: Thames and Hudson.

———. 1972. "Sorcery, Demons, and the Rise of Christianity: From Late Antiquity into the Middle Ages." In *Religion and Society in the Age of St. Augustine*, 119–46. London: Faber.

———. 1988. *The Body and Society*. New York: Columbia University Press, 1988.

———. 1992. *Power and Persuasion in Late Antiquity: Towards a Christian Empire*. The Curti Lectures 1988. Madison: University of Wisconsin Press.

———. 2000. *Augustine of Hippo*. A new edition with an epilogue. Berkeley: University of California Press.

———. 2012. *Through the Eye of a Needle: Wealth, the Fall of Rome, and the Making of Christianity in the West, 350–550 AD*. Princeton, NJ: Princeton University Press.

Brunschwig, Jacques, and Martha Craven Nussbaum, eds. 1993. *Passions and Perceptions: Studies in Hellenistic Philosophy of Mind. Proceedings of the Fifth Symposium Hellenisticum*. Cambridge: Cambridge University Press / Paris: Editions de la Maison des Sciences de l'Homme.

Buchenau, Stefanie, and Roberto Lo Presti, eds. 2017. *Human & Animal Cognition in Early Modern Philosophy*. Pittsburgh: University of Pittsburgh Press.

Burnyeat, M. F. 1992. "Is an Aristotelian Philosophy of Mind Still Credible? (A Draft)." In *Essays on Aristotle's De Anima*, edited by Martha C. Nussbaum and Amélie Oksenberg Rorty, 15–26. Oxford: Clarendon Press.

Bynum, Caroline Walker. 1995a. *The Resurrection of the Body in Western Christianity 200–1336*. New York: Columbia University Press.

———. 1995b. "Why All the Fuss about the Body? A Medievalist's Perspective." *Critical Inquiry* 22, no. 1: 1–33.

Caciola, Nancy. 2003. *Discerning Spirits: Divine and Demonic Possession in the Middle Ages*. Ithaca, NY: Cornell University Press.

Cain, Andrew. 2009. *The Letters of Jerome: Asceticism, Biblical Exegesis, and the Construction of Christian Authority in Late Antiquity*. Oxford: Oxford University Press.

Cameron, Alan. 1966. "The Date and Identity of Macrobius." *Journal of Roman Studies* 56, no. 1 and 2: 25–38.

———. 2011. *The Last Pagans of Rome*. Oxford: Oxford University Press.

Cameron, Averil. 1991. *Christianity and the Rhetoric of Empire: The Development of Christian Discourse.* Berkeley: University of California Press.

———. 1993. *The Mediterranean World in Late Antiquity, AD 395–600.* London: Routledge.

Cameron, Averil, Brian Ward-Perkins, and Michael Whitby, eds. 2000. *The Cambridge Ancient History 14: Late Antiquity: Empire and Successors, AD 425–600.* Cambridge: Cambridge University Press.

Caner, Daniel. 2002. *Wandering, Begging Monks: Spiritual Authority and the Promotion of Monasticism in Late Antiquity.* Berkeley: University of California Press.

Cañizares, Pilar Pérez. 2010. "The Importance of Having Medical Knowledge as a Layman: The Hippocratic Treatise *Affections* in the Context of the Hippocratic Corpus." In *Hippocrates and Medical Education,* edited by Manfred Horstmanshoff, 87–99. Leiden: Brill.

Cary, Phillip. 2008. *Inner Grace: Augustine in the Traditions of Plato and Paul.* New York: Oxford University Press.

Castelli, Elizabeth A. 1991. "'I Will Make Mary Male': Pieties of the Body and Gender Transformation of Christian Women in Late Antiquity." In *Body Guards: The Cultural Politics of Gender Ambiguity,* edited by J. Epstein and K. Straub, 29–49. London: Routledge.

———. 1992. "Mortifying the Body, Curing the Soul: Beyond Ascetic Dualisms in the Life of Saint Syncletica." *differences* 4, no. 2: 134–53.

Cellamare, Davide. 2017. "Renaissance Psychology: Francisco Vallesius (1524–1592) & Otto Casmann (1562–1607) on Animal & Human Souls." In *Human and Animal Cognition in Early Modern Philosophy & Medicine,* edited by Stefanie Buchenau and Roberto Lo Presti, 74–88. Pittsburgh: University of Pittsburgh Press.

Charry, Ellen T. 2010. *God and the Art of Happiness.* Grand Rapids, MI: Eerdmans, 2010.

Chin, Catherine M. 2008. *Grammar and Christianity in the Late Roman World.* Philadelphia: University of Pennsylvania Press.

Choudhury, Suparna, and Jan Slaby. 2012a. "Introduction: Critical Neuroscience—Between Lifeworld and Laboratory." In *Critical Neuroscience: A Handbook of the Social and Cultural Contexts of Neuroscience,* edited by Suparna Choudhury and Jan Slaby, 1–26. Chichester, West Sussex: Wiley-Blackwell.

———. 2012b. "Proposal for a Critical Neuroscience." In *Critical Neuroscience: A Handbook of the Social and Cultural Contexts of Neuroscience,* edited by Suparna Choudhury and Jan Slaby, 29–51. Chichester, West Sussex: Wiley-Blackwell.

Chroust, Anton-Hermann. 1995. "Legal Profession in Ancient Imperial Rome." *Notre Dame Law Review* 30, no. 4: 521–616.

Cilliers, Louise. 2005. "Vindicianus's 'Gynaecia': Text and Translation of the Codex Monacensis." *The Journal of Medieval Latin* 15: 153–236.

———. 2010. "The Didactic Letters Prefacing Marcellus' *On Drugs* as Evidence for the Expertise and Reputation of Doctors in the Late Roman Empire." In *Hippocrates and Medical Education*, edited by Manfred Horstmanshoff, 401–18. Leiden: Brill, 2010.

———. 2019. *Roman North Africa: Environment, Society and Medical Contribution.* Amsterdam: Amsterdam University Press.

Clark, Elizabeth A. 1990. "New Perspectives on the Origenist Controversy: Human Embodiment and Ascetic Strategies." *Church History* 59, no. 2: 145–62.

———. 1997. "Sane Insanity: Women and Asceticism in Late Ancient Christianity." *Medieval Encounters* 3, no. 3: 211–30.

———. 1998. "Holy Women, Holy Words: Early Christian Women, Social History, and the 'Linguistic Turn.' *Journal of Early Christian Studies* 6, no. 3: 413–30.

———. 1999. *Reading Renunciation: Asceticism and Scripture in Early Christianity.* Princeton, NJ: Princeton University Press.

Clark, Gillian. 1998a. "The Fathers and the Animals: The Rule of Reason." In *Animals on the Agenda: Questions about Animals for Theology and Ethics*, edited by Andrew Linzey and Dorothy Yamamoto, 67–79. Urbana: University of Illinois Press.

———. 1998b. "Women and Asceticism in Late Antiquity: The Refusal of Status and Gender." In *Asceticism*, edited by Vincent L. Wimbush and Richard Valantasis, 33–48. Oxford: Oxford University Press.

———. 2005. "The Health of the Spiritual Athlete." In *Health in Antiquity*, edited by Helen King, 216–29. London: Routledge.

Clarke, Edwin, and Charles D. O'Malley. 1996. *The Human Brain and Spinal Cord: A Historical Study Illustrated by Writings from Antiquity to the Twentieth Century.* 2nd ed. San Francisco: Norman Publishing.

Clarke, Edwin, and Jerry Stannard. 1963. "Aristotle on the Anatomy of the Brain." *Journal of the History of Medicine and Allied Sciences* 18, no. 2: 130–48.

Clarke, W.K. Lowther. 1918. *The Lausiac History of Palladius.* London: Society for Promoting Christian Knowledge.

Cobb, Stephanie. 2008. *Dying to Be Men: Gender and Language in Early Christian Martyr Texts.* New York: Columbia University Press.

Colish, Marcia L. 1985. *The Stoic Tradition from Antiquity to the Early Middle Ages*, vol. 1, *Stoicism in Classical Latin Literature.* Leiden: Brill.

Conrad, Lawrence I. 1995. "The Arab-Islamic Medical Tradition." In *The Western Medical Tradition: 800 BC to AD 1800*, edited by Lawrence I. Conrad, Michael Neve, Vivian Nutton, Roy Porter, and Andrew Wear, 93–138. Cambridge: Cambridge University Press.

Conrad, Peter, and Joseph W. Schneider. 1980. *Deviance and Medicalization. From Badness to Sickness.* Maryland Heights, MI: The C.V. Mosby Company.

Cooper, John M., and D.S. Hutchinson. 1997. *Plato. Complete Works.* Indianapolis: Hackett.

Corrigan, Kevin. 2009. *Evagrius and Gregory: Mind, Soul and Body in the 4th Century.* Farnham: Ashgate.

Couenhoven, Jesse. 2013. *Stricken by Sin, Cured by Christ: Agency, Necessity, and Culpability in Augustinian Theology.* New York: Oxford University Press.

Craik, Elizabeth M. 2001. "Thucydides on the Plague: Physiology of Flux and Fixation." *The Classical Quarterly (New Series)* 51, no. 1: 102–8.

———, ed. 2009. *The Hippocratic Treatise "On Glands."* Leiden: Brill.

———. 2012. "The Reception of the Hippocratic Treatise *On Glands.*" In *Blood, Sweat and Tears: The Changing Concepts of Physiology from Antiquity into Early Modern Europe,* edited by Manfred Horstmanshoff, Helen King, and Claus Zittel, 65–82. Leiden: Brill.

———. 2015. *The "Hippocratic" Corpus: Content and Context.* London: Routledge.

Cribiore, Raffaella. 2001. *Gymnastics of the Mind: Greek Education in Hellenistic and Roman Egypt.* Princeton, NJ: Princeton University Press.

Crignon, Claire. 2017. "How Animals May Help Us Understand Men: Thomas Willis's *Anatomy of the Brain* (1664) & *Two Discourses Concerning the Soules of Brutes* (1672)." In *Human and Animal Cognition in Early Modern Philosophy & Medicine,* edited by Stefanie Buchenau and Roberto Lo Presti, 173–85. Pittsburgh: University of Pittsburgh Press.

Crislip, Andrew. 2013. *Thorns in the Flesh: Illness and Sanctity in Late Ancient Christianity.* Philadelphia: University of Pennsylvania Press.

Crivellato, Enrico, Franco Mallardi, and Domenico Ribatti. 2006. "Diogenes of Apollonia: A Pioneer in Vascular Anatomy." *The Anatomical Record Part B: The New Anatomist* 289B, no. 4: 116–20.

Crockett, William R. 1989. *Eucharist: Symbol of Transformation.* Collegeville, MN: Liturgical Press.

Cunningham, Andrew. 1988. "Getting the Game Right: Some Plain Words on the Identity and Invention of Science." *Studies in History and Philosophy of Science Part A* 19, no. 3: 365–89.

Curd, Patricia, and Daniel W. Graham. 2008. Introduction to *The Oxford Handbook of Presocratic Philosophy,* edited by Patricia Curd and Daniel W. Graham, 3–24. Oxford: Oxford University Press.

Damasio, Antonio R. 1994. *Descartes' Error: Emotion, Reason, and the Human Brain.* New York: Putnam.

Davies, David O., and L. G. Westerink. 1981. *Agnellus of Ravenna, Lectures on Galen's "De Sectis."* Arethusa Monographs 8. Buffalo, NY: SUNY Buffalo.

De Lacy, Phillip, ed. 2005. *Galen's 'On the Opinions of Hippocrates and Plato' [Galeni De Placitis Hippocratis et Platonis].* CMG V 4.1.2. Berlin: Akademie-Verlag.

De Wet, Chris L. 2015. *Preaching Bondage: John Chrysostom and the Discourse of Slavery in Early Christianity.* Oakland: University of California Press.

———. 2019. "Gluttony and the Preacher's Diet: Gluttony, Regimen, and Psycho-Somatic Health in the Homilies of John Chrysostom." In *(Re)Visioning John Chrysostom: New Theories and Approaches,* edited by Chris L. De Wet and Wendy Mayer, 410–63. Leiden: Brill.

Dean-Jones, Lesley. 1994. *Women's Bodies in Classical Greek Science.* Oxford: Clarendon Press.

Debru, Armelle. 2005. "Christianisme et Galénisme: Le mouvement volontaire chez Némésius d'Émèse." In *Les pères de l'église face à la science médicale de leur temps*, edited by Véronique Boudon-Millot and Bernard Pouderon, 89–103. Paris: Beauchesne.

———. 2008. "Physiology." In *The Cambridge Companion to Galen*, edited by R.J. Hankinson, 263–81. Cambridge: Cambridge University Press.

DeLeon, Abraham Paul. 2010. "The Lure of the Animal: The Theoretical Question of the Nonhuman Animal." *Critical Education* 1, no. 2: 1–26.

Devlin, Richard, and Dianne Pothier. 2006. "Introduction: Toward a Critical Theory of Dis-Citizenship." In *Critical Disability Theory*, edited by Richard Devlin and Dianne Pothier, 1–24. Vancouver: UBC Press.

Dickson, Keith M. 1998. *Stephanus the Philosopher and Physician: Commentary on Galen's Therapeutics to Glaucon*. Leiden: Brill.

Diels, Hermann. 1879. *Doxographi Graeci*. Berlin: Weidmann.

Dillon, John. 1993. *Alcinous: The Handbook of Platonism*. Oxford: Clarendon Press.

Donini, Pierluigi. 2008. "Psychology." In *The Cambridge Companion to Galen*, edited by R.J. Hankinson, 184–209. Cambridge: Cambridge University Press.

Doody, Aude. 2010. *Pliny's Encyclopedia: The Reception of the Natural History*. Cambridge: Cambridge University Press.

Dossey, Leslie. 2013. "Watchful Greeks and Lazy Romans: Disciplining Sleep in Late Antiquity." *Journal of Early Christian Studies* 21, no. 2: 209–39.

Doty, Robert W. 2007. "Alkmaion's Discovery That Brain Creates Mind: A Revolution in Human Knowledge Comparable to That of Copernicus and of Darwin." *Neuroscience* 147, no. 3: 561–68.

Douglas, Mary. 1966. *Purity and Danger: An Analysis of Concepts of Pollution and Taboo*. London: Routledge and Kegan Paul.

Drabkin, I.E. 1951. *Caelius Aurelianus, On Acute Diseases and On Chronic Diseases*. Chicago: University of Chicago Press.

Duckworth, W.L.H., ed. 1962. *Galen. On Anatomical Procedures: De Anatomicis Administrationibus; The Later Books, IX.6–XV*. Cambridge: Cambridge University Press.

Duffy, John. 1983. *Stephanus the Philosopher: A Commentary on the Prognosticon of Hippocrates*. Berlin: Akademie-Verlag.

———. 1984. "Byzantine Medicine in the Sixth and Seventh Centuries: Aspects of Teaching and Practice." *Dumbarton Oaks Papers* 38: 21–27.

———. ed. 1997. *John of Alexandria: Commentary on Hippocrates' Epidemics VI Fragments; Commentary of an Anonymous Author on Hippocrates' Epidemics VI Fragment*. Berlin: Akademie-Verlag.

Dumit, Joseph. 2004. *Picturing Personhood: Brain Scans and Biomedical Identity*. Princeton, NJ: Princeton University Press.

Ebbeler, Jennifer. 2012. *Disciplining Christians: Correction and Community in Augustine's Letters*. Oxford: Oxford University Press.

Elm, Susanna. 1994. *Virgins of God: The Making of Asceticism in Late Antiquity*. Oxford Classical Monographs. Oxford: Clarendon Press.

———. 2012. *Sons of Hellenism, Fathers of the Church: Emperor Julian, Gregory of Nazianzus, and the Vision of Rome*. Berkeley: University of California Press.

El Refaie, Lisa. 2019. *Visual Metaphor and Embodiment in Graphic Illness Narratives*. Oxford: Oxford University Press.

Everson, Stephen. 1997. *Aristotle on Perception*. Oxford: Clarendon Press.

Ewers, Miriam. 2009. *Marcellus Empiricus: De medicamentis; Christliche Abhandlung über Barmherzigkeit oder abergläubische Rezeptsammlung?* Trier: WVT, Wissenschaftlicher Verlag Trier.

Fadiman, Anne. 1997. *The Spirit Catches You and You Fall Down: A Hmong Child, Her American Doctors, and the Collision of Two Cultures*. New York: Farrar, Straus and Giroux.

Fancy, Nahyan A. G. 2013. *Science and Religion in Mamluk Egypt: Ibn Al-Nafis, Pulmonary Transit and Bodily Resurrection*. London: Routledge.

Fine, Cordelia. 2010. *Delusions of Gender: How Our Minds, Society, and Neurosexism Create Difference*. New York: W. W. Norton.

Finger, Stanley. 2000. *Minds Behind the Brain: A History of the Pioneers and Their Discoveries*. New York: Oxford University Press.

Fitzgerald, Des, Svenja Matusall, Joshua Skewes, and Andreas Roepstorff. 2014. "What's So Critical about Critical Neuroscience? Rethinking Experiment, Enacting Critique." *Frontiers in Human Neuroscience* 8, article 365: 1–12.

Flemming, Rebecca. 2000. *Medicine and the Making of Roman Women: Gender, Nature, and Authority from Celsus to Galen*. Oxford: Oxford University Press.

———. 2005. "Empires of Knowledge: Medicine and Health in the Hellenistic World." In *A Companion to the Hellenistic World*, edited by Andrew Erskine, 449–63. Oxford: Blackwell.

Fournier, Eric. 2016. "Amputation Metaphors and the Rhetoric of Exile: Purity and Pollution in Late Antique Christianity." In *Clerical Exile in Late Antiquity*, edited by Julia Hillner, Jakob Engberg, and Jörg Ulrich, 47–65. Frankfurt am Main: Peter Lang.

Fowden, Garth. 2014. *Before and after Muhammad: The First Millennium Refocused*. Princeton, NJ: Princeton University Press.

Frampton, Michael. 2008. *Voluntary Animal Motion from Greek Antiquity to the Latin Middle Ages, 400 B.C.–A.D. 1300*. Saarbrücken: VDM Verlag.

Frank, Georgia. 2000. "Macrina's Scar: Homeric Allusion and Heroic Identity in Gregory of Nyssa's Life of Macrina." *Journal of Early Christian Studies* 8, no. 4: 511–30.

Fredriksen, Paula. 2010. *Augustine and the Jews: A Christian Defense of Jews and Judaism*. New Haven, CT: Yale University Press.

Freeman, Michael D. A., and Oliver R. Goodenough, eds. 2009. *Law, Mind and Brain*. Farnham: Ashgate.

French, Roger. 2006. *William Harvey's Natural Philosophy*. Cambridge: Cambridge University Press.

Frend, W.H.C. 1952. *The Donatist Church: A Movement of Protest in Roman North Africa*. Oxford: Clarendon Press.

Freudenthal, Gad. 1995. *Aristotle's Theory of Material Substance: Heat and Pneuma, Form and Soul*. Oxford: Clarendon Press.

Freudenthal, Jacob. 1879. *Der platoniker Albinos und der falsche Alkinoos*. Hellenistische Studien 3. Berlin: S. Calvary.

Froehlich, K. 1984. *Biblical Interpretation in the Early Church*. Philadelphia: Fortress Press.

Furley, David J., and J.S. Wilkie. 1984. *Galen On Respiration and the Arteries*. Princeton, NJ: Princeton University Press.

Gäbel, Ricarda. 2018. "Mental Illnesses in the Medical Compilations of Late Antiquity: The Case of Aëtius of Amida." In *Mental Illness in Ancient Medicine: From Celsus to Paul of Aegina*, edited by Chiara Thumiger and P.N. Singer, 315–40. Leiden: Brill.

Gaddis, Michael. 2005. *There Is No Crime for Those Who Have Christ: Religious Violence in the Christian Roman Empire*. Berkeley: University of California Press.

García-Ballester, Luis. 1988. "Soul and Body, Disease of the Soul and Disease of the Body in Galen's Medical Thought." In *Le opere psicologiche di Galeno: atti del terzo colloquio Galenico internazionale Pavia, 10–12 Settembre 1986*, edited by Paola Manuli and Mario Vegetti, 117–52. Napoli: Bibliopolis.

———. 2002. *Galen and Galenism: Theory and Medical Practice from Antiquity to the European Renaissance*. Aldershot: Ashgate.

Garofalo, Ivan. 1988. *Erasistrati fragmenta*. Biblioteca di studi antichi 62. Pisa: Giardini.

Gaskin, Richard. 2014. *Simplicius: On Aristotle Categories 9–15*. Ancient Commentators on Aristotle. London: Bloomsbury Academic.

Gersh, Stephen, and Charles Kannengiesser, eds. 1992. *Platonism in Late Antiquity*. Notre Dame, IN: University of Notre Dame Press.

Gershon, Michael D. 1999. *The Second Brain: A Groundbreaking New Understanding of Nervous Disorders of the Stomach and Intestine*. New York: HarperPerennial.

Gibbs, Raymond W., Jr. 2017. *Metaphor Wars: Conceptual Metaphors in Human Life*. Cambridge: Cambridge University Press.

Gilbert, Brent Douglas. 2014. "The Image of God, Greek Medicine and Trinitarian Polemic in Gregory of Nyssa's De Hominis Opificio." PhD diss., The Catholic University of America.

Gill, Christopher. 2006. "Psychophysical Holism in Stoicism and Epicureanism." In *Common to Body and Soul: Philosophical Approaches to Explaining Living Behaviour in Greco-Roman Antiquity*, edited by R.A.H. King, 209–31. Berlin: Walter de Gruyter.

———. 2013. "Philosophical Therapy as Preventive Psychological Medicine." In *Mental Disorders in the Classical World*, edited by William V. Harris, 339–60. Leiden: Brill.

———. 2018. "Philosophical Psychological Therapy: Did It Have Any Impact on Medical Practice?" In *Mental Illness in Ancient Medicine: From Celsus to Paul of Aegina.*, edited by Chiara Thumiger and P. N. Singer, 365–80. Leiden: Brill.

Gleason, Maud. 2009. "Shock and Awe: The Performance Dimension of Galen's Anatomy Demonstrations." In *Galen and the World of Knowledge*, edited by Christopher Gill, Tim Whitmarsh, and John Wilkins, 85–114. Cambridge: Cambridge University Press.

Goff, Barbara, ed. 2005. *Classics and Colonialism*. London: Duckworth.

Goldhill, Simon. 2007. "What Is Ekphrasis For?" *Classical Philology* 102, no. 1: 1–19.

Goldstein, M. 1994. "Decade of the Brain: An Agenda for the Nineties." *Western Journal of Medicine* 161, no. 3: 239–41.

Gomory, Tomi, David Cohen, and Stuart A. Kirk. 2013. "Madness or Mental Illness? Revisiting Historians of Psychiatry." *Current Psychology* 32, no. 2: 119–35.

Goss, Charles Mayo. 1968. "On the Movement of Muscles by Galen of Pergamum." *American Journal of Anatomy* 123: 1–26.

Gould, Stephen Jay. 1996. *The Mismeasure of Man*. New York: W. W. Norton.

Gourevitch, Danielle, and Michel Gourevitch. 1998. "Le phrénétique chez Augustin." In *Augustin prédicateur (315–411): Actes du colloque international de Chantilly (5–7/09/96)*, edited by Goulven Madec, 505–17. Paris: Institut d'Études Augustiniennes.

Grant, Mark. 1997. *Dieting for an Emperor: A Translation of Books 1 and 4 of Oribasius' Medical Compilations with an Introduction and Commentary*. Leiden: Brill.

Graver, Margaret. 2007. *Stoicism and Emotion*. Chicago: University of Chicago Press.

Green, Christopher D. 2003. "Where Did the Ventricular Localization of Mental Faculties Come From?" *Journal of the History of the Behavioral Sciences* 39, no. 2: 131–42.

Greenwood, Emily. 2010. *Afro-Greeks: Dialogues between Anglophone Caribbean Literature and Classics in the Twentieth Century*. Oxford: Oxford University Press.

Gregoric, Pavel, and Martin Kuhar. 2014. "Aristotle's Physiology of Animal Motion: On *Neura* and Muscles." *Apeiron* 47: 94–115.

Grey, Cam. 2005. "Demoniacs, Dissent, and Disempowerment in the Late Roman West: Some Case Studies from the Hagiographical Literature." *Journal of Early Christian Studies* 13, no. 1: 39–69.

Gross, Charles G. 1995. "Aristotle on the Brain." *The Neuroscientist* 1, no. 4: 245–50.

———. 1998. "Galen and the Squealing Pig." *The Neuroscientist* 4, no. 3: 216–21.

———. 1999. *Brain, Vision, Memory: Tales in the History of Neuroscience*. Cambridge, MA: MIT Press.

Gross, Sky. 2015. "A Stone in a Spaghetti Bowl: The Biological and Metaphorical Brain in Neuro-Oncology." *Sociological Reflections on the Neurosciences* 13: 99–119.

Gruen, Lori, and Kari Weil. 2012. "Animal Others—Editors' Introduction." *Hypatia* 27, no. 3: 477–87.

Grunert, Peter. 2002. "Die Bedeutung der Hirnkammer in der antiken Naturphilosophie und Medizin." *Antike Naturwissenschaft und ihre Rezeption* 12: 151–82.

Hahm, David E. 1977. *The Origins of Stoic Cosmology*. Columbus: Ohio State University Press.

Halton, Thomas P. 1989. "The Five Senses in Nemesius, *De Natura Hominis* and Theodoret, *De Providentia*." *Studia Patristica*, no. 20: 94–101.

Hankinson, R. J. 1991. "Galen's Anatomy of the Soul." *Phronesis* 36, no. 2: 197–233.

———. 2006. "Body and Soul in Galen." In *Common to Body and Soul: Philosophical Approaches to Explaining Living Behaviour in Greco-Roman Antiquity*, edited by R. A. H. King, 232–58. Berlin: Walter de Gruyter.

Hanson, Ann Ellis. 1975. "Hippocrates: 'Diseases of Women 1.'" *Signs* 1, no. 2: 567–84.

Harmless, William. 1995. *Augustine and the Catechumenate*. Collegeville, MN: Liturgical Press.

———. 2004. *Desert Christians: An Introduction to the Literature of Early Monasticism*. Oxford: Oxford University Press.

Harris, Charles R. S. 1973. *The Heart and the Vascular System in Ancient Greek Medicine: From Alcmaeon to Galen*. Oxford: Clarendon Press.

Harrison, Peter. 2006. "'Science' and 'Religion': Constructing the Boundaries." *Journal of Religion* 86, no. 1: 81–106.

———. 2015. *The Territories of Science and Religion*. Chicago: University of Chicago Press.

Harrison, Victoria S. 2007. *Religion and Modern Thought*. London: SCM Press.

Harvey, Susan Ashbrook. 2006. *Scenting Salvation: Ancient Christianity and the Olfactory Imagination*. Berkeley: University of California Press.

Hatfield, Gary. 2000. "Descartes' Naturalism About the Mental." In *Descartes' Natural Philosophy*, edited by Stephen Gaukroger, John Andrew Schuster, and John Sutton, 630–58. London: Routledge.

Henderson, John. 2006. *The Renaissance Hospital: Healing the Body and Healing the Soul*. New Haven, CT: Yale University Press.

Henne, Kathryn, and Matt Ventresca. 2020. "A Criminal Mind? A Damaged Brain? Narratives of Criminality and Culpability in the Celebrated Case of Aaron Hernandez." *Crime, Media, Culture: An International Journal* 16, no. 3: 395–413.

Hill, Edmund. 1995. *Augustine. Sermons (341–400) on Various Subjects*. Edited by John E. Rotelle. Vol. 3 of 10. Hyde Park, NY: New City Press.

———. 2002. *Augustine. On Genesis*. Hyde Park, NY: New City Press, 2002.

Hokowhitu, Brendan. 2004. "Tackling Māori Masculinity: A Colonial Genealogy of Savagery and Sport." *The Contemporary Pacific* 16, no. 2: 259–84.

Holmes, Brooke. 2009. "Medicine." In *The Oxford Handbook of Hellenic Studies*, edited by George Boys-Stones, Barbara Graziosi, and Phiroze Vasunia, 552–68. Oxford: Oxford University Press.

———. 2010. *The Symptom and the Subject: The Emergence of the Physical Body in Ancient Greece*. Princeton, NJ: Princeton University Press.

———. 2012. *Gender. Antiquity and Its Legacy*. Oxford: Oxford University Press.

———. 2013. "Causality, Agency, and the Limits of Medicine." *Apeiron* 46, no. 3: 1–25.

Hombert, Pierre-Marie. 2000. *Nouvelles recherches de chronologie Augustinienne*. Paris: Institut d'Études Augustiniennes.

Horden, Peregrine. 2013. "Introduction." In *The Body in Balance: Humoral Medicines in Practice*, edited by Peregrine Horden and Elisabeth Hsu, 1–21. New York: Berghahn Books.

Hunt, Hannah. 2012. *Clothed in the Body: Asceticism, the Body, and the Spiritual in the Late Antique Era*. Farnham: Ashgate.

Hunter, David. 1989. "Libanius and John Chrysostom: New Thoughts on an Old Problem." *Studia Patristica* 22: 129–35.

Inglebert, Hervé. 2012. "Introduction: Late Antique Conceptions of Late Antiquity." In *The Oxford Handbook of Late Antiquity*, edited by Scott Fitzgerald Johnson, 3–28. Oxford: Oxford University Press.

Innes, Doreen. 2003. "Metaphor, Simile, and Allegory as Ornaments of Style." In *Metaphor, Allegory, and the Classical Tradition: Ancient Thought and Modern Revisions*, edited by George Boys-Stones, 7–27. Oxford: Oxford University Press.

Insel, Thomas R. 2007. "From Animal Models to Model Animals." *Biological Psychiatry* 62: 1337–39.

Ireland, S., and F. L. D. Steel. 1975. "Φρένες as an Anatomical Organ in the Works of Homer." *Glotta* 53: 183–95.

Iskandar, A. Z. 1976. "An Attempted Reconstruction of the Late Alexandrian Medical Curriculum." *Medical History* 20, no. 3: 235–58.

Jacobs, Andrew. 2000. "Writing Demetrias: Ascetic Logic in Ancient Christianity." *Church History* 69, no. 4: 719–48.

James, Edward. 2008. "The Rise and Function of the Concept 'Late Antiquity.'" *Journal of Late Antiquity* 1, no. 1: 20–30.

Jaeger, Werner. 1914. *Nemesios von Emesa*. Berlin: Wiedmannsche Buchhandlung.

———. 1961. *Early Christianity and Greek Paideia*. Cambridge, MA: Belknap Press of Harvard University Press.

Johnson, Christopher D. L. 2014. "'Base, but Nevertheless Holy': Lessons in Liminality from Symeon the Holy Fool." *Studies in Religion/Sciences Religieuses* 43, no. 4: 592–612.

Johnson, J. Cale. 2017. "The Stuff of Causation: Etiological Metaphor and Pathogenic Channeling in Babylonian Medicine." In *The Comparable Body—Analogy and Metaphor in Ancient Mesopotamian, Egyptian, and Greco-Roman Medicine*, edited by John Z. Wee, 72–121. Leiden: Brill.

Johnson, Monte R. 2005. *Aristotle on Teleology*. Oxford: Clarendon Press.

Johnston, Ian. 2006. *Galen on Diseases and Symptoms*. Cambridge: Cambridge University Press.

Jones, Allen E. 2009. *Social Mobility in Late Antique Gaul: Strategies and Opportunities for the Non-Elite*. Cambridge: Cambridge University Press.

Jones, William H. S. 1931. *Hippocrates*, vol. 4. Loeb Classical Library 150. Cambridge, MA: Harvard University Press.

Jordan-Young, Rebecca M. 2011. *Brain Storm*. Cambridge, MA: Harvard University Press.

Jouanna, Jacques. 2012a. "Air, Miasma and Contagion in the Time of Hippocrates and the Survival of Miasmas in Post-Hippocratic Medicine (Rufus of Ephesus, Galen and Palladius)." In *Greek Medicine from Hippocrates to Galen: Selected Papers*, 119–36. Leiden: Brill.

———. 2012b. "Rhetoric and Medicine in the Hippocratic Corpus: A Contribution to the History of Rhetoric in the Fifth Century." In *Greek Medicine from Hippocrates to Galen: Selected Papers*, 39–53. Leiden: Brill.

Kahn, Charles H. 2001. *Pythagoras and the Pythagoreans*. Cambridge: Hackett.

Kapetanaki, Sophia, and R. W. Sharples, eds. 2006. *Pseudo-Aristoteles (Pseudo-Alexander), Supplementa problematorum*. Peripatoi 20. Berlin: Walter de Gruyter.

Kapp, Steven K., ed. 2020. *Autistic Community and the Neurodiversity Movement: Stories from the Frontline*. Singapore: Palgrave Macmillan.

Karfíková, Lenka. 2012. *Grace and the Will According to Augustine*. Supplements to *Vigiliae Christianae* 115. Leiden: Brill.

Kaster, Robert. 2011. *Macrobius: Saturnalia*, vols. 1–3. Loeb Classical Library 510–12. Cambridge, MA: Harvard University Press.

Keenan, Mary E. 1936. "Augustine and the Medical Profession." *Transactions of the American Philological Association* 67: 168–90.

———. 1939. "St. Augustine and the Biological Sciences." *Osiris* 7: 588–608.

———. 1941. "St. Gregory of Nazianzus and Early Byzantine Medicine." *Bulletin of the History of Medicine* 9: 8–30.

Kimmerer, Robin Wall. 2020. *Braiding Sweetgrass: Indigenous Wisdom, Scientific Knowledge and the Teachings of Plants*. London: Penguin Books.

King, Helen. 1998. *Hippocrates' Woman*. London: Routledge.

———. 2013. *The One-Sex Body on Trial: The Classical and Early Modern Evidence*. Farnham: Ashgate.

———. 2019. *Hippocrates Now: The 'Father of Medicine' in the Internet Age*. London: Bloomsbury Academic.

Knuuttila, Simo. 2005. "The Organ of the Soul: The Brain or the Heart?" In *Sphinx: 2004–2005; Yearbook of the Finnish Society of Sciences and Letters*, 45–50. Helsingfors: Multiprint.

Kolbet, Paul R. 2010. *Augustine and the Cure of Souls: Revising a Classical Ideal*. Notre Dame, IN: University of Notre Dame Press.

König, Jason. 2012. *Saints and Symposiasts: The Literature of Food and the Symposium in Greco-Roman and Early Christian Culture*. Cambridge: Cambridge University Press,.

Kornmeier, Uta, ed. 2016. *The Soul Is an Octopus. Ancient Ideas of Life and the Body*. Berlin: Berliner Medizinhistorisches Museum der Charité.

Krell, David Farrell. 1987. "Paradoxes of the Pineal: From Descartes to Georges Bataille." *Royal Institute of Philosophy Lecture Series* 21:215–28.

Krueger, Derek. 1996. *Symeon the Holy Fool: Leontius's Life and the Late Antique City.* Berkeley: University of California Press.

Kurdock, Anne. 2007. "*Demetrias Ancilla Dei:* Anicia Demetrias and the Problem of the Missing Patron." In *Religion, Dynasty, and Patronage in Early Christian Rome, 300–900,* edited by Kate Cooper and Julia Hillner, 190–224. Cambridge: Cambridge University Press.

Kuriyama, Shigehisa. 1999. *The Expressiveness of the Body and the Divergence of Greek and Chinese Medicine.* New York: Zone Books.

Ladner, Gerhart B. 1958. "The Philosophical Anthropology of Saint Gregory of Nyssa." *Dumbarton Oaks Papers* 12: 59–94.

Laín Entralgo, Pedro. 1970. *The Therapy of the Word in Classical Antiquity.* Translated by L. J. Rather and John M. Sharp. New Haven, CT: Yale University Press.

Laird, Raymond J. 2013. "John Chrysostom and the Anomoeans: Shaping an Antiochene Perspective on Christology." In *Religious Conflict from Early Christianity to the Rise of Islam,* edited by Wendy Mayer and Bronwen Neil, 129–49. Berlin: De Gruyter.

Lakoff, George, and Mark Johnson. 1980. *Metaphors We Live By.* Chicago: University of Chicago Press.

Laks, André. 1999. "Soul, Sensation, and Thought." In *The Cambridge Companion to Early Greek Philosophy,* edited by Anthony A. Long, 250–70. Cambridge: Cambridge University Press.

———. 2002. "Philosophes présocratiques: Remarques sur la construction d'une catégorie de l'historigraphie philosophique." In *Qu'est-ce que la philosophie présocratique?,* edited by André Laks and Claire Louguet, 17–38. Cahiers de philologie 20. Villeneuve d'Ascq (Nord): Presses Universitaires du Septentrion.

———, ed. 2008a. *Diogène d'Apollonie: Édition, traduction et commentaire des fragments et témoignages.* 2nd ed. International Pre-Platonic Studies 6. Sankt Augustin: Academia Verlag.

———. 2008b. "Speculating about Diogenes of Apollonia." In *The Oxford Handbook of Presocratic Philosophy,* edited by Patricia Curd and Daniel W. Graham, 353–64. Oxford: Oxford University Press.

Lamberton, Robert. 1989. *Homer the Theologian: Neoplatonist Allegorical Reading and the Growth of the Epic Tradition.* Berkeley: University of California Press.

Lancel, Serge. 2002. *St. Augustine.* Translated by Antonia Nevill. London: Hymns Ancient & Modern Ltd.

Laskaris, Julie. 2002. *The Art Is Long: "On the Sacred Disease" and the Scientific Tradition.* Leiden: Brill.

Leduc, Francis. 1969. "Le thème de la vaine gloire chez Saint Jean Chrysostome." *Proche-Orient Chretien* 19: 3–32.

Lesses, Glenn. 1998. "Content, Cause, and Stoic Impressions." *Phronesis* 43, no. 1: 1–25.

Lewis, Orly. 2017. *Praxagoras of Cos on Arteries, Pulse and Pneuma: Fragments and Interpretation.* Leiden: Brill.

Leyerle, Blake. 1993. "John Chrysostom on the Gaze." *Journal of Early Christian Studies* 1, no. 2: 159–74.

———. 2001. *Theatrical Shows and Ascetic Lives: John Chrysostom's Attack on Spiritual Marriage*. Berkeley: University of California Press.

———. 2009. "Refuse, Filth, and Excrement in the Homilies of John Chrysostom." *Journal of Late Antiquity* 2, no. 2: 337–56.

Lim, Richard. 1990. "The Politics of Interpretation in Basil of Caesarea's 'Hexaemeron.'" *Vigiliae Christianae* 44, no. 4: 351–70.

Lindberg, David C. "The Fate of Science in Patristic and Medieval Christendom." In *The Cambridge Companion to Science and Religion*, edited by Peter Harrison, 21–38. Cambridge: Cambridge University Press, 2010.

Litwa, David M. 2016. *Refutation of All Heresies, Translated with an Introduction and Notes*. Writings from the Greco-Roman World 40. Atlanta: Society of Biblical Literature.

Lizzi Testa, Rita. 2017. Introduction to *Late Antiquity in Contemporary Debate*, edited by Rita Lizzi Testa, vii–xlix. Cambridge: Cambridge Scholars Publishing.

Lloyd, G. E. R. 1975. "Alcmaeon and the Early History of Dissection." *Sudhoffs Archiv für die Geschichte der Medicin* 59, no. 2: 113–47.

———. 1991. "The Invention of Nature." In *Methods and Problems in Greek Science*, 417–34. Cambridge: Cambridge University Press.

———. 2003. *In the Grip of Disease: Studies in the Greek Imagination*. Oxford: Oxford University Press.

———. 2007. "Pneuma between Body and Soul." *Journal of the Royal Anthropological Institute* 13:135–46.

Lock, Margaret. 1993. *Encounters with Aging: Mythologies of Menopause in Japan and North America*. Berkeley: University of California Press.

Long, A. A. 1982. "Soul and Body in Stoicism." *Phronesis* 27, no. 1: 34–57.

———. 1986. *Hellenistic Philosophy: Stoics, Epicureans, Sceptics*. Berkeley: University of California Press.

Longrigg, James. 1988. "Anatomy in Alexandria in the Third Century BC." *The British Journal for the History of Science* 21, no. 4: 455–88.

———. 1993. *Greek Rational Medicine: Philosophy and Medicine from Alcmaeon to the Alexandrians*. London: Routledge.

Lonie, Iain M. 1981. *The Hippocratic Treatises, "On Generation," "On the Nature of the Child," "Diseases IV": A Commentary*. Ars Medica 7.2. Berlin: Walter de Gruyter.

Lo Presti, Roberto. 2008. *In forma di senso: l'Encefalocentrismo del trattato Ippocratico Sulla malattia sacra nel suo contesto epistemologico*. Roma: Carocci.

———. 2015. "'For Sleep, in Some Way, Is an Epileptic Seizure' (*Somn. Vig.* 3, 457a9–10)." In *The Frontiers of Ancient Science: Essays in Honor of Heinrich von Staden*, edited by Brooke Holmes and Klaus-Dietrich Fischer, 339–96. Berlin: Walter de Gruyter.

Lovejoy, A. O. 1936. *The Great Chain of Being: A Study of the History of an Idea.* Cambridge, MA: Harvard University Press.
Ludlow, M. 2009. "Science and Theology in Gregory of Nyssa's De Anima et Resurrectione: Astronomy and Automata." *Journal of Theological Studies* 60, no. 2: 467–89.
Ludwig, David, and Stéphanie Ruphy. 2021. "Scientific Pluralism." *The Stanford Encyclopedia of Philosophy*, edited by Edward N. Zalta. Winter 2021 Edition. https://plato.stanford.edu/archives/win2021/entries/scientific-pluralism/.
MacDonald, Dennis R. 1994. *Christianizing Homer: The Odyssey, Plato, and the Acts of Andrew.* New York: Oxford University Press.
Maciver, Calum Alasdair. 2012. *Quintus Smyrnaeus' Posthomerica: Engaging Homer in Late Antiquity.* Mnemosyne, Supplements 343. Leiden: Brill.
Magee, Joseph M. 2000. "Sense Organs and the Activity of Sensation in Aristotle." *Phronesis* 45, no. 4: 306–30.
Malabou, Catherine. 2008. *What Should We Do with Our Brain?* New York: Fordham University Press.
Malosse, Pierre-Louis. 2008. "Jean Chrysostome a-t-il été l'élève de Libanios?" *Phoenix* 62, no. 3 and 4: 273–80.
Mansfeld, Jaap. 1989. "Chrysippus and the 'Placita.'" *Phronesis* 34, no. 3: 311–42.
Mansfeld, Jaap, and David T. Runia. 1997. *Aëtiana: The Method and Intellectual Context of a Doxographer.* Philosophia Antiqua 73. Leiden: Brill.
Manuli, Paola, and Mario Vegetti. 1977. *Cuore, sangue e cervello: Biologia e antropologia nel pensiero antico.* Milano: Episteme.
Manzoni, Tullio. 1998. "The Cerebral Ventricles, the Animal Spirits and the Dawn of Brain Localization of Function." *Archives Italiennes de biologie* 136: 103–52.
Marrou, Henri I. 1956. *A History of Education in Antiquity.* Translated by George Lamb. New York: Sheed and Ward.
Martens, Peter W. 2008. "Revisiting the Allegory/Typology Distinction: The Case of Origen." *Journal of Early Christian Studies* 16, no. 3: 283–317.
Martensen, Robert L. 2004. *The Brain Takes Shape: An Early History.* Oxford: Oxford University Press.
Martin, Dale B. 1995. *The Corinthian Body.* New Haven: Yale University Press.
———. 2004. *Inventing Superstition. From the Hippocratics to the Christians.* Cambridge, MA: Harvard University Press.
Martin, Emily. 1991. "The Egg and the Sperm: How Science Has Constructed a Romance Based on Stereotypical Male-Female Roles." *Signs* 16, no. 3: 485–501.
———. 2010. "Self-Making and the Brain." *Subjectivity* 3, no. 4: 366–81.
Martin, Thomas F. 2001. "Paul the Patient." *Augustinian Studies* 32, no. 2: 219–56.
Martin, Troy W. 2006. "Paul's Pneumatological Statements and Ancient Medical Texts." In *The New Testament and Early Christian Literature in Greco-Roman Context: Studies in Honor of David E. Aune*, edited by John Fotopoulos, 105–26. Leiden: Brill.
Marx-Wolf, Heidi. 2015. "Medicine." In *Late Ancient Knowing: Explorations in Intellectual History*, edited by Catherine M. Chin and Moulie Vidas, 80–98. Oakland: University of California Press.

———. 2017. "The Good Physician: Imperial Doctors and Medical Professionalization in Late Antiquity." *Studia Patristica* 81: 79–90.

———. 2018. "Religion, Medicine, and Health." In *A Companion to Religion in Late Antiquity*, edited by Josef Lössl and Nicholas J. Baker-Brian, 511–28. Hoboken, NJ: Wiley.

Marx-Wolf, Heidi, and Kristi Upson-Saia. 2015. "The State of the Question: Religion, Medicine, Disability, and Health in Late Antiquity." *Journal of Late Antiquity* 8, no. 2: 257–72.

Mattern, Susan P. 2008. *Galen and the Rhetoric of Healing*. Baltimore: Johns Hopkins University Press.

———. 2013. *Prince of Medicine: Galen in the Roman World*. New York: Oxford University Press.

Maxwell, Jaclyn L. 2006. *Christianization and Communication in Late Antiquity: John Chrysostom and His Congregation in Antioch*. Cambridge: Cambridge University Press.

May, Margaret Tallmadge. 1968. *Galen: On the Usefulness of the Parts of the Body*. Ithaca, NY: Cornell University Press.

Mayer, Emeran A., Rob Knight, Sarkis K. Mazmanian, John F. Cryan, and Kirsten Tillisch. 2014. "Gut Microbes and the Brain: Paradigm Shift in Neuroscience." *Journal of Neuroscience* 34, no. 46: 15490–96.

Mayer, Wendy. 2015a. "Medicine in Transition: Christian Adaptation in the Later Fourth-Century East." In *Shifting Genres in Late Antiquity*, edited by Geoffrey Greatrix, Hugh Elton, and Lucas McMahon, 11–26. Farnham: Ashgate.

———. 2015b. "Shaping the Sick Soul: Reshaping the Identity of John Chrysostom." In *Christians Shaping Identity from the Roman Empire to Byzantium: Studies Inspired by Pauline Allen*, edited by Wendy Mayer and Geoffrey D. Dunn, 140–64. Leiden: Brill.

———. 2015c. "The Persistence in Late Antiquity of Medico-Philosophical Psychic Therapy." *Journal of Late Antiquity* 8, no. 2: 337–51.

———. 2018. "Medicine and Metaphor in Late Antiquity: How Some Recent Shifts Are Changing the Field." *Studies in Late Antiquity* 2, no. 4: 440–63.

McCoskey, Denise Eileen. 2018. "Beware of Greeks Bearing Gifts: How Neo-Nazis and Ancient Greeks Met in Charlottesville." *Origins: Current Events in Historical Perspective* 11, no. 11. https://origins.osu.edu/article/beware-greeks-bearing-gifts-how-neo-nazis-and-ancient-greeks-met-charlottesville.

McDonald, Glenda. 2009a. "Concepts and Treatments of Phrenitis in Ancient Medicine." PhD diss., University of Newcastle.

———. 2009b. "Mapping Madness: Two Medical Responses to Insanity in Later Antiquity." In *Mania: Madness in the Greco-Roman World*, edited by Philip Bosman, 106–29. Pretoria: Classical Association of South Africa.

McGill, Scott, and Edward J. Watts. 2018. Introduction to *A Companion to Late Antique Literature*, edited by Scott McGill and Edward J. Watts, 3–8. Hoboken, NJ: John Wiley & Sons.

McGuckin, John Anthony. 2001. *St. Gregory of Nazianzus: An Intellectual Biography.* Crestwood, NY: St. Vladimir's Seminary Press.

Meconi, David Vincent. 2014. "Recapitulative Tropes in Augustine's Sermons." *New Blackfriars* 95, no. 1060: 689–97.

Meid, Wolfgang. 1996. *Heilpflanzen und Heilsprüche: Zeugnisse gallischer Sprache bei Marcellus von Bordeaux.* Innsbruck: Institut für Sprachwissenschaft der Universität Innsbruck.

Menakem, Resmaa. 2017. *My Grandmother's Hands: Racialized Trauma and the Pathways to Mending Our Hearts and Bodies.* Las Vegas: Central Recovery Press.

Merideth, Anne Elizabeth. 1999. "Illness and Healing in the Early Christian East." PhD diss., Princeton University.

Metzger, Nadine. 2018. "'Not a *Daimōn*, but a Severe Illness': Oribasius, Posidonius and Later Ancient Perspectives on Superhuman Agents Causing Disease." In *Mental Illness in Ancient Medicine: From Celsus to Paul of Aegina,* edited by Chiara Thumiger and P. N. Singer, 79–106. Leiden: Brill.

Metzl, Jonathan M., and Kenneth T. MacLeish. 2015. "Mental Illness, Mass Shootings, and the Politics of American Firearms." *American Journal of Public Health* 105, no. 2: 240–49.

Meyer, Robert T. 1965. *Palladius: The Lausiac History.* Ancient Christian Writers 34. Westminster, MD: The Newman Press.

Miller, Patricia Cox. 1993. "The Blazing Body: Ascetic Desire in Jerome's Letter to Eustochium." *Journal of Early Christian Studies* 1, no. 1: 21–45.

———. 2018. *In the Eye of the Animal: Zoological Imagination in Ancient Christianity.* Philadelphia: University of Pennsylvania Press.

Mitchell, Margaret M. 1991. *Paul and the Rhetoric of Reconciliation: An Exegetical Investigation of the Language and Composition of 1 Corinthians.* Tübingen: Mohr Siebeck.

———. 2009. "Christian Martyrdom and the 'Dialect of the Holy Scriptures': The Literal, the Allegorical, the Martyrological." *Biblical Interpretation* 17, no. 1: 177–206.

Mitchell, Paul Wolff, and John S. Michael. 2019. "Bias, Brains, and Skulls: Tracing the Legacy of Scientific Racism in the Nineteenth-Century Works of Samuel George Morton and Friedrich Tiedemann." In *Embodied Difference: Divergent Bodies in Public Discourse,* edited by Jamie A. Thomas and Christina Jackson, 77–98. Lanham, MD: Lexington Books.

Momigliano, Arnaldo. 1985. "History between Medicine and Rhetoric." *Annali della Scuola Normale Superiore di Pisa: Classe di lettere e filosofia* III, 15, no. 3: 767–80.

Morison, Ben. 2008. "Language." In *The Cambridge Companion to Galen,* edited by R. J. Hankinson, 116–56. Cambridge: Cambridge University Press.

Mudrik, Liad, and Uri Maoz. 2015. "'Me & My Brain': Exposing Neuroscience's Closet Dualism." *Journal of Cognitive Neuroscience* 27, no. 2: 211–21.

Musgrove, C. J. 2017. "Oribasius' Woman: Medicine, Christianity and Society in Late Antiquity." PhD diss., University of Cambridge.

Niehoff, Maren R., ed. 2012. *Homer and the Bible in the Eyes of Ancient Interpreters.* Leiden: Brill.

North, Robert. 1993. "Brain and Nerve in the Biblical Outlook." *Biblica* 74, no. 4: 577–97.

Nussbaum, Martha C. 1978. *Aristotle's* De Motu Animalium: *Text with Translation, Commentary, and Interpretive Essays.* Princeton, NJ: Princeton University Press.

———. 1994. *The Therapy of Desire: Theory and Practice in Hellenistic Ethics.* Princeton, NJ: Princeton University Press.

Nussbaum, Martha C., and Hilary Putnam. 1995. "Changing Aristotle's Mind." In *Words and Life,* edited by James Conant, 22–61. Cambridge, MA: Harvard University Press.

Nutton, Vivian. 1984. "From Galen to Alexander, Aspects of Medicine and Medical Practice in Late Antiquity." *Dumbarton Oaks Papers* 38: 1–14.

———. 2012. *Ancient Medicine.* 2nd ed. London: Routledge.

———. 2013. "Galenic Madness." In *Mental Disorders in the Classical World,* edited by William V. Harris, 119–28. Leiden: Brill.

Nyord, Rune. 2017. "Analogy and Metaphor in Ancient Medicine and the Ancient Egyptian Conceptualisation of Heat in the Body." In *The Comparable Body—Analogy and Metaphor in Ancient Mesopotamian, Egyptian, and Greco-Roman Medicine,* edited by John Z. Wee, 12–42. Leiden: Brill.

Ochs, Sidney. 2004. *A History of Nerve Functions: From Animal Spirits to Molecular Mechanisms.* Cambridge: Cambridge University Press.

O'Daly, Gerald J. P. 1987. *Augustine's Philosophy of Mind.* London: Duckworth.

O'Donnell, James J. 2005. *Augustine: A New Biography.* New York: HarperCollins.

O'Meara, Dominic J. 1981. *Neoplatonism and Christian Thought.* Norfolk, VA: International Society for Neoplatonic Studies.

Osborne, Catherine. 1987. *Rethinking Early Greek Philosophy: Hippolytus of Rome and the Presocratics.* Ithaca, NY: Cornell University Press.

Panagiotidou, Olympia. 2016. "Asclepius: A Divine Doctor, A Popular Healer." In *Popular Medicine in Graeco-Roman Antiquity: Explorations,* edited by William V. Harris, 86–104. Leiden: Brill.

Parker, Robert. 1983. *Miasma: Pollution and Purification in Early Greek Religion.* Oxford: Clarendon Press.

Patterson, Charles. 2002. *Eternal Treblinka: Our Treatment of Animals and the Holocaust.* New York: Lantern Books.

Pender, Stephen. 2005. "Between Medicine and Rhetoric." *Early Science and Medicine* 10, no. 1: 36–64.

Penella, Robert J. 1990. *Greek Philosophers and Sophists in the Fourth Century A.D.: Studies in Eunapius of Sardis.* ARCA, Classical and Medieval Texts, Papers, and Monographs 28. Leeds: F. Cairns.

Penniman, John David. 2015. "'The Health-Giving Cup': Cyprian's Ep. 63 and the Medicinal Power of Eucharistic Wine." *Journal of Early Christian Studies* 23, no. 2: 189–211.

Perkins, Judith. 1995. *The Suffering Self: Pain and Narrative Representation in the Early Christian Era.* London: Routledge.

Pigeaud, Jackie. 1987. *Folies et cures de la folie chez les médecins de l'antiquité Gréco-Romaine: La manie*. L'âne d'or 32. Paris: Les Belles Lettres.

Pinault, Jody Rubin. 1992. *Hippocratic Lives and Legends*. Leiden: Brill.

Pitts-Taylor, Victoria. 2016. *The Brain's Body: Neuroscience and Corporeal Politics*. Durham, NC: Duke University Press.

Plastira-Valkanou, Maria. 2003. "AP 11.281: A Satirical Epitaph on Magnus of Nisibis." *L'Antiquité Classique* 72: 187–94.

Polansky, Ronald M. 2007. *Aristotle's De Anima*. New York: Cambridge University Press.

Pormann, Peter E. 2004. *The Oriental Tradition of Paul of Aegina's Pragmateia*. Leiden: Brill.

———. 2010. "Medical Education in Late Antiquity: From Alexandria to Montpellier." In *Hippocrates and Medical Education*, edited by Manfred Horstmanshoff, 419–42. Leiden: Brill.

Pormann, Peter, and Emilie Savage-Smith. 2007. *Medieval Islamic Medicine*. Edinburgh: Edinburgh University Press.

Potter, Paul. 1988. *Hippocrates*, vol. 5. Loeb Classical Library 472. Cambridge, MA: Harvard University Press.

Rafter, Nicole Hahn. 2008. *The Criminal Brain: Understanding Biological Theories of Crime*. New York: New York University Press.

Raj, Kapil. 2013. "Beyond Postcolonialism . . . and Postpositivism: Circulation and the Global History of Science." *Isis* 104, no. 2: 337–47.

Rees, Brinley R. 1998. *Pelagius: Life and Letters*. Suffolk: Boydell & Brewer.

Reeve, C. D. C. 2019. *Aristotle—Generation of Animals & History of Animals I, Parts of Animals I*. Indianapolis: Hackett.

Reid, Shelley Annette. 2008. "'The First Dispensation of Christ Is Medicinal': Augustine and Roman Medical Culture." PhD diss., University of British Columbia.

Retief, François P. 2010. "St. Augustine and Medical Science." *Acta Patristica et Byzantine* 21, no. 1: 94–101.

Rich, Audrey. 1963. "Body and Soul in the Philosophy of Plotinus." *Journal of the History of Philosophy* 1, no. 1: 1–15.

Rippon, Gina. 2019. *Gender and Our Brains: How New Neuroscience Explodes the Myths of the Male and Female Minds*. New York: Pantheon Books.

Robbins, Frank Egleston. 1912. *The Hexaemeral Literature: A Study of the Greek and Latin Commentaries on Genesis*. Chicago: University of Chicago Press.

Rocca, Julius. 2003. *Galen on the Brain: Anatomical Knowledge and Physiological Speculation in the Second Century AD*. Leiden: Brill.

———. 2008. "Anatomy." In *The Cambridge Companion to Galen*, edited by R. J. Hankinson, 242–62. Cambridge: Cambridge University Press.

———. 2012. "From Doubt to Certainty: Aspects of the Conceptualisation and Interpretation of Galen's Natural Pneuma." In *Blood, Sweat, and Tears: The Changing Concepts of Physiology from Antiquity into Early Modern Europe*, edited by Manfred Horstmanshoff, Helen King, and Claus Zittel, 629–60. Leiden: Brill.

Rose, Nikolas. 2003. "Neurochemical Selves." *Society* 41, no. 1: 46–59.

Rose, Nikolas S, and Joelle M. Abi-Rached. 2013. *Neuro: The New Brain Sciences and the Management of the Mind.* Princeton, NJ: Princeton University Press.

Roskam, Geert. 2014. "John Chrysostom on Pagan Euergetism: A Reading of the First Part of De Inani Gloria et de Educandis Liberis." *Sacris Erudiri* 53: 147–70.

Rotelle, John E., ed. 2000. *Augustine: Expositions of the Psalms 1–32.* Translated by Maria Boulding. Hyde Park, NY: New City Press.

Rousseau, Philip. 1994. *Basil of Caesarea.* Berkeley: University of California Press.

Rousselle, Aline. 1988. *Porneia: On Desire and the Body in Antiquity.* Translated by F. Pheasant. Oxford: Blackwell.

Ruddy, Deborah Wallace. 2004. "The Humble God: Healer, Mediator, and Sacrifice." *Logos: A Journal of Catholic Thought and Culture* 7, no. 3: 87–108.

Runia, David T. 1995. *Philo and the Church Fathers: A Collection of Papers.* Leiden: Brill.

———. 1999a. "The Placita Ascribed to Doctors in Aëtius' Doxography on Physics." In *Ancient Histories of Medicine: Essays in Medical Doxography and Historiography in Classical Antiquity,* edited by Philip J. van der Eijk, 189–250. Leiden: Brill.

———. 1999b. "What Is Doxography?" In *Ancient Histories of Medicine: Essays in Medical Doxography and Historiography in Classical Antiquity,* edited by Philip J. van der Eijk, 33–55. Leiden: Brill.

———, ed. 2001. *Philo: On the Creation of the Cosmos According to Moses.* Philo of Alexandria Commentary Series 1. Leiden: Brill.

———. 2008. "The Sources for Presocratic Philosophy." In *The Oxford Handbook of Presocratic Philosophy,* edited by Patricia Curd and Daniel W. Graham, 27–54. Oxford: Oxford University Press.

Russell, D. A., and David Konstan, eds. 2005. *Heraclitus: Homeric Problems.* Atlanta: Society of Biblical Literature.

Rylaarsdam, David. 2014. *John Chrysostom on Divine Pedagogy: The Coherence of His Theology and Preaching.* Oxford: Oxford University Press.

Sabra, A. I. 1987. "The Appropriation and Subsequent Naturalization of Greek Science in Medieval Islam: A Preliminary Statement." *History of Science* 25, no. 3: 223–43.

Sambursky, S. 1959. *Physics of the Stoics.* London: Routledge and Kegan Paul.

Sandnes, Karl Olav. 2011. *The Gospel "According to Homer and Virgil": Cento and Canon.* Leiden: Brill.

Sandwell, Isabella. 2011. "How to Teach Genesis 1.1–19: John Chrysostom and Basil of Caesarea on the Creation of the World." *Journal of Early Christian Studies* 19, no. 4: 539–64.

Sanlon, Peter T. 2014. *Augustine's Theology of Preaching.* Augsburg Fortress, MN: Fortress Press.

Savage, John J. 1961. *Saint Ambrose. Hexameron, Paradise, and Cain and Abel.* New York: Fathers of the Church.

Scarborough, John. 2010. "Teaching Surgery in Late Byzantine Alexandria." In *Hippocrates and Medical Education,* edited by Manfred Horstmanshoff, 235–60. Leiden: Brill.

Scheck, Thomas P. 2008. *St. Jerome. Commentary on Matthew.* Washington, DC: Catholic University of America Press.

Schiefsky, Mark. 2007a. "Art and Nature in Ancient Mechanics." In *The Artificial and the Natural: An Evolving Polarity,* edited by Bernadette Bensaude-Vincent and William R. Newman, 67–108. Cambridge, MA: MIT Press.

———. 2007b. "Galen's Teleology and Functional Explanation." *Oxford Studies in Ancient Philosophy* 33: 369–400.

———. 2012. "Galen and the Tripartite Soul." In *Plato and the Divided Self,* edited by Rachel Barney, Tad Brennan, and Charles Brittain, 331–49. Cambridge: Cambridge University Press.

Schmitz, Sigrid, and Grit Höppner. 2014. "Neurofeminism and Feminist Neurosciences: A Critical Review of Contemporary Brain Research." *Frontiers in Human Neuroscience* 8, article 546: 1–10.

Schopp, Ludwig, ed. 1948. *Saint Augustine. The Happy Life, Answer to Skeptics, Divine Providence and the Problem of Evil, Soliloquies.* New York: CIMA Publishing.

Schwartz, Jeffrey, and Sharon Begley. 2003. *The Mind and the Brain: Neuroplasticity and the Power of Mental Force.* New York: Regan Books.

Secord, Jared. 2013. "Medicine and Sophistry in Hippolytus' *Refutatio.*" *Studia Patristica* 65: 217–24.

Sedley, David. 1993. "Chrysippus on Psychophysical Causality." In *Passions and Perceptions: Studies in Hellenistic Philosophy of Mind; Proceedings of the Fifth Symposium Hellenisticum,* edited by J. Brunschwig and M. Nussbaum, 313–31. Cambridge: Cambridge University Press / Paris: Editions de la Maison des Sciences de l'Homme.

Sharples, R. W., and Philip J. van der Eijk, eds. 2008. *Nemesius: On the Nature of Man.* Liverpool: Liverpool University Press.

Shaw, Brent D. 1992. "African Christianity: Disputes, Definitions, and 'Donatists.'" In *Orthodoxy and Heresy in Religious Movements: Discipline and Dissent,* edited by Malcolm R. Greenshields and Thomas A. Robinson, 5–34. Lewiston, NY: Edwin Mellen Press.

———. 2011. *Sacred Violence: African Christians and Sectarian Hatred in the Age of Augustine.* Cambridge: Cambridge University Press.

———. 2015. "Augustine and Men of Imperial Power." *Journal of Late Antiquity* 8, no. 1: 32–61.

Shaw, Teresa M. 1998. *The Burden of the Flesh: Fasting and Sexuality in Early Christianity.* Minneapolis: Fortress Press.

Shepardson, Christine. 2014. *Controlling Contested Places: Late Antique Antioch and the Spatial Politics of Religious Controversy.* Berkeley: University of California Press.

Sheppard, Anne. 2000. "Philosophy and Philosophical Schools." In *The Cambridge Ancient History Volume 14: Late Antiquity: Empire and Successors, AD 425–600,* edited by Averil Cameron, Bryan Ward-Perkins, and Michael Whitby, 835–54. Cambridge: Cambridge University Press.

Sherry, Mark. 2013. *If I Only Had a Brain: Deconstructing Brain Injury.* New York: Routledge.

Siebers, Tobin. 2008. *Disability Theory*. Corporealities: Discourses of Disability. Ann Arbor: University of Michigan Press.

Siegel, Rudolph E. 1970. *Galen on Sense Perception: His Doctrines, Observations and Experiments on Vision, Hearing, Smell, Touch and Pain, and Their Historical Sources*. Basel: Karger.

———. 1976. *Galen on the Affected Parts: Translation from the Greek Text with Explanatory Notes*. Basel: Karger.

Sigerist, Henry E. 1958. "The Latin Medical Literature of the Early Middle Ages." *Journal of the History of Medicine and Allied Sciences* 13, no. 2: 127–46.

Singer, P.N. 1997. *Galen: Selected Works*. Oxford: Oxford University Press.

———. 2013. *Galen: Psychological Writings*. Cambridge Galen Translations. New York: Cambridge University Press.

———. 2018. "Galen's Pathological Soul: Diagnosis and Therapy in Ethical and Medical Texts and Contexts." In *Mental Illness in Ancient Medicine: From Celsus to Paul of Aegina*, edited by Chiara Thumiger and P.N. Singer, 381–420. Leiden: Brill.

Singer, P.N., Philip van der Eijk, and Piero Tassinari. 2018. *Galen: Works on Human Nature*, vol. 1, *Mixtures (De Temperamentis)*. Cambridge Galen Translations. New York: Cambridge University Press.

Siraisi, Nancy G. 1990. *Medieval & Early Renaissance Medicine: An Introduction to Knowledge and Practice*. Chicago: University of Chicago Press.

———. 1997. "Vesalius and the Reading of Galen's Teleology." *Renaissance Quarterly* 50, no. 1: 1–37.

Skard, E. 1936. "Nemesiosstudien: 1, Nemesios und die Genesisexegese von Origen." *Symbolae Osloenses* 16: 23–43.

———. 1937. "Nemesiosstudien: 2, Nemesios und Galenus." *Symbolae Osloenses* 17: 9–25.

———. 1938. "Nemesiosstudien: 3, Nemesios und die Elementenlehre des Galenos." *Symbolae Osloenses* 18: 31–41.

———. 1939. "Nemesiosstudien: 4, Nemesios und die Physiologie des Galenos." *Symbolae Osloenses* 19: 46–56.

———. 1942. "Nemesiosstudien: 5, Galens Lehre von Tierischer und menschlicher Intelligenz." *Symbolae Osloenses* 22: 40–48.

Smith, Andrew. 2004. *Philosophy in Late Antiquity*. London: Routledge.

Smith, C.U.M. 2010. "The Triune Brain in Antiquity: Plato, Aristotle, Erasistratus." *Journal of the History of the Neurosciences: Basic and Clinical Perspectives* 19, no. 1: 1–14.

———. 2014. "Beginnings: Ventricular Psychology." In *Brain, Mind and Consciousness in the History of Neuroscience*, edited by C.U.M. Smith and Harry Whitaker, 1–20. Dordrecht: Springer.

Smith, Gregory A. 2008. "How Thin Is a Demon?" *Journal of Early Christian Studies* 16, no. 4: 479–512.

Smith, Justin E.H. 2017. "Between Language, Music, & Sound: Birdsong as a Philosophical Problem from Aristotle to Kant." In *Human & Animal Cognition in Early*

Modern Philosophy, edited by Stefanie Buchenau and Roberto Lo Presti, 127–46. Pittsburgh: University of Pittsburgh Press.

Smith, J. Warren. 2000. "Macrina, Tamer of Horses and Healer of Souls: Grief and the Therapy of Hope in Gregory of Nyssa's *De Anima et Resurrectione*." *Journal of Theological Studies* 52: 37–60.

Smith, Linda Tuhiwai. 1999. *Decolonizing Methodologies: Research and Indigenous Peoples*. London: Zed Books.

Smith, Mark S. 1998. "The Heart and Innards in Israelite Emotional Expressions: Notes from Anthropology and Psychobiology." *Journal of Biblical Literature* 117, no. 3: 427–36.

Smith, Wesley D. 1979. *The Hippocratic Tradition*. Ithaca, NY: Cornell University Press.

Solignac, A., ed. 1962. *Les Confessions*. Translated by E. Tréhorel and G. Bouisson. Bibliothèque Augustinienne 13–14. Paris: Desclée de Brouwer.

Solmsen, Friedrich. 1957. "The Vital Heat, the Inborn Pneuma and the Aether." *Journal of Hellenic Studies* 77: 119–34.

———. 1961. "Greek Philosophy and the Discovery of the Nerves." *Museum Helveticum* 18, no. 3: 150–67, 169–97.

Sorabji, Richard. 1974. "Body and Soul in Aristotle." *Philosophy* 49, no. 187: 63–89.

———. 1993. *Animal Minds and Human Morals*. Ithaca, NY: Cornell University Press.

———. 2000. *Emotion and Peace of Mind: From Stoic Agitation to Christian Temptation*. Oxford: Oxford University Press.

Stannard, Jerry. 1973. "Marcellus of Bordeaux and the Beginnings of Medieval Materia Medica." *Pharmacy in History* 15, no. 2: 47–53.

Steckerl, Fritz, ed. 1958. *The Fragments of Praxagoras of Cos and His School*. Leiden: Brill.

Stefaniw, Blossom. 2007. "Reading Revelation: Allegorical Exegesis in Late Antique Alexandria." *Revue de l'histoire des religions* 224, no. 2: 231–51.

———. 2016. "A Disciplined Mind in an Orderly World: Mimesis in Late Antique Ethical Regimes." In *Metaphor—Narratio—Mimesis—Doxologie*, edited by Ulrich Volp, Friedrich Horn, and Ruben Zimmermann, 235–56. Wissenschaftliche Untersuchungen zum Neuen Testament 356. Tübingen: Mohr Siebeck.

Stratton, George M. 1931. "Brain Localization by Albertus Magnus and Some Earlier Writers." *American Journal of Psychology* 43, no. 1: 128–31.

Streck, Martin. 2001. "Aristotelische und neuplatonische Elemente in der Anthropologie des Nemesius von Emesa." *Studia Patristica* 34:559–64.

Stump, Eleanore. 1996. "Libertarian Freedom and the Principle of Alternative Possibilities." In *Faith, Freedom, and Rationality: Philosophy of Religion Today*, edited by Jeff Jordan and Daniel Howard-Snyder, 73–88. Lanham, MD: Rowman & Littlefield.

Sullivan, Shirley D. 1988. *Psychological Activity in Homer: A Study of Phrēn*. Ottawa: Carleton University Press.

Sutton, John. 2000. "The Body and the Brain." In *Descartes' Natural Philosophy*, edited by Stephen Gaukroger, John Andrew Schuster, and John Sutton, 697–722. London: Routledge.

Swaab, D. F. 2015. *We Are Our Brains: From the Womb to Alzheimer's*. Translated by Jane Hedley-Prôle. New York: Spiegel & Grau.

Tallbear, Kim. 2013. *Native American DNA: Tribal Belonging and the False Promise of Genetic Science*. Minneapolis: University of Minnesota Press.

Taylor, Charles. 1983. "The Arguments in the Phaedo Concerning the Thesis That the Soul Is a Harmonia." In *Essays in Ancient Greek Philosophy II*, edited by J. P. Anton and A. Preus, 217–31. Albany, NY: SUNY Press.

Telfer, William. 1955. *Cyril of Jerusalem and Nemesius of Emesa*. London: SCM Press.

Temkin, Owsei. 1935. "Studies on Late Alexandrian Medicine." *Bulletin of the History of Medicine* 3: 404–30.

———. 1962. "Byzantine Medicine: Tradition and Empiricism." *Dumbarton Oaks Papers* 16:95, 97–115.

———. 1973. *Galenism*. Ithaca, NY: Cornell University Press.

———. 1991. *Hippocrates in a World of Pagans and Christians*. Baltimore: Johns Hopkins University Press.

Thomas, Rosalind. 2002. *Herodotus in Context: Ethnography, Science and the Art of Persuasion*. Cambridge: Cambridge University Press.

Thumiger, Chiara. 2017. *A History of the Mind and Mental Health in Classical Greek Medical Thought*. Cambridge: Cambridge University Press.

———. 2018a. "Stomachikon, Hydrophobia and Other Eating Disturbances: Volition and Taste in Late-Antique Medical Discussions." In *Mental Illness in Ancient Medicine: From Celsus to Paul of Aegina*, edited by Chiara Thumiger and P. N. Singer, 245–68. Leiden: Brill.

———. 2018b. "'A Most Acute, Disgusting and Indecent Disease': Satyriasis and Sexual Disorders in Ancient Medicine." In *Mental Illness in Ancient Medicine. From Celsus to Paul of Aegina*, edited by Chiara Thumiger and P. N. Singer, 269–84. Leiden: Brill.

———. 2020. "Therapy of the Word and Other Psychotherapeutic Approaches in Ancient Greek Medicine." *Transcultural Psychiatry* 57, no. 6: 741–52.

Thumiger, Chiara, and P. N. Singer. 2018. "Introduction: Disease Classification and Mental Illness: Ancient and Modern Perspectives." In *Mental Illness in Ancient Medicine: From Celsus to Paul of Aegina*, edited by Chiara Thumiger and P. N. Singer, 1–32. Leiden: Brill.

Tieleman, Teun. 1996. *Galen and Chrysippus on the Soul: Argument and Refutation in the* De Placitis, *Books II–III*. Philosophia Antiqua 68. Leiden: Brill.

———. 1998. "Plotinus on the Seat of the Soul: Reverberations of Galen and Alexander in 'Enn.' IV, 3 [27], 23." *Phronesis* 43, no. 4: 306–25.

———. 2003. *Chrysippus "On Affections": Reconstruction and Interpretation*. Philosophia Antiqua 94. Leiden: Brill.

Tilby, Angela. 2005. "From Evil Thoughts to Deadly Sins: Evagrius of Pontus's Psychology of Sin." In *Wilderness: Essays in Honour of Frances Young,* edited by R. S. Sugirtharajah. London: T&T Clark.

Tilley, Maureen A. 1996. *Donatist Martyr Stories: The Church in Conflict in Roman North Africa.* Liverpool: Liverpool University Press.

———. 1997. *The Bible in Christian North Africa.* Minneapolis: Fortress Press.

———. 2006. "Devotion, Discipline and Dissent: The Practice of Christianity in North Africa." *Studia Patristica,* no. 29: 121–26.

———. 2007. "2006 NAPS Presidential Address: When Schism Becomes Heresy in Late Antiquity: Developing Doctrinal Deviance in the Wounded Body of Christ." *Journal of Early Christian Studies* 15, no. 1: 1–21.

Toner, Jerry. 2015. "Smell and Christianity." In *Smell and the Ancient Senses,* edited by Mark Bradley, 158–70. London: Routledge.

Tonias, Demetrios E. 2014. *Abraham in the Works of John Chrysostom.* Minneapolis: Fortress Press.

Totelin, Laurence M. V. 2015. "Smell as Sign and Cure in Ancient Medicine." In *Smell and the Ancient Senses,* edited by Mark Bradley, 17–29. London: Routledge.

Tracy, Theodore J. 1976. "Plato, Galen, and the Center of Consciousness." *Illinois Classical Studies* 1: 43–52.

Trentin, Lisa. 2013. "Exploring Visual Impairment in Ancient Rome." In *Disabilities in Roman Antiquity: Disparate Bodies, a capite ad calcem,* edited by Christian Laes, C. F. Goodey, and Martha L. Rose, 89–114. Leiden: Brill.

Trompeter, Julia. 2016. "Die gespannte Seele: Tonos bei Galen." *Phronesis* 61, no. 1: 82–109.

Tuana, Nancy. 2008. "Viscous Porosity: Witnessing Katrina." In *Material Feminisms,* edited by S. Alaimo and S.J. Hekman, 323–33. Bloomington: Indiana University Press.

Upson-Saia, Kristi. 2018. "Guest Editor Foreword: Rethinking Medical Metaphors in Late Ancient Christianity." *Studies in Late Antiquity* 2, no. 4: 437–39.

Urso, Anna Maria. 2018. "Mental Derangement in Methodist Nosography: What Caelius Aurelianus Had to Say." In *Mental Illness in Ancient Medicine: From Celsus to Paul of Aegina.,* edited by Chiara Thumiger and P. N. Singer, 285–314. Leiden: Brill.

Valantasis, Richard. 1995. "Constructions of Power in Asceticism." *Journal of the American Academy of Religion* 63, no. 4: 775–821.

Van Dam, Raymond. 1996. "Governors of Cappadocia during the Fourth Century." *Medieval Prosopography* 17, no. 1: 7–93.

———. 2002. *Kingdom of Snow: Roman Rule and Greek Culture in Cappadocia.* Philadelphia: University of Pennsylvania Press.

van der Eijk, Philip J. 1997. "The Matter of Mind: Aristotle on the Biology of 'Psychic' Processes and the Bodily Aspects of Thinking." In *Aristotelische Biologie: Intentionen, Methoden, Ergebnisse,* edited by Wolfgang Kullmann and Sabine Föllinger, 231–58. Stuttgart: F. Steiner Verlag.

———. 2005a. "The Heart, the Brain, the Blood and the Pneuma: Hippocrates, Diocles and Aristotle on the Location of Cognitive Processes." In *Medicine and Philosophy in Classical Antiquity*, 119–38. Cambridge: Cambridge University Press.

———. 2005b. "The 'Theology' of the Hippocratic Treatise *On the Sacred Disease*." In *Medicine and Philosophy in Classical Antiquity*, 45–73. Cambridge: Cambridge University Press.

———. 2010. "Principles and Practices of Compilation and Abbreviation in the Medical 'Encyclopaedias' of Late Antiquity." In *Condensing Texts—Condensed Texts*, edited by M. Horster and C. Reitz, 519–54. Palingenesia 98. Stuttgart: Franz Steiner Verlag.

———. 2015. "Galen on the Assessment of Bodily Mixtures." In *The Frontiers of Ancient Science: Essays in Honor of Heinrich von Staden*, edited by Brooke Holmes and Klaus-Dietrich Fischer, 675–98. Berlin: Walter de Gruyter.

van der Kolk, Bessel A. 2014. *The Body Keeps the Score: Mind, Brain and Body in the Transformation of Trauma*. New York: Viking.

van Hoof, Lieve, and Peter van Nuffelen, eds. 2014. *Literature and Society in the Fourth Century AD: Performing Paideia, Constructing the Present, Presenting the Self*. Leiden: Brill.

van Tilburg, Cornelis. 2015. *Streets and Streams: Health Conditions and City Planning in the Graeco-Roman World*. Leiden: Primavera Press.

Vasunia, Phiroze. 2013. *Classics in Colonial India*. Oxford: Oxford University Press.

Verbeke, G. 1945. *L'évolution de la doctrine du pneuma, du Stoicisme à s. Augustin: Étude philosophique*. Paris: D. de Brouwer.

Vidal, Fernando. 2009. "Brainhood, Anthropological Figure of Modernity." *History of the Human Sciences* 22, no. 1: 5–36.

———. 2016. "Frankenstein's Brain, 'The Final Touch.'" *SubStance* 45, no. 2: 88–117.

Vidal, Fernando, and Francisco Ortega. 2017. *Being Brains: Making the Cerebral Subject*. New York: Fordham University Press.

Vivian, Tim, ed. 2004. *Four Desert Fathers: Pambo, Evagrius, Macarius of Egypt, and Macarius of Alexandria: Coptic Texts Relating to the Lausiac History of Palladius*. Crestwood, NY: St. Vladimir's Seminary Press.

Vogt, Kari. 1993. "'Becoming Male': A Gnostic, Early Christian and Islamic Metaphor." In *Women's Studies of the Christian and Islamic Traditions: Ancient, Medieval and Renaissance Foremothers*, edited by Kari Elisabeth Børresen and Kari Vogt, 217–42. Dordrecht: Springer.

von Staden, Heinrich. 1989. *Herophilus: The Art of Medicine in Early Alexandria*. Cambridge: Cambridge University Press.

———. 1992. "The Discovery of the Body: Human Dissection and Its Cultural Contexts in Ancient Greece." *The Yale Journal of Biology and Medicine* 65, no. 3: 223–41.

———. 1995. "Anatomy as Rhetoric: Galen on Dissection and Persuasion." *Journal of the History of Medicine and Allied Sciences* 50, no. 1: 47–66.

———. 1997a. "Galen and the 'Second Sophistic.'" *Bulletin of the Institute of Classical Studies, supplement*, no. 68, *Aristotle and After*, 33–54.

———. 1997b. "Teleology and Mechanism: Aristotelian Biology and Early Hellenistic Medicine." In *Aristotelische Biologie: Intentionen, Methoden, Ergebnisse*, edited by Wolfgang Kullmann and Sabine Föllinger. Stuttgart: F. Steiner Verlag.

———. 1999. "Rupture and Continuity: Hellenistic Reflections on the History of Medicine." In *Ancient Histories of Medicine: Essays in Medical Doxography and Historiography in Classical Antiquity*, edited by Philip J. van der Eijk, 143–88. Leiden: Brill.

———. 2000. "Body, Soul, and Nerves: Epicurus, Herophilus, Erasistratus, the Stoics, and Galen." In *Psyche and Soma: Physicians and Metaphysicians on the Mind-Body Problem from Antiquity to Enlightenment*, edited by John P. Wright and Paul Potter, 79–116. Oxford: Clarendon Press.

———. 2005. "Early European Conceptions of the Brain and the Nerves: Classical Intuitions and Hellenistic Discoveries." In *Sphinx: 2004–2005; Yearbook of the Finnish Society of Sciences and Letters*, 11–32. Helsingfors: Multiprint.

Wagner, Ellen. 2001. "Supervenience and the Thesis That the Soul Is a Harmonia." In *Essays on Plato's Psychology*, edited by Ellen Wagner, 69–88. Lanham, MD: Lexington Books.

Wagner, Kim A. 2018. "Savage Warfare: Violence and the Rule of Colonial Difference in Early British Counterinsurgency." *History Workshop Journal* 85:217–37.

Watts, Edward J. 2006. *City and School in Late Antique Athens and Alexandria*. Berkeley: University of California Press.

———. 2009. "The Enduring Legacy of the Iatrosophist Gessius." *Greek, Roman, and Byzantine Studies* 49, no. 1: 113–33.

———. 2012. "Speaking, Thinking, and Socializing: Education in Late Antiquity." In *The Oxford Handbook of Late Antiquity*, edited by Scott Johnson, 467–86. Oxford: Oxford University Press.

———. 2015. "Ordering Intellectual Life." In *The Cambridge Companion to the Age of Atiila*, edited by Michael Maas, 376–93. Cambridge: Cambridge University Press.

Webb, Ruth. 2009. *Ekphrasis, Imagination and Persuasion in Ancient Rhetorical Theory and Practice*. Farnham: Ashgate.

Wee, John Z. 2017. "Earthquake and Epilepsy: The Body Geologic in the Hippocratic Treatise *On the Sacred Disease*." In *The Comparable Body—Analogy and Metaphor in Ancient Mesopotamian, Egyptian, and Greco-Roman Medicine*, edited by John Z. Wee, 142–67. Leiden: Brill.

Wellmann, M. 1929. "Alkmaion von Kroton." *Archeion* 10: 156–69.

Wendt, Heidi. 2016. *At the Temple Gates: The Religion of Freelance Experts in the Roman Empire*. New York: Oxford University Press.

Wessel, Susan. 2009. "The Reception of Greek Science in Gregory of Nyssa's 'De Hominis Opificio.'" *Vigiliae Christianae* 63, no. 1: 24–46.

———. 2010. "Human Action and the Passions in Nemesios of Emesa." *Studia Patristica* 48: 3–13.

Wetzel, James. 2012. "Augustine on the Origin of Evil: Myth and Metaphysics." In *Augustine's City of God. A Critical Guide*, edited by James Wetzel, 167–85. Cambridge: Cambridge University Press.

Wicher, Helen Brown. 1986. "Nemesius Emesenus." In *Catalogus Translationum et Commentariorum: Mediaeval and Renaissance Latin Translations and Commentaries*, edited by Paul Oskar Kristeller and F. Edward Cranz, 31–72. Washington, DC: Catholic University of America Press.

Willis, Geoffrey G. 2005. *Saint Augustine and the Donatist Controversy*. Eugene, OR: Wipf and Stock Publishers.

Wilson, Elizabeth. 2004a. "Gut Feminism." *differences* 15, no. 3, 66–94.

———. 2004b. *Psychosomatic: Feminism and the Neurological Body*. Durham, NC: Duke University Press.

Woloschak, Gayle. 2011. "The Broad Science-Religion Dialogue: Maximus, Augustine, and Others." In *Science and the Eastern Orthodox Church*, edited by Daniel Buxhoeveden and Gayle Woloschak, 133–40. Farnham: Ashgate.

Woolgar, C.M. 2006. *The Senses in Late Medieval England*. New Haven, CT: Yale University Press.

Wright, Jessica. 2015. "Between Despondency and the Demon: Diagnosing and Treating Spiritual Disorders in John Chrysostom's Letter to Stageirios." *Journal of Late Antiquity* 8, no. 2: 352–67.

———. 2016. "Brain and Soul in Late Antiquity." PhD diss., Princeton University.

———. 2017. "John Chrysostom and the Rhetoric of Cerebral Vulnerability." Edited by Jared Secord, Heidi Marx-Wolf, and Christoph Markschies. *Studia Patristica* 81, no. 7: 109–24.

———. 2018. "The Brain as Treasury and as Aqueduct: Metaphors of the Brain in Theodoret of Cyrrhus." *Studies in Late Antiquity* 2, no. 4: 542–66.

———. 2019. "Brain, Nerves, and Ecclesial Membership in John Chrysostom." In *(Re) Visioning John Chrysostom: New Theories and Approaches*, edited by Chris L. De Wet and Wendy Mayer, 361–409. Leiden: Brill.

———. 2020. "Preaching Phrenitis: Augustine's Medicalization of Religious Difference." *Journal of Early Christian Studies* 28, no. 4: 525–53.

Young, Frances. 2003. "Alexandrian and Antiochene Exegesis." In *A History of Biblical Interpretation*, vol. 1, *The Ancient Period*, edited by Alan J. Hauser and Duane F. Watson, 334–52. Grand Rapids, MI: Eerdmans.

Young, Robert M. 1970. *Mind, Brain, and Adaptation in the Nineteenth Century: Cerebral Localization and Its Biological Context from Gall to Ferrier*. Oxford: Oxford University Press.

Young, Robin D. 1993. "Gregory of Nyssa's Use of Theology and Science in Constructive Theological Anthropology." *Pro Ecclesia* 2, no. 3: 345–63.

Zucconi, Laura M. 2019. *Ancient Medicine: From Mesopotamia to Rome*. Grand Rapids, MI: Eerdmans.

INDEX